Neurodevelopmental Problems
in Early Childhood

Assessment and Management

Neurodevelopmental Problems in Early Childhood

Assessment and Management

Edited by

C. M. Drillien MD FRCPE DCH

*Senior Lecturer, Department of Child Health, University of Dundee
and Honorary Consultant Paediatrician, Armitstead
Child Development Centre, Dundee*

M. B. Drummond MB CHB DCH

*Senior Research Fellow, Department of Child Health,
University of Dundee*

BLACKWELL SCIENTIFIC PUBLICATIONS

OXFORD LONDON EDINBURGH MELBOURNE

© 1977 Blackwell Scientific Publications

Osney Mead, Oxford, OX2 0EL
8 John Street, London WC1N 2ES
9 Forrest Road, Edinburgh EH1 2QH
P.O. Box 9, North Balwyn, Victoria, Australia

British Library Cataloguing in Publication Data

Neurodevelopmental problems in early childhood.
1. Children – Diseases   2. Nervous system – Diseases
I. Drillien, Cecil Mary   II. Drummond, M B
618.9'28   RJ486
ISBN 0–632–00409–6

Distributed in the United States of America by
J. B. Lippincott Company, Philadelphia
and in Canada by
J. B. Lippincott Company of Canada Ltd, Toronto

Printed in Great Britain by
Billing & Sons Limited
Guildford, London and Worcester

CONTENTS

Section 3. Presentation, Investigation and Management of the Commoner Mental, Neurological, Sensory and Behavioural Disorders

PREFACE

Over the past decade an increasing interest in the developmental, social and educational aspects of paediatrics has been reflected in the many reports on this subject from government and other official bodies. Ten years ago the Sheldon report (Child Welfare Centres, 1967) anticipated the changing pattern of paediatric practice in concluding that 'the early detection of physical, mental and emotional defect is a major function of the modern Child Health Service. Its efficient performance turns on the knowledge and training of the doctor.' More recently the Court report (*Fit for the Future*, 1976) considered comprehensive services for children in great detail. In a post-publication interview (*British Medical Journal*, 1977, **3**, 1522) Professor Court said, 'while acute illness and injury remain, the emphasis of paediatrics has changed. Nowadays we need to look at malformation, the residual hazards of birth, physical handicap, mental handicap and psychiatric disorder in childhood.'

In this book we have attempted to produce a working manual for the increasing number of family doctors, paediatricians, allied specialists and professionals in other disciplines who are concerned with the development and health of pre-school children in the community and who staff the growing number of child development centres and assessment units.

Miss Woodburn has asked us to say that the opinions expressed in Chapter 11 are personal and in no way represent the opinions of the Scottish Education Department.

Figures 3.6 and 3.11, 5.1–6, 17.1–6, 18.2, 19.1–5, 20.1–2 and 22.2–6 were provided by the authors of those chapters, whom we thank.

We are indebted to Miss E. M. Fairgrieve, Head Occupational Therapist, Handicapped Child Services, Dundee for the Appendix to Chapter 14; to Mr. D. M. Anderson and Ms. E. C. Gilchrist, Research Superintendent Physiotherapist and Research Social Worker, White Top Foundation, University of Dundee for Appendices to Chapters 10 and 11, and to Mr. T. King, Photographic Unit, Ninewells Hospital, Dundee for providing the photograph for the book jacket.

It is also a pleasure to thank Mr. N. Palmer of Blackwell Scientific Publications for his ready availability and advice throughout the period of preparation and Mrs. N. Small who typed most of the manuscript and assisted in many other ways. Finally we would like to express our gratitude to the Trustees of the White Top Foundation, whose regard for the needs of young handicapped children led to the establishment of the Armitstead Child Development Centre, Dundee for the investigation, management and study of neurodevelopmental problems in early childhood.

CONTRIBUTORS

F.D. Bowles, D.A. *Senior Lecturer in charge of Vocational Art and Design, College of Commerce, Dundee.*

K.M. Bryant, M.B., B.S., F.R.C.S. *Consultant Orthopaedic Surgeon, St. James and Bolingbroke Hospitals, London; Senior Lecturer, St. George's Hospital Medical School, University of London.*

C.E. Cooper, O.B.E., M.A., M.B. B.Chir., F.R.C.P., D.C.H. *Senior Lecturer, Department of Child Health, University of Newcastle; Consultant Paediatrician, Royal Victoria, General and Babies Hospitals, Newcastle.*

G. Curtis-Jenkins, M.A., M.B., B.Chir., D.Obst. R.C.O.G. *Family Doctor, Ashford Middlexex.*

P.A. Davies, M.D., F.R.C.P., D.C.H. *Senior Lecturer, Institute of Child Health, University of London; Consultant Children's Physician, Hammersmith Hospital, London.*

C.M. Drillien, M.D., F.R.C.P.E., D.C.H. *Senior Lecturer, Department of Child Health, University of Dundee; Honorary Consultant Paediatrician, Armitstead Child Development Centre, Dundee.*

M.B. Drummond, M.B. Ch.B., D.C.H. *Senior Research Fellow, Department of Child Health, University of Dundee.*

J. Mulhall Egan, D.B.A.O.T. *Head Occupational Therapist, Cheyne Centre for Spastic Children, London.*

J. Foley, M.D., F.R.C.P. *Consultant Physician, Cheyne Centre for Spastic Children, London; Consultant Neurologist, West Sussex Area Health Authority.*

J. Francis-Williams (Late), M.A. (Psychology) A.B.Ps.S. *Clinical Psychologist (research), Newcomen Centre, London and Children's Assessment Unit, Guildford; lately Consultant Psychologist, Guy's Hospital, London.*

B. Harcourt, M.A., M.B., B.Chir., F.R.C.S. *Consultant Ophthalmic Surgeon, Leeds General Hospital; Clinical Lecturer in Paediatric Ophthalmology, University of Leeds.*

S. Goodwin, L.C.S.T. *Senior Speech Therapist, Chelmsford District; lately Senior Speech Therapist, Child Development Unit, Dorchester.*

N.S. Gordon, M.D., F.R.C.P. *Consultant Paediatric Neurologist, Royal Manchester and Booth Hall Children's Hospitals and Duchess of York Hospital for Babies, Manchester.*

P.J. Graham, M.B., B.Chir., F.R.C.P., F.R.C.Psych. *Walker Professor of Child Psychiatry, Institute of Child Health, University of London.*

M.I. Griffiths, M.D., M.R.C.P., D.C.H. *Honorary Senior Research Fellow, Institute of Child Health, University of Birmingham; lately Consultant Associate in Developmental Paediatrics, The Children's Hospital, Birmingham.*

J. Lorber, M.D., F.R.C.P. *Reader in Paediatrics, University of Sheffield; Consultant Paediatrician, The Children's Hospital, Sheffield.*

E. McKay, M.D., F.R.C.P.E., M.R.C.Psych. *Consultant in Development Paediatrics, Grampian Health Board; Medical Director, Raeden Centre, Aberdeen.*

J.A.M. Martin, M.B., B.S., F.R.C.S., D.L.O. *Director, Nuffield Hearing and Speech Centre, Royal National Throat, Nose and Ear Hospital, London.*

R.G. Mitchell, M.D., F.R.C.P.E., D.C.H. *Professor of Child Health, University of Dundee.*

A. Moosa, M.D., M.R.C.P. *Senior Lecturer, Department of Paediatrics and Child Health, University of Cape Town; Senior Paediatrician, Somerset Hospital.*

M.I. Nash, M.C.S.P. *Superintendent Physiotherapist, Highbury Hospital, Nottingham; lately Research Superintendent Physiotherapist, Department of Child Health, University of Dundee.*

M.J. Noronha, M.R.C.S., F.R.C.P. *Consultant Paediatric Neurologist, Booth Hall and Royal Manchester Children's Hospitals.*

N. O'Doherty, M.D., F.R.C.P., D.C.H. *Associate Professor of Paediatrics, University College, Dublin; Consultant Paediatrician, The Children's Hospital, Dublin.*

R.J. Purvis, M.B. Ch.B., M.R.C.P.E., D.C.H. *Consultant Paediatrician, Dorset Area Health Authority.*

M.D. Sheridan, O.B.E., M.A., M.D., D.C.H. *Honorary Senior Lecturer, Institute of Child Health, University of London; Consultant Paediatrician Emeritus, Guy's Hospital, London.*

M.F. Woodburn, A.I.M.S.W. *Social Work Adviser, Social Work Services Group, Scottish Education Department, Edinburgh.*

J.A. Young, M.B. Ch.B., M.R.C.P. *Consultant Paediatrician (Developmental Neurology), Tayside Area Health Board; Honorary Senior Lecturer, Department of Child Health, University of Dundee.*

CHAPTER 1

The Nature and Causes
of Disability in Childhood

Disability and Handicap

Variation is a fundamental characteristic of living things and people vary widely
in their mental and physical abilities. For example, there is a great difference in
manual dexterity between the concert pianist and the unskilled labourer, yet
both are within the range accepted as normal. However, if this range is projected
in the direction of diminishing dexterity, an area of clumsiness is reached where
it is difficult to define normality and with further projection the lack of skill
becomes manifestly abnormal, i.e. a disability.

It is easier to estimate the extent of functional impairment in some disabilities
than in others: for example, the ability to walk can be determined more readily
than the ability to perceive spatial relationships. Nevertheless, disability is
something that can be measured objectively and, where more than one function
is impaired, the extent of the total disability can be stated, thus allowing individual
and group comparisons to be made.

A child is said to be handicapped when a disability puts him at a disadvantage
in his particular environmental circumstances. Such a disability of body, intellect
or personality may adversely affect the child's development and capacity to
learn and to adjust to life. The extent of the consequent handicap will obviously
depend not only on the nature of the disability but also on what is expected of
him and on the personal qualities and abilities which will help him to meet the
challenge. The aspirations of the parents, the tolerance of teachers, the rivalry
of other children, the nature of the physical surroundings and the demands made
by the society in which he lives will all influence the severity of his handicap.
For example, mild mental retardation and physical clumsiness may not be very
great disadvantages to a farm child in a rural community, because little is
required of him intellectually and his disabilities may be compatible with
performing unskilled farm work reasonably adequately. The same degree of
disability in the child of professional parents in a large city is likely to constitute
a considerable handicap, because expectations and pressures are so much greater.
In technologically developed countries these pressures are increasing all the
time as society becomes more complex.

Social deprivation and an inadequate home and parents tend to increase
handicap whereas it is lessened by a warm supporting family. Thus a child's
strengths and weaknesses, the resources and deficiencies of his home background,

and the impact of his surrounding environment must all be considered in determining the degree of his handicap.

There is virtually always a social component in the genesis of handicap, but it must also be appreciated that adverse socioeconomic conditions alone may impose a handicap without any associated mental or physical disability. However, data from the National Child Development Study (Wedge and Prosser, 1973) showed that 23 per cent of 11-year-old children came from large or one-parent families, 23 per cent were or had been in poor housing, and 14 per cent were living on a low income. Altogether more than one-third (36 per cent) of British children had one or more of these disadvantages. Thus to include social deprivation as a separate category of chronic handicap in childhood would so broaden the concept that it would lose all value as a basis for study and action.

Clearly disability can only be considered a handicap in relation to circumstances. In practice the words 'disability' and 'handicap' are often used loosely and even interchangeably, but this can give rise to misunderstanding and confusion of thought, and it is preferable to preserve the distinctions outlined above as far as possible. They have been adopted widely, though not universally, by writers on the subject of handicap in childhood, (e.g. Holt, 1977) but there has not yet been international agreement on definitions.

Prevalence

We cannot measure the amount of handicap in a community or compare the numbers of handicapped children in two areas, except as an approximate estimate, since what constitutes a handicap in one may not do so in the other and the degree of handicap can vary in the same child with changes in his environment. Indeed, as Kirman (1972) has said, handicap is not really a thing in itself but involves the notion of how society reacts to its less able citizens. We can, however, try to determine the frequency and severity of various kinds of disability in a population of children. In any such survey, the period covered and the nature of the population studied, especially its age structure, must be clearly defined. The continuing survey of 1000 families in Newcastle-upon-Tyne has shown how the pattern of disability varies at different stages of childhood as disabilities recognized early are treated or resolve spontaneously and as new ones arise or are recognized for the first time (Miller *et al.*, 1974). Estimating the prevalence of disability presents difficulties not only of ascertainment but also of deciding what should be included. If disability is defined too narrowly, many children with significant handicap may be excluded, while too broad a definition may bring in a large proportion of the total child population. Bradshaw (1975) has estimated that there are between 85 and 108 thousand children with very severe mental and/or physical disability in Britain, i.e. about 0.8 per cent of the childhood population. On the assumption that there are about three moderately severely affected children for every very severe one, there may be 3 to 4 hundred thousand seriously handicapped children in the country, or about 3 per cent of the child population. In about two-thirds of these mental retardation will be the major or only disability.

The prevalence will be even higher if all degrees of severity are included. Thus Mattsson (1972) stated that 30–40 per cent of American children had some degree of disability and that of these 7–10 per cent had physical disorders. Talbot (1965) reported that roughly 23 per cent of all children under 17 years of age in the United States had a chronic physical condition of some sort, but only 2 per cent were so severely handicapped as to be limited in play or school work or both. In Britain, Davie, Butler and Goldstein (1972) concluded that 8 per cent of 7-year-old children had mental or physical disability, and that the figure would have been substantially higher if educational and psychiatric disabilities had been included. Miller and his colleagues (1974) reported that at 15 years of age not less than one in five children in Newcastle-upon-Tyne had residual disability, defined very broadly as physical handicap, recurrent illness, intellectual limitation, poor educational performance or severe difficulties of emotional or social adaptation. The prevalence will be much less when only neurodevelopmental disability is considered, though even here the problem of definition is a very real one. On the basis of medical examination at school entry, Bax and Whitmore (1973) estimated that 6 per cent of children in the Isle of Wight had neurodevelopmental disorders likely to lead to difficulties in later childhood.

Such approximations may be of some practical help in planning services but depend so much on whether all chronic disabilities are included or only neurodevelopmental disorders and on the degree of disability considered significant, that their value is limited. For example, if asthma is included, with an estimated prevalence of 5 per cent (Dawson *et al.*, 1969), the total prevalence will be substantially increased but only a small proportion of all children with asthma can be considered to have a disability sufficient to cause handicap and the borderline is difficult to define in population studies.

More reliable data on prevalence can be gained by considering individual disabilities, especially when these can be precisely defined. There have been many community studies of mental retardation and 27 of these have recently been critically reviewed by Abramowicz and Richardson (1975). They define severe mental retardation as an Intelligence Quotient (I.Q.) of less than 50 and concluded that the prevalence amongst older children was about 4 per 1000 of the population at risk, being somewhat higher in males than in females and independent of social class. About one-half of all severely mentally retarded children have associated disabilities causing handicap, according to this composite report. If less stringent criteria of mental retardation are adopted, the number of children included will be proportionately higher, the precise percentage depending on the nature of the tests applied. Thus Drillien, Jameson and Wilkinson (1966) found that 1.13 per cent of Edinburgh children aged $7\frac{1}{2}$–$14\frac{1}{2}$ years had an I.Q. of less than 70. Kirman (1972) reported that if all children scoring less than I.Q. 75 on some tests are counted, about 3 per cent of the population will be included. These estimates correspond well with Talbot's statement (1965) that 2–3 per cent of children in the United States are diagnosed as mentally retarded by the time they reach 15–19 years of age, about one-sixth of these having an I.Q. below 50 and the rest in the range 50–75.

Ascertainment of disorders of the special senses usually presents no great difficulty, since there are reasonably precise methods of measurement. However, problems do arise in the mentally subnormal and in very young children.

Blindness in childhood, about 70 per cent now being of congenital origin, has diminished from the peak in 1953 caused by retrolental fibroplasia. There may have been a slight increase recently due to a rise in the incidence of optic atrophy (Taylor, 1975). About 22 children per 100 000 are registered as blind in England and Wales.

In a study of 12 772 11-year-old children from the National Child Development Study (Peckham and Adams, 1975), 78 per cent were found to have optimal or near-optimal vision, i.e. at least 6/9 in each eye. Of the 12 per cent with defective vision, 3.3 per cent had marked impairment (visual acuity of 6/24 or worse in both eyes).

A careful study in Buffalo, USA, showed that deafness of all degrees, including mild high-frequency loss, affected about 4 per cent of all children (Anderson, 1967). Estimates in Britain vary widely, ranging from 1.2–49 per 1000 if the less severely hearing-impaired are included (Dinnage, 1972). Only about 2 per 1000 require a hearing aid (Rutter *et al.*, 1970).

In the National Child Development Study, between 10 and 13 per cent of children at 7 years of age were considered to have an appreciable degree of speech impairment, while 1–2 per cent had a marked impairment which reassessment at 11 years of age showed to have been a clear indication of the likelihood of continued backwardness in verbal communication, social maturity and scholastic attainment (Butler *et al.*, 1973; Sheridan and Peckham, 1975). Mac Keith and Rutter (1972) concluded that 7–8 school children per 10 000 had severe language retardation.

There are special problems in estimating the incidence of spina bifida and related malformations of the central nervous system, for it varies greatly with geographical area, social class and season. Thus in Britain the incidence varies from 4.1 per 1000 total births in South Wales to 1.6 in East Anglia; the average number born alive in the whole country is about 2 per 1000 live births. The number born per month between December and May is higher than between June and November, and the incidence is lower in Social Classes I and II than in IV and V (Brocklehurst, 1976). The number of older children with spina bifida depends not only on incidence at birth but also on the severity of the malformation, the extent of associated abnormalities and the policy of medical care. At present about 40 per cent of children born with spina bifida in Britain reach school age but the recent trend towards a more conservative approach when the quality of life is likely to be very low is reducing the proportion of survivors.

Determining the prevalence of epilepsy presents difficulties of definition and of knowing what to include. Thus decisions have to be made whether to consider all children who have ever had a convulsion or to include only those who have had recurrent fits or those who are still having fits. Van den Berg and Yerushalmy (1969) followed up a cohort of 18 500 newborn infants and found that, by the age of 5 years, 2 per cent had had one or more febrile convulsions and 1 per cent had had non-febrile convulsions. In their study of a total population of 3271 children aged 10–12 years, Rutter, Tizard and Whitmore (1970) defined epilepsy as having had a definite fit since starting school *and* a fit or regular anticonvulsant medication during the previous year. They reported that epilepsy affected 8.9 children per 1000 or 6.4 per 1000 if children with coexisting brain disorders of other kinds were excluded.

In the 1950s, when interest in cerebral palsy was growing rapidly, many population surveys were carried out (Mair, 1961) indicating that the prevalence among British children of school age was between 2.0 and 2.5 per 1000. More recently advances in medical science, with the consequently greater chances of surviving serious brain damage, have roused fears of an increase in prevalence. There may indeed be more cerebral palsy as a sequel of head injury or certain forms of meningitis, notably neonatal meningitis (Fitzhardinge *et al.*, 1974), but this has been more than offset by the diminution in cerebral palsy in children who were of low weight at birth. Thus a survey of 560 Swedish children with cerebral palsy born in 1954–70 showed that the incidence per 1000 live births had fallen from 2.24 in 1954–8 to 1.34 in 1967–70. The main decrease was in spastic and ataxic diplegia, especially in those cases associated with a birth weight of less than 2500 g (Hagberg *et al.*, 1975). While this Swedish experience is not necessarily applicable to Britain, the encouraging results of intensive care of newborn infants (*Lancet*, 1974; Roberton and Tizard, 1975) make it probable that the prevalence of cerebral palsy has diminished correspondingly in this country. This is certainly the impression of many people working with handicapped children and is borne out by the report of Davies and Tizard (1975) that the incidence of diplegia in infants of very low birth-weight at Hammersmith Hospital declined between 1961–4 and 1965–70.

During the past decade there has been increasing awareness that minor degrees of motor disability may cause clumsy, awkward behaviour not amounting to overt cerebral palsy. These and other borderline disorders of brain function have been included under the general term 'minimal cerebral dysfunction' (Chapter 16). They are believed to affect about 4–5 per cent of the school population but much depends on the experience of the observer and his views on what should be included (Bax and Mac Keith, 1963; Paine, 1966; Mitchell, 1967).

When we consider the prevalence of disabilities which are less clearly of organic origin, it is even more difficult to be precise about where definitive lines should be drawn. Thus overactive behaviour is known to be a sequel of brain damage but we cannot assume that its frequency is an index of the prevalence of neurological impairment, since there are many other reasons for hyperactivity in childhood (Mac Keith, 1974; *British Medical Journal*, 1975). It is commonly recognized as a symptom, being found in about 5 per cent of school children in North America (Stephenson, 1975). Teachers in the Isle of Wight reported overactivity in more than half of all children with behaviour disturbances (Rutter *et al.*, 1970). On the other hand, the hyperkinetic syndrome, characterized by extreme hyperactivity of primary origin, is rare (Bax, 1972). Rutter and his colleagues (1970) diagnosed it in only two of 118 disturbed 11-year-old children, although they pointed out that hyperactivity is age-related and an adequate estimate of incidence would require a study of a younger age group.

In the National Study of nearly 8000 7-year-old children born during one week in 1958 (Pringle *et al.*, 1966), a total of 13 per cent were receiving or would have benefited from special help because of educational or mental backwardness. Three per cent of the sample were non-readers and 24 per cent were poor readers. Rutter and his co-workers reported that 12.0 per cent of 10-year-old children in the Isle of Wight had psychiatric and behavioural disturbances, while 3.9 per cent had specific reading retardation and 8.3 per cent were generally backward in reading. Corresponding figures for children in an inner London borough were 25.4, 9.9. and 19.0 respectively. The difficulty in interpreting these data is that, while physical impairment is known to be a cause of behavioural disorder and educational difficulty, environmental causes operating after birth are probably responsible for a greater number of cases, while often the origin is multifactorial. Thus Rutter reported that social disadvantage, family discord, parental deviance and certain adverse characteristics of the school (e.g. a high turnover rate amongst teachers) were major factors in determining the higher rate of these disorders in London (Rutter *et al.*, 1975a and b; Berger *et al.*, 1975).

Causes of Disability

Any malformation or disease process which alters mental, physical or emotional behaviour can give rise to disability. For example, chronic pulmonary or renal disease, cardiac malformation and congenital metabolic disorders may all impair function in the organ or tissue concerned or cause secondary effects in other parts of the body. Serious disease, and malignant neoplasia in particular, carries such a grave prognosis that the anxiety generated and the consequent changes in attitude often increase the handicap.

While many conditions may thus cause handicapping disability in childhood by far the most important causative disorders are those affecting the central nervous system. This is because they are common, because their relative frequency is increasing as the incidence of other diseases diminishes and because the nervous system controls so many bodily functions. Moreover, in infancy and early childhood the central nervous system is developing very rapidly and is so intimately concerned with general growth and development that neurological disturbance has profound and far-reaching effects on all behaviour.

Child development centres, assessment units and other resources of the services for handicapped children are principally concerned with neurodevelopmental disability, for acute neurological disease is treated in paediatric hospital units, psychiatric disorder is dealt with by the psychiatric services and chronic diseases of other systems are usually managed in specialist clinics. Further consideration of aetiology will therefore be confined to neurodevelopmental disorders.

The immense complexity of the human brain means that any disturbance of its development can produce many different kinds of abnormal behaviour. For descriptive purposes they can be classified in broad groups, viz. diminished intelligence (mental subnormality); motor disorders; sensory disorders, including disorders of the special senses; paroxysmal disorders resulting from abnormal electrical discharges from the affected brain (epilepsy), and disorders of the emotions and personality. In practice these manifestations of disturbed function can and often do occur together, in varying combinations and degrees of severity, so that the clinical patterns of disordered cerebral function show considerable variety. When discussing aetiology, however, it is generally inappropriate to consider individual conditions, since the same aetiological agents may produce quite different functional disorders in different patients. It is true that character-istic congeries of symptoms may commonly occur after certain kinds of insult (for example, the sequelae of kernicterus) but even then there is wide variation in the possible nature and combinations of symptoms. It is preferable therefore to consider the aetiology of neurodevelopmental disorder as a whole rather than in terms of particular functional disturbances.

The central nervous system, being so complex, is susceptible to many kinds of adverse influence. A mutant gene or chromosomal aberration may ensure that the brain of the new individual is abnormal from the very start, or a hostile embryonic environment may distort the early formation of the central nervous system. During later intrauterine life various noxious influences may affect the fetal brain; some of them, such as iso-immunization, can also cause damage during birth or in the few days after delivery. Three groups of causes can therefore be considered: those operating in the early organogenetic period, those in the perinatal period, and postnatal causes, i.e. those affecting the infantile central nervous system after the perinatal period. Strictly speaking, there is overlap between the terms 'perinatal' and 'postnatal', because the former does not end until the 7th day of extrauterine life and the latter starts at birth. If definition is required, it may be appropriate to consider the postnatal period as starting after the 7th day, since the later causes of neurodevelopmental disorder are usually different in their nature as well as in their effect. However, in considering aetiology, we are less concerned with timing than with the nature of the insult and its relationship to the happenings of later pregnancy and delivery. Thus intraventricular haemorrhage occurring on the 8th day of extrauterine life as the culminating event in pre-term birth and respiratory distress would properly be considered as a perinatal cause, whereas gastroenteritis with hypernatraemic brain damage arising in a previously healthy 6-day-old infant would clearly be postnatal in origin.

Such factors in aetiology as genetic inheritance, epidemic infection, or standards of medical practice show considerable temporal and geographical variation and so their relative importance will vary greatly in different com-munities and at different times. It cannot therefore be assumed that there is any 'true' pattern of causation or that, when two published reports differ, one of them is necessarily wrong. At any time noxious agents may be identified and eliminated or disappear spontaneously while new ones may arise, so that the aetiological background to neurodevelopmental disorder is constantly changing.

Another possible source of error is failure to distinguish between those instances where a causal relationship has been established between an agent and neurodevelopmental disorder and those where there is merely an association between the two.

With these preliminary caveats, the aetiology of neurodevelopmental disorder will now be considered under three main headings.

Organogenetic period
Genetic and chromosomal factors. Certain rare diseases of the central nervous system are transmitted by single gene inheritance, usually autosomal recessive but sometimes dominant and in a few instances sex-linked. In most of these conditions the pathological process is progressive and so they are not normally included among the neurodevelopmental disorders causing chronic disability. However, their variable age of onset and clinical course, sometimes characterized by long periods of arrest, mean that they frequently present as retarded development and it may be some time before the progressive nature of the disease is recognized. In other familial neurological disorders aetiology may be polygenic or multifactorial; in the latter, genetic influences may be important but the role they play often cannot readily be elucidated.

Chromosomal anomalies have been identified as concomitants of a variety of developmental disorders. The more common varieties are described elsewhere (p. 246). Recently trisomies 8 and 9p have been described (Cassidy *et al.*, 1975; Centerwall and Beatty-de Sana, 1975), and it is likely that in the next few years an increasing number of structural alterations to chromosomes will be associated with clinical syndromes. While in such cases it is tempting to accept the chromosomal anomaly as the cause of the neurological disorder, it is more accurate to say that it initiates the mechanism of malformation (Poswillo, 1976) and that the cause of both must be sought.

Environmental factors. When the conceptus is genetically and chromosomally normal, disturbances of nidation or early embryogenesis could theoretically give rise to fetal malformation, though they are more likely to cause abortion. Subsequently, as the major organs are forming, a number of agents are known to cause abnormalities. Thus maternal rubella, maternal medication with thalidomide or cytotoxic drugs, environmental chemicals such as lead (Beattie *et al.*, 1975) and mercury, and therapeutic radiation to the maternal pelvis may all produce major malformation of the infant. Many other things have been thought to damage the embryo, mostly on the basis of animal experiment or circumstantial evidence; nutritional factors, especially vitamin deficiency, infections other than rubella and drugs other than thalidomide or cytotoxic agents, diagnostic radiation, and toxins of various sorts have all been incriminated at one time or another (Smithells, 1976).

While there is thus a large variety of possible causes of early malformation of the central nervous system, aetiological agents are identified in only a small proportion of all cases, perhaps no more than 10 per cent, and in the great majority the cause is quite unknown.

Perinatal period
Asphyxia. The most important single cause of neurodevelopmental disorder arising in the perinatal period is asphyxia, accounting for at least half of all

cases. The term 'asphyxia' includes the fall in oxygen tension and pH and the rise in carbon dioxide tension which occur in the blood and tissues when gaseous exchange through the placenta or lungs is interfered with. It has been shown in fetal monkeys that asphyxia sets in train a cycle of brain swelling and impaired cerebral blood flow which can lead on to cortical necrosis (Brann and Myers, 1975).

Many different circumstances give rise to perinatal asphyxia, including toxaemia, antepartum haemorrhage and reduced utero-placental circulation in late pregnancy; pressure on the umbilical cord, premature separation of the placenta and faulty anaesthesia during labour and delivery, and failure to establish satisfactory respiration after birth. The last may have many causes, among the most important being cerebral birth injury during prolonged or difficult delivery, intrapartum asphyxia (which thus precipitates more severe asphyxia after birth), excessive sedation of the infant, and the various disorders causing respiratory distress.

Brown and his colleagues (1974) reported that about 5 per cent of liveborn infants were asphyxiated at birth and that the cause was antepartum in 51 per cent of these, intrapartum in 40 per cent and postpartum in 9 per cent. They estimated that seven infants per 1000 were likely to be at risk of permanent brain damage.

While the importance of asphyxia as a cause of brain damage is established, the exact role of the different constituents is not yet clear; for example, it is not known whether hypoxia causes direct injury to cerebral tissue or produces its effect indirectly by associated metabolic disturbance. Moreover, there does not seem to be any critical level of hypoxia, hypercapnia or acidaemia at which brain injury is certain, and it may only be precipitated by a combination of adverse factors, no one of which would cause damage when acting alone. Thus hypoglycaemia with moderate asphyxia may cause brain damage where severe asphyxia occurring alone would not; a degree of hypoxia unlikely to injure brain cells may do so if there is associated circulatory disturbance and so on.

Trauma. When the standard of obstetric practice is high, direct trauma during delivery is not a frequent cause of cerebral damage, though it may occur when unexpected difficulty arises. When the fetus is already suffering from intrauterine asphyxia, prolonged or difficult instrumental delivery is particularly liable to cause direct cerebral damage. In breech delivery, hyperextension of the head or stretching of the vertebral column may give rise to spinal cord injury, as may rotational torsion from forceps in cephalic delivery (Byers, 1975). However, the great improvement in antenatal care and the wider use of elective caesarean section and other procedures have diminished the relative importance of traumatic delivery in most western countries.

Biochemical disorders. The newly born infant is at risk of various biochemical disorders as he adjusts to extrauterine life and to the environmental hazards that confront him. Hypoglycaemia may be a cause of brain damage, especially when acting with another adverse factor, such as hypoxia, but the relationship between the level of plasma glucose and the degree of injury is not close and indeed transient hypoglycaemia may even, in certain circumstances, protect against the effects of hypoxia (Griffiths and Laurence, 1974). The role of hypocalcaemia and hypomagnesaemia in the genesis of neurodevelopmental disorder is also far from clear. They may cause convulsions between the 5th and 8th days of extrauterine life but these have not the same sinister prognostic significance as convulsions occurring within the first 3 days, which are usually indicative of cerebral birth trauma (Brown *et al.*, 1972). Nevertheless, convulsions at any stage can harm the brain, for Wasterlain (1975) has shown that a reduction in the number of brain cells results from seizures in the neonatal period.

Low birth-weight. It is sometimes said that prematurity is a major cause of cerebral birth injury, but this is not an acceptable statement because birth before term *per se* is not the cause. Certainly the correlation between low birth-weight and subsequent neurodevelopmental disorder is close (Drillien, 1964; McDonald, 1967; Drorbaugh *et al.*, 1975), for the pre-term infant has anatomical and physiological disadvantages which predispose him to cerebral damage, but the relationship is not a direct causal one and the reason why a pre-term infant has sustained brain injury should always be determined and recorded if possible.

Cerebral diplegia is one of the principal neurological sequelae of birth before term, although the incidence has fallen in recent years along with that of other forms of cerebral palsy. While it may be difficult to identify the particular agents which have damaged the brain of an affected infant, there is little doubt that intraventricular haemorrhage is usually the most important finding (Churchill *et al.*, 1974; Davies and Tizard, 1975). The frequency of bleeding into the cerebral ventricles increases with diminishing gestational age at birth. Its pathogenesis is poorly understood but there is recent evidence that raised venous pressure following myocardial failure due to asphyxia is important (Cole *et al.*, 1974) and that hypothermia is probably a contributory factor (Davies and Tizard, 1975).

Pre-term infants are more liable than those born at term to respiratory distress and to disorders such as hyperbilirubinaemia, hypoglycaemia and coagulation defects. While the adverse effects of these on the brain may be prevented or reduced by modern methods of treatment, their occurrence significantly increases the liability of low birth-weight infants to cerebral damage.

About one-third of low birth-weight infants are inappropriately light for their gestational age at birth (light for date). Like pre-term infants of appropriate weight for age, they show an increased incidence of neurological disability in childhood but the causes are different. Thus the infant may be light for date because he is genetically abnormal, and therefore more likely to have a malformed brain, or because he was malnourished *in utero*, and therefore predisposed to mild mental retardation and other minor neurological abnormalities (Drillien, 1972).

While in individual infants it may thus be difficult to be certain of the particular combination of adverse factors which has caused brain damage, it is clear that, in low birth-weight infants as a group, 'when serious perinatal complications occur, the incidence of major handicap in survivors is significantly greater than among infants without such complications' (Davies and Stewart, 1975).

Postnatal period
Infection. When the hazards of birth are past, the greatest threat to the child's central nervous system is infection. Despite the advent of powerful antibiotics, pyogenic meningitis is still a common and dangerous disease. Failure to make the diagnosis early or to treat meningitis vigorously and effectively may result in widespread tissue damage. This is especially the case with staphylococci and pneumococci, with their invasive and necrotizing tendencies, but may occur in any type of bacterial meningitis. Tuberculous meningitis, formerly nearly always fatal, is now amenable to treatment but recovery may be at the cost of permanent neurological sequelae (Steiner and Portugaleza, 1973). In western countries it has become rare as tuberculosis has declined in frequency, but it is still often encountered in the developing countries. Viral infections less often have lasting effects but encephalitis of any type may give rise to disability. Even viruses not usually considered as potentially brain-damaging can have such an effect. For example, Sells, Carpenter and Ray (1975) have shown that enterovirus infections of the central nervous system during the first year of life may result in neurological impairment.

Trauma. A cause of brain damage in young children which has been attracting increasing attention is assault by a parent or other adult (Mitchell, 1975). Such non-accidental injury frequently leads to diffuse cerebral contusion, sometimes accompanied by subdural or retinal haemorrhage, the results either of direct trauma or of vigorous shaking with whiplash effects. Follow-up studies have shown that neurological sequelae such as epilepsy, cerebral palsy and blindness are common. Up to one-half of abused children subsequently show retarded development, although it is not always easy to distinguish between the effects of non-accidental injury and of the emotional and physical deprivation which nearly always accompany it (Sarsfield, 1974).

As the child grows older and ventures outside the home, opportunities for accidental injury increase. Young children involved in serious falls or motor vehicle accidents frequently sustain head injuries and many die as a result. With modern methods of treatment, however, survival rates are increasing but often the survivor shows signs of cerebral dysfunction which do not clear up (Heiskanen and Kaste, 1974).

Other causes. Less common conditions which can result in chronic disability are intracranial haemorrhage, usually from vascular anomalies such as congenital aneurysms, scarring from removal of a cerebral neoplasm, metabolic diseases which only become manifest after birth, and the toxic effects of drugs and of poisons such as lead. The brain may be injured in hypernatraemic dehydration, a real danger when an infant fed with a high-solute dried milk develops an infection such as gastroenteritis (Department of Health and Social Security, 1974; Chambers, 1975). Certain hypersensitivity reactions, such as post-vaccinial states, can result in demyelinating encephalopathy, and although this ceases to progress or is arrested by treatment, the residual effects may persist.

From this list, which is by no means exhaustive, it will be apparent that many different diseases can cause permanent neurological sequelae, given the right circumstances. Moreover, agents which are unlikely by themselves to injure nervous tissue may do so when they act in combination. Thus infection or trauma insufficient to affect a normal brain may damage the malformed nervous system. An inherited tendency to brain injury is not a clearly defined entity but it is likely that there are varying degrees of susceptibility to noxious influences and that genetic predisposition may play a part.

The relative frequency of causes

While the antecedents and other broad associations of neurodevelopmental disorder can be determined, it is often impossible to be certain of the aetiology of disability in a particular child. Probability may point strongly to one agent, such as perinatal asphyxia or postnatal infection, but frequently there is more than one possible factor in the history and it may be little more than speculation to attribute the result to one or another. It is therefore not feasible to do more than indicate broad trends. Thus it may be said that causes associated with low birth-weight are tending to fall, sequelae of road accidents may be increasing, and so on, but there is little scientific basis for determining precisely the frequency of each cause.

There may, however, be some practical purpose in trying to estimate the relative importance of causes at a particular time in one area, recognizing that judgment will to some extent be subjective. In Dundee all children known or suspected of neurodevelopmental disability are referred to the Armitstead Child Development Centre; in 100 consecutive cases of children with definite neurodevelopmental abnormality, the presumed aetiology was determined as accurately as possible, taking account of data from a full history and assessment. It was concluded that 44 per cent of disability was of genetic or embryonic origin, 36 per cent was due to perinatal events and 7 per cent arose in infancy. In the remaining 13 per cent, no aetiological association could be identified (Drillien, unpublished data). Perinatal factors were implicated in 62 per cent of cases of cerebral palsy compared with 7 per cent of cases of simple mental retardation without physical disability. In the latter group there was evidence of genetic or embryonic factors in 60 per cent, while in 30 per cent there was no apparent cause.

These figures give an indication of the contribution made by different aetiological factors, but they can be no more than an approximation, based as they are on referrals to one assessment centre and on clinical impression. Nevertheless, prevention of future disability depends on general understanding of the aetiology, and action need not wait until full data are available, for much could be done now to reduce the total of neurodevelopmental disability, especially those forms associated with perinatal and postnatal disorders (Mitchell, 1971).

References

ABRAMOWICZ H.K. and RICHARDSON S.A. (1975) Epidemiology of severe mental retardation in children: community studies. *American Journal of Mental Deficiency*, **80**, 18.

ANDERSON U.M. (1967) The incidence and significance of high-frequency deafness in children. *American Journal of Diseases in Children*, **113**, 560.

BAX M. (1972) The active and the over-active school child. *Developmental Medicine and Child Neurology*, **14**, 83.

BAX M. and MAC KEITH R. (1963) *Minimal Cerebral Dysfunction. Clinics in Developmental Medicine No. 10.* London: Heinemann.

BAX M. and WHITMORE K. (1973) Neurodevelopmental screening in the school-entrant medical examination. *Lancet*, **ii**, 368.

BEATTIE A.D., MOORE M.R., GOLDBERG A., FINLAYSON M.J.W., GRAHAM J.F., MACKIE E.M., MAIN J.C., MCLAREN D.A., MURDOCH R.M. and STEWART G.T. (1975) Role of chronic low-level lead exposure in the aetiology of mental retardation. *Lancet*, **i**, 589.

BERGER M., YULE W. and RUTTER M. (1975) Attainment and adjustment in two geographical areas: II. the prevalence of specific reading retardation. *British Journal of Psychiatry*, **126**, 510.

BRADSHAW J. (1975) Research and the Family Fund. *Concern*, **16**, 28.

BRANN A.W. and MYERS R.E. (1975) Central nervous system findings in the newborn monkey following severe in utero partial asphyxia. *Neurology*, **25**, 327.

BRITISH MEDICAL JOURNAL (1975) Hyperactivity in children. *British Medical Journal*, **4**, 123.

BROCKLEHURST G. (1976) *Spina Bifida for the Clinician. Clinics in Developmental Medicine No. 57.* London: Heinemann.

BROWN J.K., COCKBURN F. and FORFAR, J.O. (1972) Clinical and chemical correlates in convulsions of the newborn. *Lancet*, **i**, 135.

BROWN J.K., PURVIS R.J., FORFAR J.O. and COCKBURN F. (1974) Neurological aspects of perinatal asphyxia. *Developmental Medicine and Child Neurology*, **16**, 567.

BUTLER N.R., PECKHAM C. and SHERIDAN M. (1973) Speech defects in children aged 7 years: a national study. *British Medical Journal*, **1**, 253.

BYERS R.K. (1975) Spinal-cord injuries during birth. *Developmental Medicine and Child Neurology*, **17**, 103.

CASSIDY S.B., MCGEE B.J., VAN EYS J., NANCE W.E. and ENGEL E. (1975) Trisomy 8 syndrome. *Pediatrics*, **56**, 826.

CENTERWALL W.R. and BEATTY-DE SANA J.W. (1975) The trisomy 9p syndrome. *Pediatrics*, **56**, 748.

CHAMBERS T.L. (1975) Hypernatraemia: a preventable cause of acquired brain damage. *Developmental Medicine and Child Neurology*, **17**, 91.

CHURCHILL J.A., MASLAND R.L., NAYLOR A.A. and ASHWORTH M.R. (1974) The etiology of cerebral palsy in pre-term infants. *Developmental Medicine and Child Neurology*, **16**, 143.

COLE V.A., DURBIN G.M., OLAFFSON A., REYNOLDS E.O.R., RIVERS R.P.A. and SMITH J.F. (1974) Pathogenesis of intraventricular haemorrhage in newborn infants. *Archives of Disease in Childhood*, **49**, 722.

DAVIE R., BUTLER N.R. and GOLDSTEIN H. (1972) *From Birth to Seven.* London: Longmans.

DAVIES P.A. and STEWART A.L. (1975) Low-birth-weight infants: neurological sequelae and later intelligence. *British Medical Bulletin*, **31**, 85.

DAVIES P.A. and TIZARD J.P.M. (1975) Very low birthweight and subsequent neurological defect. *Developmental Medicine and Child Neurology*, **17**, 3.

DAWSON B., HOROBIN G., ILLSLEY R. and MITCHELL R. (1969) A survey of childhood asthma in Aberdeen. *Lancet*, **i**, 827.

DEPARTMENT OF HEALTH AND SOCIAL SECURITY (1974) *Present-day Practice in Infant Feeding.* London: Her Majesty's Stationery Office.

DINNAGE R. (1972) *The Handicapped Child. Research Review* Vol. II. London: Longmans.

DRILLIEN C.M. (1964) *The Growth and Development of the Prematurely Born Infant.* Edinburgh: Livingstone.

DRILLIEN C.M., JAMESON S. and WILKINSON E.M. (1966) Studies in mental handicap. *Archives of Disease in Childhood*, **41**, 528.

DRILLIEN C.M. (1972) Aetiology and outcome in low-birth-weight infants. *Developmental Medicine and Child Neurology*, **14**, 563.

DRORBAUGH J.E., MOORE D.M. and WARRAM J.H. (1975) Association between gestational and environmental events and central nervous system function in 7-year-old children. *Pediatrics*, **56**, 529.

FITZHARDINGE P.M., KAZEMI M., RAMSAY M. and STERN L. (1974) Long-term sequelae of neonatal meningitis. *Developmental Medicine and Child Neurology*, **16**, 3.

GRIFFITHS A.D. and LAURENCE K.M. (1974) The effect of hypoxia and hypoglycaemia on the brain of the newborn human infant. *Developmental Medicine and Child Neurology*, **16**, 308.

HAGBERG B., HAGBERG G. and OLOW I. (1975) The changing panorama of cerebral palsy in Sweden 1954-1970. *Acta paediatrica Scandinavica*, **64**, 187.

HEISKANEN O. and KASTE M. (1974) Late prognosis of severe brain injury in children. *Developmental Medicine and Child Neurology*, **16**, 11.

HOLT K.S. (1977) *Developmental Paediatrics*. London: Butterworth.

KIRMAN B.H. (1972) *The Mentally Handicapped Child*. London: Nelson.

LANCET (1974) Intensive care of the newborn. *Lancet*, i, 969.

MCDONALD A. (1967) *Children of Very Low Birth Weight. Research Monograph No. 1*. London: Spastics Society/Heinemann.

MAC KEITH R. (1974) High activity and hyperactivity. *Developmental Medicine and Child Neurology*, **16**, 543.

MAC KEITH R. and RUTTER M. (1972) A note on the prevalence of language disorders in young children. In *The Child with Delayed Speech*. eds. Rutter M. and Martin J.A.M. *Clinics in Developmental Medicine No. 43*. London: Heinemann.

MAIR A. (1961) In *Cerebral Palsy in Childhood and Adolescence*, ed. Henderson J.L. Edinburgh: Livingstone.

MATTSSON A. (1972) Long-term physical illness in childhood: a challenge to psycho-social adaptation. *Pediatrics*, **50**, 801.

MILLER F.J.W., COURT S.D.M., KNOX E.G. and BRANDON S. (1974) *The School Years in Newcastle-upon-Tyne*. London: Oxford University Press.

MITCHELL R.G. (1967) Hidden handicap. *Journal of the Irish Medical Association*, **60**, 79.

MITCHELL R.G. (1971) The prevention of cerebral palsy. *Developmental Medicine and Child Neurology*, **13**, 137.

MITCHELL R.G. (1975) The incidence and nature of child abuse. *Developmental Medicine and Child Neurology*, **17**, 641.

PAINE R.S. (1966) Neurological grand rounds: minimal chronic brain syndrome. *Clinical Proceedings of the Children's Hospital (Washington)*, **22**, 21.

PECKHAM C. and ADAMS B. (1975) Vision screening in a national sample of 11-year-old children *Child care, health and development*, **1**, 93.

POSWILLO D. (1976) Mechanisms and pathogenesis of malformation. *British Medical Bulletin* **32**, 59.

PRINGLE M.L.K., BUTLER N.R. and DAVIE R. (1966) *11,000 Seven-Year-Olds*. London: Longmans.

ROBERTON N.R.C. and TIZARD J.P.M. (1975) Prognosis for infants with idiopathic respiratory distress syndrome. *British Medical Journal*, **3**, 271.

RUTTER M., TIZARD J. and WHITMORE K. (1970) *Education, Health and Behaviour*. London: Longmans.

RUTTER M., COX A., TUPLING C., BERGER M. and YULE W. (1975a) Attainment and adjustment in two geographical areas: I. The prevalence of psychiatric disorder. *British Journal of Psychiatry*, **126**, 493.

RUTTER M., YULE B., QUINTON D., ROWLANDS O., YULE W. and BERGER M. (1975b) Attainment and adjustment in two geographical areas: III. Some factors accounting for area differences. *British Journal of Psychiatry*, **126**, 520.

SARSFIELD J.K. (1974) The neurological sequelae of non-accidental injury. *Developmental Medicine and Child Neurology*, **16**, 826.

SELLS C.J., CARPENTER R.L. and RAY C.G. (1975) Sequelae of central-nervous-system entero-virus infections. *New England Journal of Medicine*, **293**, 1.

SHERIDAN M.D. and PECKHAM C. (1975) Follow-up at 11 years of children who had marked speech defects at 7 years. *Child care, health and development*, **1**, 157.

SMITHELLS R.W. (1976) Environmental teratogens of man. *British Medical Bulletin*, **32**, 27.

STEINER P. and PORTUGALEZA C. (1973) Tuberculous meningitis in children. *American Review of Respiratory Disease*, **107**, 22.

STEPHENSON P.S. (1975) The hyperkinetic child: some misleading assumptions. *Canadian Medical Association Journal*, **113**, 764.

TALBOT N.B. (1965) Pediatric frontiers in developmental medicine. *American Journal of Diseases of Children*, **110**, 287.

TAYLOR D. (1975) The prevalence of visual handicap in children in England and Wales. *Child care, health and development*, **1**, 291.

VAN DEN BERG B.J., and YERUSHALMY J. (1969) Studies on convulsive disorders in young children. *Pediatric Research*, **3**, 298.

WASTERLAIN C.G. (1975) Developmental brain damage after chemically induced epileptic seizures. *European Neurology*, **13**, 495.

WEDGE P. and PROSSER H. (1973) *Born to Fail?* London: Arrow Books.

CHAPTER 2

The Multidisciplinary Approach to Assessment and Treatment

The recent increase in the provision for multidisciplinary assessment of handicapped children followed the publication of the Sheldon report (Ministry of Health, 1967). The traditional approach to this problem, in which a hospital paediatric out-patient clinic visit is followed by referral to other specialists, may or may not lead to a complete assessment, but is time-consuming and exhausting for the child and his parents and often results in conflicting advice being given.

The comprehensive approach to assessment accepts that the problems are multiple and provides for the examination of the child by experts in different disciplines while he remains in one place for a given period of time. This means that the child is tested in the optimal behavioural state, in an environment with which he has become familiar and in the company of those whom he has come to trust. There is no doubt, however, that the greatest advantages of the comprehensive approach are the informal contacts between members of staff and between parents and staff during the assessment period. The therapeutic value of the assessment procedure must not be overlooked. Without fail the parents of a handicapped child appreciate the detailed examination of their child and the time given to listening to and discussing their problems and their fears. Even if the assessment leads to the introduction of no new treatment much has been gained.

TABLE 2.1. Common problems existing alone or in combination in handicapped children.

Motor defects	Language and speech defects
Mental retardation	Feeding problems and malnutrition
Convulsions	Incontinence
Visual defects	Poor concentration
Hearing defects	Emotional problems
Other sensory loss	Learning disorders
Disorders of perception	

The range of problems that may exist in any combination in a handicapped child is shown in Table 2.1. The team at the assessment centre that is required to deal with these problems is shown in Table 2.2. Each member of the team has an important role in liaison with colleagues in his own discipline who will care for the child in the community.

TABLE 2.2. The assessment team.

Team at assessment centre	Available for consultation
Paediatrician	Orthopaedic surgeon
Community paediatrician	Orthotist
Dental surgeon	Ophthalmologist
Psychologist	Otorhinolaryngologist
Physiotherapist	Audiometrician
Occupational therapist	Child psychiatrist
Speech therapist	Teacher of the handicapped
Social worker	Teacher of the blind
Nurses	Teacher of the deaf
Health visitors	
Secretary	
Receptionist	

It must be stressed that the goal of assessment, particularly in the early years of life, is not prediction; rather it is the construction of a profile of the child's strengths and weaknesses on which to base a programme of management which will be consistent with his capabilities and yet will promote development to the full. Assessment must include the medical, emotional, educational and social needs and incorporate provision for all of these in the treatment plan that results from the case conference. Continuing reassessment and modification of the programme should be automatic.

Age of assessment
It is not yet known at what age comprehensive assessment should begin. For the 3–4 years age group there are many well-standardized tests of intellectual and language development (Chapters 6, 9), and of vision and hearing (Chapter 8) and it is much easier to make confident statements about the child. It is, however, often essential that comprehensive management start long before this. It is the author's opinion that infants with delay or disorder of development should have a full examination by a paediatrician, with involvement of other disciplines as required, so that a programme of management can be started, and that from the second year of life onwards routine multi-disciplinary assessment becomes increasingly appropriate.

Assessment procedure
The physician in charge should be a paediatrician with a special knowledge of developmental neurology or a paediatric neurologist with a wide knowledge of general paediatrics. His role is to make a general medical, developmental and neurological assessment and to arrange ancillary investigations. His relationship to the rest of the team is as a conductor's to an orchestra. He need not play all

the instruments but he must understand the potential of each and ensure that each is used to maximum effect and blended with the others to make the final · product a well-balanced whole.

Assessment should begin with a home visit by a health visitor or social worker. The purpose of this visit is to explain the nature of the assessment procedure, to answer any preliminary questions that the parents may have and to observe the child in his home environment in order to assess the physical and emotional adequacy of that environment. In this way any necessary modification of the domestic situation can be arranged and unrealistic suggestions about home care will not be made.

Routine testing of vision and hearing should be performed early in the assessment period so that allowance for any deficit can be made in the further testing of the child. This may be carried out by a Senior Medical Officer (Child Health) with special training using methods described elsewhere (Chapter 8). Any child in whom a defect is identified or suspected is referred to the appropriate specialist department, where more complex examination techniques are available. Alternatively, the initial assessments may be performed by an ophthalmologist and otorhinolaryngologist or audiometrician who have experience in dealing with young handicapped children and who can set aside sufficient time to allow for limited co-operation from such children. If defects of the special senses are present the help of special educational advisers for the visually handicapped or hearing impaired will be sought.

Psychological, speech and language, physical and occupational therapists' assessments are carried out in accordance with the principles outlined elsewhere. The physiotherapist's assessment can well be complemented by an expert in orthotics so that the provision of mobility aids and other appliances can be integrated into the programme. The roles of clinical and educational psychologists will depend on local conditions. In general it becomes increasingly important that an educational psychologist is involved as the child approaches school entry.

Prophylactic and conservative dentistry is important in handicapped children, so a dental examination should be part of the assessment. Orthodontic management may help the speech therapist.

A community paediatrician should be included in the team for the purpose of providing a link with the range of community services that will be utilized and to have responsibility for the continuing supervision of these services.

A method of assessment of proven value is for the child to join a nursery group of three to five children in the care of two nurses (and these can be children's trained or nursery nurses). The child's nurse provides a report of his behaviour, play activities, spontaneous speech and achievements in self-help skills and also how he relates to other children and strange adults in the nursery situation. This supplements the home report and the more formal assessments of the other members of the team.

In most cases it is possible to make a reliable assessment in a period of 1 or 2 weeks and to construct a useful programme of management. The nature of some children's problems is such that a longer term of assessment is required, often in a continuing treatment situation. Facilities for this should also be available, preferably in the form of a nursery group within the assessment centre. It is surprising how often the child whose retardation is due in large part to environmental deprivation acquires a range of new skills even during a 2-week assessment period.

The assessment case conference
This is attended by all members of staff and by those who have been, or will be, caring for the child professionally at home and in his local community. The object of the conference is to provide a statement of the child's current condition and to make a plan for his continuing care. One person must be clearly seen to be in charge of the co-ordination and execution of this plan.

The parents of a handicapped child are usually searching for answers to five questions:

'Has it really happened?'
'Why did it happen to me?'
'What can be done about it?'
'What does the future hold?'
'Will it happen again?'

At his meeting with the parents after the case conference, the paediatrician should be in a position to give at least partial answers to these questions.

Later management
A range of treatment situations should be available in each Health Area to suit the varying needs of different families. The extremes of the range are on the one hand the admission of the child to a handicapped nursery situation where therapy is given on a daily basis, on the other a system of home management with daily care provided by the parents and periodic visits to follow-up clinics and therapists. These possibilities were discussed by Rosenbaum (1974), who found that one group of parents, predominantly in the lower social classes, preferred a nursery situation with little travelling or parent responsibility while another group, mainly in the higher social classes, preferred to travel to a centre where a range of expert help was available but where frequency of visits was such that heavy parent involvement in treatment was required. However, these are not the only options; nursery placement does not and should not preclude active involvement of parents.

Nursery facilities should be strategically placed to suit the local variations in population density, staffed by traditional nursery personnel and visited frequently by members of the team from the assessment centre. This will ensure that each child's therapy programme is taught to those who are dealing with him day by day. One such nursery group should be sited in the assessment centre itself, to provide for the daily therapy and intensive sensori-motor stimulation that a selected group of children will require. It will also provide the environment for the assessment of each new group of children.

The advantages of a nursery facility are many. Daily attendance ensures the required frequency of treatment sessions. The children become familiar with their surroundings and attendants and are seen to enjoy themselves. The various therapies can be assimilated into the day's activities and the therapist can treat the children when they are in a receptive mood. Day attendance benefits most mothers by allowing them time for shopping and other activities.

Great care must be taken, however, to involve and instruct the parents in the child's management because even in this therapy situation they must remain the major source of help for their own child.

Throughout the process it should be remembered that the whole family must be supported and the child treated through his parents (Mitchell, 1975). Maintenance of family stability, prevention of neglect or exploitation of siblings and provision of practical as well as emotional support are among the most important aspects of the management plan. This family support may be provided through a parents' group organized, for example, by a social worker. A successful way of guiding parents in making provision for their handicapped child is the use of a toy library where an occupational therapist or psychologist gives specific advice about which toys and activities are most appropriate to each child's needs.

The physical environment
The physical provision is probably less important than the personnel of the unit. In many areas purpose-built accommodation is not provided and available accommodation must be adapted. The basic provision should always include an informal but efficient reception area and a large comfortable waiting room equipped with a wide range of toys. One wall should be adapted so that it is suitable for drawing on and for the display of pictures and other works of art by the children. If the centre serves the dual purpose of longer-term assessment and treatment, as well as short-term assessment, some nursery accommodation will be required. This may be in the form of a series of rooms to accommodate 'families' of four to six children, or a single large room to accommodate the whole group.

The whole range of traditional nursery equipment will be required, together with whatever is especially appropriate to the children's sensori-motor stimulation or other therapy. One or two rooms should be equipped as medical consulting rooms and should include small size tables and chairs and other equipment appropriate for developmental assessment of young children. One consulting room should be quiet enough to allow reliable testing of hearing, but since more detailed examination will usually be carried out in an ENT department the more stringent requirements for formal audiometry need not be satisfied. The other room, if it allows a testing distance of ten feet, may be furnished for vision-testing. Psychological examination requires a suite of two rooms joined by a one-way window and a two-way intercommunication system. A similar facility suitably sound-proofed should be available for speech therapy. Physical and occupational therapy require a large room capable of accommodating the necessary equipment, with wall-mirrors and a suitable floor covering. The usual range of office accommodation should be provided, together with one room that is suitable for social work interviews. The waiting-room may usefully double up as a seminar room and may also provide accommodation for meetings of the parents' group. A wide range of storage accommodation is required and this should include provision for a toy library. Dining and toiletting facilities must accommodate the special needs of the handicapped children and their parents, as well as the regular members of staff.

The site of the assessment centre has been much debated (Jackson, 1973). Whether it is part of the paediatric out-patient department or geographically separate from the hospital matters less than the atmosphere that prevails within. The unit should, however, be a separate and complete entity. Most writings on the subject, including the Brotherston report (Scottish Home and Health Department, 1973) seem to imply that these units should be part of district general hospitals, although the possible use of health centres is mentioned. The main advantage of the hospital site is the ready availability of a full range of specialist and diagnostic services. The main disadvantage is the clinical atmosphere that prevails in most hospitals. Another disadvantage in parts of the country where the population is scattered over a wide area is the distance that patients have to travel each day. It seems that children and their parents prefer and are more relaxed and co-operative in an informal friendly atmosphere that does not resemble a hospital in any way and this is what must be provided, no matter what site is chosen.

J.A. YOUNG

The Organization of a Day Nursery for Young Handicapped Children

Selection of patients
While it is generally agreed that it is never ideal to separate a young child of less than 3 years from his mother for more than occasional short periods, admission to a specialized day nursery may best serve the needs of the young handicapped child and his family. In particular, the multiply handicapped child can constitute a full time commitment for the mother if she is mainly responsible for sensori-motor and language stimulation, reinforcement of physiotherapy and care-taking activities (which are likely to be complicated by practical difficulties in feeding and handling), leaving her with little time or energy for the legitimate claims of husband and siblings and little respite or relaxation for herself. If progress is very slow, providing little reward or motivation to persevere, the burden may become intolerable. Unfortunately, in few areas is there adequate home help support for mothers, domiciliary therapy services, or day facilities for all young handicapped children. Moreover some parents, who would accept day placement in an active therapy environment, may not wish to take advantage of a facility that offers little more than baby-minding. Since demand usually exceeds supply, some system of priorities may be inevitable including the concentration of resources where response to therapy is most likely to be expected.

At the Armitstead Child Development Centre, Dundee it is not general policy to deny nursery placement to the more severely handicapped (if a vacancy is available) but a child is not retained for a prolonged period if progress is imperceptible. Admission for a few months during which full investigation is carried out and intensive intervention is attempted, demonstrates to parents that their child has not been 'written off' and that a fair trial of specialized management has been given. This period also enables medical, social work and therapy staff to develop closer relations with the family than is likely in an outpatient situation—relations which it is hoped will continue after alternative arrangements are made. In addition, occasionally one is surprised by the response to an intensive stimulation programme of an overtly unpromising child.

The young child with a single handicap such as hemiplegia, mild to moderate mental retardation or a sensory defect, may be well managed at home, perhaps with attendance at play group or at a later age in nursery class. Another child with a more severe or complicated problem may also be well managed at home if he is the only young child in the family, if domestic help and other support (as from an active grandmother) is available to mother, and if she has access to transport so that regular outpatient therapy sessions can be attended easily. Even in these circumstances an initial period of a few months' daily attendance may be valuable for establishing programmes and instructing parents. Other children, passing through the negative stage, may benefit from a short period of attendance if over-anxiety of parents, exacerbated by negative reactions of the child, is hampering effective home management.

A prolonged period of daily attendance (for 12 months or longer) may provide maximum benefit for the child with multiple problems who requires intensive sustained sensori-motor stimulation as well as daily physiotherapy and regular speech therapy, particularly when the physical environment of the home, other commitments of parents and the emotional health of unhandicapped family members make effective management difficult to achieve at home.

Physical environment and nursery staffing
After trials of different dispositions of nursing staff and children in different environmental settings, it was concluded that young children settle more quickly, feel more secure and are seen to be happier, when they are included in a small family group, have a recognized and restricted home base in which most activities (including play therapy, meals, toileting and resting) take place and are in daily contact with two permanent staff members (nursery nurse/'house mother' and nursing assistant). A number of separate rooms to accommodate family groups of 5 children is preferable to one or two large rooms. However, if available accommodation only provides the latter, room dividers can be used to establish separate areas; this arrangement is less successful in reducing noise level and more disturbance is caused to children by through traffic.

It is easier to arrange the children's daily programmes if those with similar types of disability and of similar mental age are grouped together. However, this might be hard on those nursing staff who, over a prolonged period, were called upon to undertake the management of children with the most severe handicaps, as they are generally less rewarding than children who are seen to make more progress. For this reason each family of five children includes an age range (both chronological and mental) and a variety of physical disabilities.

However, it is a good idea to try to ensure that all children over a mental age of $2\frac{1}{2}$–3 years have in their family group a congenial companion of like age. While younger members spend most of their day in their 'house', older children meet with friends from other 'houses' for group activities.

General aims of management

The general aims of management are:

that throughout the therapy day (0915 to 1445 hours) each child should be actively and enjoyably involved with an adult or activity at all times as far as is possible;

that each child should be encouraged towards a maximum of independence in self-help skills and play activities and that no help should be given to any child in any activity that, given reasonable time, he could achieve himself;

that nursing staff should adhere at all times to instructions from therapists and psychologist about language stimulation, posture and movement, hand function and cognitive development training and that these instructions are incorporated into all planned play activities.

Staff relationships

Implementing the management programme for a handicapped child requires a total team effort and in this situation 'no man is an island'. Each member of the team should be aware of the advice given by the other members and should incorporate it into their own area of expertise. For example, the physiotherapist should know what current aims have been set for cognitive and language stimulation and should reinforce these aims in her handling of and conversations with the child. Similarly the speech therapist should be aware of helpful and unhelpful postures and use the former in formal therapy sessions. Above all it must be remembered that those who spend most time with the child (i.e. their parents and their own nurses) are the most important influences in effective management.

For these reasons the hierarchical staffing structures, appropriate in a hospital situation, are not suitable for the ongoing therapy environment of a day nursery for handicapped children. Here, a horizontal staffing structure is essential with each member of the therapy team, including parents and the nurses in daily contact with the children, acknowledged to be working together on the same level, with free interchange of observations, suggestions and instructions, although for efficient organization and implementation of the common purpose, one or more senior staff members will be seen to be in a central or pivotal position.

Case conferences

After 4 weeks' attendance a case conference is held with all staff members who have personal contact with the child. This session is used for discussion of the child's behaviour and happiness and any difficulties in implementing the initial programme. Concrete aims in different areas of functioning are redefined and recorded.

Thereafter a full reassessment and restatement of therapy aims is carried out 6-monthly. In an attempt to combine the reporting, parent involvement and educational aspects of these meetings, a two-part system has evolved. In the first half all interested members of staff (and outside professionals) attend for a more formal presentation of reassessment reports and general discussion. The parents (and other close friends or near relatives if the parents so desire) are included in the second part of the meeting for which only those staff members closely involved with the child remain. Each area of the child's development is discussed again with active involvement of the parents and with medical terminology kept to a minimum. A free flow of information between parents and staff facilitates evaluation of progress, reveals new achievements, provides an early warning system about emerging problems and encourages reinforcement of management programmes at home.

Not all situations call for parent involvement in such a case conference and all parents do not find it helpful. When a child is making very little progress, and particularly if discharge from the nursery is under consideration, it is less traumatic for parents to talk to the paediatrician alone or with a familiar social worker present. Other parents find a case conference too stressful to be helpful, even when staff members present are all well known to them. In a survey of parental attitudes to case conferences it was found that four-fifths thought these helpful or very helpful and one-fifth preferred to talk with the paediatrician and various therapists separately. There was general agreement among parents that if progress in some or all areas of functioning was slow, this should be discussed with parents alone well before the case conference so that immediate disappointment would not militate against the practical assistance which most felt they derived from the conference itself.

The local Senior Medical Officer (Child Health) with special responsibility for handicap and, when possible, the health visitor and the family practitioner should attend the conferences. When children reach the age of about 4 years the educational psychologist who will be involved in discussions about schooling and in making pre-entry assessments should also be present.

C.M. DRILLIEN, M.B. DRUMMOND

References

JACKSON A.D.M. (1973) A hospital service for the comprehensive assessment of handicapped children. *Redbridge Medical Journal*, **Aug. 1.**

MINISTRY OF HEALTH. Standing Medical Advisory Committee (1967) *Child Welfare Centres.* London: Her Majesty's Stationery Office.

MITCHELL R.G. (1975) Habilitation in childhood. *Health Bulletin* **33,** 245.

ROSENBAUM P. (1974) Delivery of services for young handicapped children: a look at two treatment centres. *Community Health* **5,** 193.

SCOTTISH HOME AND HEALTH DEPARTMENT JOINT WORKING PARTY SUB-GROUP ON THE CHILD HEALTH SERVICE (1973) *Towards an Integrated Child Health Service.* Edinburgh: Her Majesty's Stationery Office

CHAPTER 3

Neurological Examination of the Newborn

Systematic physical examination of the newborn infant is one of the most important routine examinations of a lifetime because so much is discovered that requires action and explanation. Its desirability is now generally accepted although many have reservations about the usefulness of the neurological component of the examination on the grounds that this is time-consuming, unrewarding and may cause unnecessary anxiety to families. However, the procedure described below has proved to be a reliable and brief method of neurological examination. It is easily learnt and practised, applicable by doctors providing primary care in the routine nursery service and is predictive of later neurological dysfunction.

Methods of neurological examination appropriate for older children and adults are unsuitable for the newborn infant because he has only a minuscule amount of definitive function which will be retained and developed in the course of time. He has, however, a large repertoire of strong automatic primitive responses that are easily evoked in the first weeks of life before they begin to fade away. In many ways these responses are parodies or previews of definitive motor abilities such as prehension (palmar grasp) and locomotion (primary walking). Two eminent authorities have made perceptive observations about these primitive responses:

'It is as if Nature had put them there so that we could test if the circuits are properly laid and expect that things would work satisfactorily when the current is subsequently switched on.' (M.D. Sheridan)

'For this brief time there is available a diagnostic window which will soon close.' (R.C. Mac Keith)

The existence of the primitive responses gives us a diagnostic tool for the easy assessment of neurological performance in the newborn and provides one effective method of 'at risk' registration based on reliable first-hand assessment.

Explanation and consideration of the origins and significance of the primitive responses on which the examination is based are not considered here. Instead, emphasis is laid on the simple mechanics of how to position and handle the baby so that reliable observations and responses are obtained, while minimizing potential errors due to various pitfalls. It is painfully obvious that this is not greatly different from a set of written instructions on how to knot a bow tie. Text and diagrams are poor tutors and nothing replaces first-hand clinical instruction. However, this method of examination has been portrayed in a ciné film* which should prove a useful visual aid for teacher and pupil.

Evolution of the examination method

The first full description of a practicable, comprehensive examination of the newborn came from André-Thomas and Saint-Anne Dargassies (1952), with emphasis on the pre-term infant and the sequential maturation of responses. Subsequently André-Thomas and colleagues (1955) wrote a shorter text more appropriate to the term infant and this, in translation (1960), became the first manual for the English-speaking paediatrician. Disappointly, this rewarding method of examination was so dependent on the subjective nuances of alterations in *passivité* and *extensibilité* that its widespread use was precluded.

Later Prechtl and Beintema (1964) described the method used at Groningen in which the infant's responses were scrupulously standardized and quantified and thus made more objective for the examiner. The authors emphasized the importance of selecting a time for examination when level of arousal (state) was optimal. The states described were:

(I) deep sleep; (II) light sleep; (III) awake, slight movement of extremities; (IV) awake, large movements, and (V) awake, crying. The optimal dominant level of arousal during examination is state IV and peak performance is expected on or close to the 6th day. This excellent research tool is far too time-consuming and over-sensitive to have relevance in the routine nursery service. Some judicious selection and modification would be needed to fashion an examination capable of general application.

Experience of a similar kind of examination was obtained by O'Doherty in the Johns Hopkins Perinatal Study in 1960–61 and from 1962 a modified form was applied in the nurseries at Guy's Hospital. Subsequently the form of examination outlined below was developed in co-operation with Zinkin. The main objective was to devise a series of easily taught items, with clear-cut responses or evaluations, to be tested and then recorded on a standard form within a time-limit of 5 minutes for a normal performance. Eventually a total of 15 items was selected. These are ordered in ascending levels of disturbance and also arranged in the sequence that best suits the easy flow of performance. Thus, items such as rooting are tested early, while primary walking comes late in the examination, and the sequence of placing/extensor thrust/walking is taught so that the performance is a single uninterrupted passage and not the three separate items that the form records.

It was found that willing junior medical staff could be trained within one week to the level of competence where they could recognize perhaps 90 per cent of the normal performances with assurance. However, neurological examination of the newborn (and routine developmental assessment of older children) should be practised by medical staff at all levels. As is the case with other routine examinations, junior staff respond to the example of their seniors. In practice we found that when senior doctors participate in regular allocated routine sessions, this keeps their own skills intact and encourages other staff by example.

* N. O'Doherty (1970) *Neurological Examination of the Full Term Neonate*. ICEM Ltd. Obtainable from Guild Sound and Vision Ltd., Woodstone House, Oundle Road, Peterborough.

In addition this is such a new area of clinical application that it offers an exciting prospect of important discovery to the prepared mind.

The setting for the examination
Optimal performance is most easily obtained at the end of the first week. If the baby goes home earlier the examination is scheduled as close as is convenient to the time of discharge. When the occasional 24 or 48 hour stay baby is examined one is struck by the difficulty arising from the fact that the limbs have not unwound from the effects of intrauterine compression, the level of tone and responsiveness is relatively depressed and the eyes are not opened easily.

The well baby has two routine examinations: the first is on delivery or within 24 hours of birth and the second is as described above. Initially neurological observations are fairly cursory while in the second examination they are much more comprehensive but are always accompanied by a full repeat of the general systematic physical examination. The work load for full neurological examination therefore runs at about 3 babies per day for each 1000 deliveries per annum.

The best time to expect a good level of arousal is when the baby is waking up, 60–30 minutes before a feed is due. Usually the most convenient time is before the 10 am feed. Nursery staff appreciate having this routine work dealt with early in the day and if any queries arise a second opinion or special tests can be expeditiously arranged. The doctor may arrive to find that of three babies one is asleep, the second awake and moving about, while the third is crying. In this event he goes first to one who is crying (state V) to attempt to quieten him so that a satisfactory examination is possible. At the same time he asks the mother to undress the baby who is sleeping (state I or II), to let him wake up naturally. In this way one can usually bring most of the babies to the starting-point in state IV and then with a little effort shepherd them through the examination in this dominant state. If sleepiness or inconsolable crying prevails the examination must be deferred.

The best place to work is the general nursery area, using a slightly yielding surface such as a table top covered with a cellular blanket. Lighting should be diffuse and fairly subdued. The mother is present and is given an explanation of the performance. Most of the recording on the standard form is done by the willing nurses or midwives who are always quickly discovered when these interesting activities are introduced into the nursery service.

The Standard Form; Explanation of Test Items

The standard recording form is illustrated in Table 1 and should be read in conjunction with the explanations given below. 'Normal responses' refers to the normal term infant.

POSTURE
Method. The baby is laid supine on a slightly yielding surface with his body axis centred on the main source of light. Posture and motor activity are observed

TABLE 3.1. The standard form for neurological examination.

	Surname	Day of life:
	Given name:	Time since feed:
	Examiner:	Dominant state:

Posture
- (i)   normal/deflexed/hyperextended/other
- (ii) scissors: no/yes
- (iii) lateral preference: no/R/L
- (iv) strong ATNR: no/R/L

Motor activity
- (i)   amount: normal/excessive/reduced
- (ii) symmetry: equal/R reduced/L reduced
- (iii) focal twitching: no/R/L
- (iv) jittery/clonic: no/R worse/L worse
- (v)   tremulous: no/yes

Head and Face
- (i)   shape: symmetrical/R compression/L compression
- (ii) cephalhaematoma: no/yes
- (iii) VII palsy: no/R/L
- (iv) rooting: normal/poor/absent
- (v)   sucking: normal/poor/absent/strong

Eyes
- (i)   straight/squint/constant deviation
- (ii) subconjunctival haemorrhage: no/yes
- (iii) VI palsy: no/R/L
- (iv) other:

Upright suspension: normal/slips/flops/ R worse/L worse

Ventral suspension: normal/floppy/hyperextended

Neck traction: normal/slight reduction/severe reduction

Palmar grasp
- (i)   response: normal/excessive/reduced
- (ii) symmetry: equal/R reduced/L reduced
- (iii) fisting: mild/strong

Hip abduction resistance: normal/increased/decreased

Placing
- (i)   response: normal/poor
- (ii) symmetry: equal/R reduced/L reduced

Extensor Thrust: normal/reduced/excessive

Primary walking
- (i)   response: normal/excessive/reduced
- (ii) scissors: no/plantigrade/tiptoe
- (iii) symmetry: equal/R abnormal/L abnormal

Moro
- (i)   threshold: normal/low/high
- (ii) symmetry: equal/R abnormal/L abnormal

Cry
- (i)   amount: normal/excessive/reduced
- (ii) cerebral: no/yes
- (iii) monotonous: no/yes

Tone
- (i)   amount: normal/increased/decreased
- (ii) symmetry: equal/R abnormal/L abnormal
- (iii) distribution: generalized/UL worse/LL worse

together. He usually assumes one lateral position and is observed in it for 30 seconds and is then put in the opposite lateral position for a further 30 seconds and finally for a similar period either in the centred position or else back in the the first lateral position.

Normal responses. The dominant posture is one of flexion with the limbs supported off the examining surface most of the time; if limbs are passively deflexed by the examiner, on release they quickly return to the resting position. The hands open and close intermittently and fairly symmetrically. The baby lies with equal ease in either lateral position and in doing so may show a transient asymmetrical tonic neck response (ATNR). In this the mental limbs extend with the hand open and the occipital limbs flex with the hand closed, the so-called 'fencer' position (Fig. 3.1).

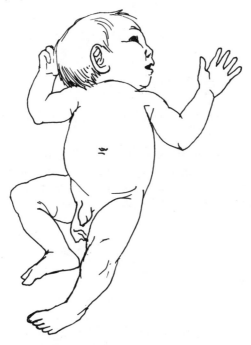

FIG. 3.1. Asymmetrical tonic neck reflex.

Deviations. In the '*pithed frog*' *posture* the limbs lie spreadeagled on the examining surface due to weakness and/or hypotonia (there is usually markedly reduced motor activity) and the hands fall open (Fig. 3.2).

Hypertonic babies may show excess fisting, scissors posture of the lower limbs and/or spinal hyperextension.

Strong lateral preference may be such as to make it difficult to posture the baby to the opposite side, or in a milder degree he gradually works his way back to the preferred side during the period of observation.

Monoparesis is the result of a peripheral lesion of nerve, bone or muscle.

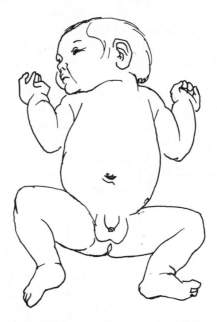

FIG. 3.2. Pithed frog posture (infant of a diabetic mother).

The classical brachial plexus lesions are Erb's, affecting the upper cervical roots (posture of a waiter expecting a tip) and Klumpke's affecting the lower roots to give weak palmar grasp and sometimes Horner's syndrome. The hemi-diaphragm may be paralysed through phrenic nerve involvement.

Pitfalls. Effects of ATNR. Some normal babies are 'hypertonic' in state V. Hyperextended postures follow face or brow presentation.

MOTOR ACTIVITY
Method. As for Posture and observed simultaneously.

Normal responses. Movements are smooth, symmetrical and appropriate to the state of arousal. The level of activity in particular is a most important observation and $1\frac{1}{2}$ minutes is in itself too brief a period of deliberate observation. However, an extended cumulative impression is gleaned indirectly during the remainder of the examination.

Deviations. Excessive, reduced and asymmetrical responses are self-explanatory. In routine practice milder deviations are given the benefit of the doubt and scored normal, so that infants scored excessive or reduced would show at least a moderate deviation in the eyes of a more expert observer.
Focal twitching means fine rapid fibrillary movement in the periphery (foot, hand, corner of eye or mouth) commonly unilateral and probably often representing mild focal fitting.

Jittery/clonic movements are slower, coarser, alternating movements in the limbs basically at rest (commonly symmetrical) and often involve the jaw. Tremulous movements are similar coarse movements imposed on the limbs in motion so that they waver unsteadily.

Pitfalls. Some babies are jittery/clonic or tremulous in state V. Motor activity is reduced in the extended mental limbs during ATNR.

HEAD AND FACE

Method. To inspect the head and face the baby is supported semi-recumbent on the flexor surface of the examiner's forearm and hand while the tips of index and middle fingers spread in a V support the occiput and the abducted thumb hooks the baby's arm to the side. His second hand holds the baby's free upper limb by its hand to keep it under control and prevent interference.

Rooting is elicitied by touching the pad of the index finger of the second hand on the crown of the baby's cheek and drawing the finger lightly but firmly across to the corner of the mouth, this leads the head round to that side (Fig. 3.3). The manoeuvre is then repeated on the other cheek and the response leads the head back to the mid-line. The finger tip is introduced into the mouth to touch the tip of the tongue; sucking is induced.

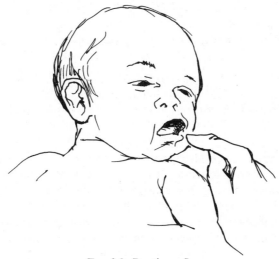

FIG. 3.3. Rooting reflex.

Normal responses. These are as described above for rooting and sucking. Minor degrees of intrauterine compression are quite common and are scored normal.

Deviations. Intrauterine ear-to-shoulder compression causes distortion of the anatomy of the neck, jaw and ear. For simplicity, the indicator of compression is a crooked mandible obviously out of line from being pushed upwards on the side of compression.

Seventh nerve (facial) palsy is most obvious in state V; the inequality of eye opening and depth of nasolabial grooves are important indices. Possible lateral confusion is avoided by remembering, apropos the mouth, 'the stem of the pear is to the side of the paralysis'. In the more complete forms of seventh nerve palsy, eye closure is also affected (Fig. 3.4).

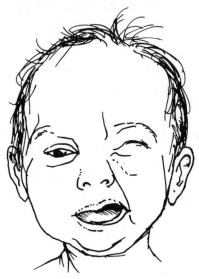

FIG. 3.4. Right-sided seventh nerve (facial) palsy in a crying infant.

Pitfalls. Rooting and sucking may be frustrated by crude rough technique. One testing is enough as these responses habituate quickly.

Ear-to-shoulder compression may mimic seventh nerve palsy.

EYES

Method. The baby is suspended upright with the major source of light at his back. A slight forward tilt promotes eye opening and if necessary this can be enhanced by induced sucking. If the eyes are straight the corneal light reflections are symmetrical. Held at arm's length the baby is carried at medium pace about 30° to the examiner's right and then a similar degree to the left to test the labyrinthine response; one manoeuvre to each side is enough.

Normal responses. The eyes are parallel and look straight ahead at rest. In the labyrinthine response the main movement of the eyes is a conjugate deviation to the leading side.

Deviations. In sixth nerve palsy the affected eye will not turn to its leading side in the labyrinthine response. The palsy may be bilateral.

Pitfalls. If the main source of light is asymmetrical this can cause normal deviation that might be misconstrued.

UPRIGHT SUSPENSION

Method. The baby is supported upright on the crotch of the examiner's hands held under the humeral necks. The quality of the response is judged immediately, as soon as the baby is stressed by weight bearing.

Normal response. The baby supports his weight with the arms below the horizontal for some seconds before the arms yield symmetrically.

Deviations. Babies slip through if they yield slowly from the very onset. Babies flop through if there is an almost total absence of resistance.

Pitfalls. Failure to appreciate that the response is judged in the very first moments of weight bearing.

VENTRAL SUSPENSION

Method. The baby is supported in the prone position on the palm of one hand held under the abdomen.

Normal response. The baby droops a little under the force of gravity (Fig. 3.5a)

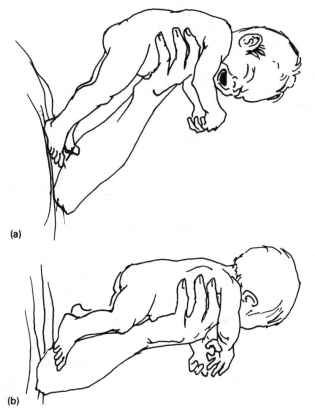

(a)

(b)

FIG. 3.5a and b. Normal postures in ventral suspension.

but extends his neck from time to time so that the head intermittently intersects the extended line of the thoracic spinous processes (Fig. 3.5b).

Deviations. The floppy baby's posture is too much that of an inverted U. He rarely or never brings his head above the line. The reverse is characteristic of the hyperextended baby (Fig. 3.6).

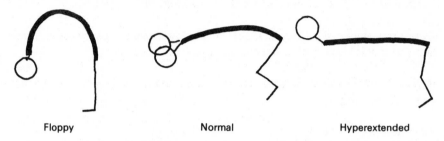

| Floppy | Normal | Hyperextended |

FIG. 3.6. Normal and abnormal postures in ventral suspension.

Pitfalls. Postural hyperextension is seen after face or brow presentation.

NECK TRACTION
Method. The baby is grasped by the hands. and drawn forwards and upwards from the supine position.

Normal response. Supportive response by flexion of the upper limbs and neck. There is a mild degree of head lag from the start and this becomes more marked within seconds.

Deviations. Too little support is commoner than too much. Asymmetry is usually due to a peripheral lesion.

Pitfalls. Postural hyperextension is seen after face or brow presentation.

PALMAR GRASP
Method. The examiner's index fingers are brought simultaneously into the baby's palms to exert gentle pressure and traction at the level of the metacarpal heads. Fisting may have to be overcome by gentle thumb pressure on the dorsum of the metacarpo-phalangeal joints while the examiner's middle fingers roll the baby's digits open with a sweeping action distally along the length of the palm.

Normal response. The baby's fingers close quite firmly and symmetrically on the examiner's index fingers.

Deviations. There is usually little problem in deciding excess or reduction, especially if there is asymmetry.
    The thumb is held in the palm with more excessive forms of fisting.

Pitfalls. Effects of ATNR.

HIP ABDUCTION

Method. In the supine position with knee and hip flexed to 90° the baby's legs are held lightly (like drumsticks) and a quick light movement of abduction is made.

Normal response. There is an initial catch due to the stretch reflex in the adductors, then the muscles yield till the thighs are easily taken to about 80° from the vertical.

Deviations. With increased resistance there is a strong catch after which it is not easy to continue abduction.

With reduced resistance there is little or no catch, the hips flop down on the surface, like a book with a broken spine.

PLACING

Method. The baby is suspended upright with the lower limbs deflexed and the dorsum of the forefoot is brought up lightly against an obstacle such as the table edge.

Normal response. The baby steps up smartly over the obstacle, often with a minor degree of asymmetry. Passive neck extension promotes a stronger response.

Deviations. These usually consist of reduced, sluggish, absent or asymmetrical responses. To be considered significant asymmetry is more than minimal and reproducible, e.g. three times out of three.

The exaggerated response is very quick and often overshoots jerkily.

Pitfalls. An exaggerated response may sometimes cause the baby's feet to catch under the obstacle.

EXTENSOR THRUST

Method. Once the baby has placed his feet on the examining surface after overcoming the obstacle, the degree of weight support is reduced so that he is allowed to sag a little through flexion in hips, knees and ankles; he is then jostled gently and the degree of weight support is increased tentatively.

Normal response. Hips, knees and ankles extend so that the baby stands upright briefly with only mild flexion at hip and knee.

Deviations. With a reduced response the lower limb flexion is excessive and little or no straightening can be produced; usually one finds that this is associated with poor head control and shoulder girdle support as the extensor response is sought. When extensor thrust is excessive it is difficult to get the baby to sag out of what would normally be the end-point of the manoeuvre; he 'stands to attention' unduly.

Pitfalls. A normal response may be masked by the postural effects of breech presentation with flexed or extended lower limbs.

PRIMARY WALKING

Method. Immediately after the extensor thrust response, the baby is leaned forward slightly. The examiner may need to let the heels come up a little off the surface while being careful not to lift too much of the body weight.

Normal response. The baby walks strongly and automatically if he is carried forward with only slight support of his body weight (Fig. 3.7). The response is a combination of progression and weight-bearing in a series of alternating unilateral extensor thrust responses. The strides are of large amplitude and there may be mild plantigrade scissors gait. The response is facilitated by passive neck extension.

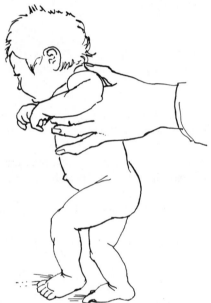

FIG. 3.7. Primary walking.

Deviations. Absent, asymmetrical, tiptoe or scissors gait are most common; with experience many milder degrees of asymmetry can be noted.

MORO

Method. Controlled head drop is used (Fig. 3.8a). The baby is semi-recumbent, the examiner supporting up to shoulder level with one forearm and hand while the head is cupped in the opposite hand. When the baby is symmetrically controlled, head drop of only a few centimetres is allowed by a quick release of the examiner's wrist. The Moro reflex should not be attempted in infants suspected of having Erb's palsy or cervical spinal lesion.

Normal responses. Abduction and extension of the upper limbs with finger spreading, then circumduction and flexion with finger closure (Fig. 3.8b).

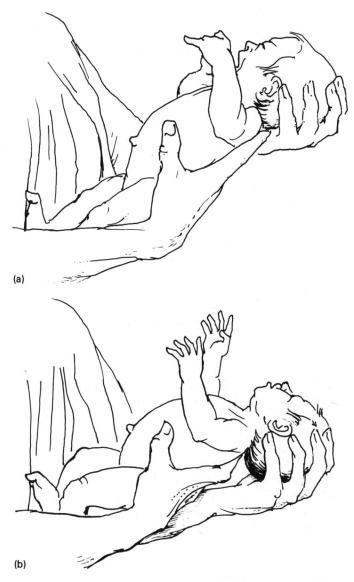

(a)

(b)

FIG. 3.8a and b. Moro response.

Deviations. The threshold is scored low if the response is inadvertently obtained during the earlier items, high if the examiner feels he has to work hard for a modest response to the stimulus. The low-threshold responses are often tremulous, the high threshold often circumscribed or partial. The former may be lightning-quick and these responses tend to be partial, i.e. only abduction and extension. Asymmetry should be reproducible, e.g. three times out of three.

Pitfalls. Effects of ATNR.

CRY
Normal behaviour. The normal baby cries towards the end of the examination in protest at this modest intrusion on his usual pattern of quietly surfacing fully before his feed.

Deviations. The cerebral cry is high-pitched and shrill.

Pitfalls. One should remember to think beyond the serious shrill cerebral cry. Other variations are common in forms of neurological dysfunction.

TONE
This is the cumulative impression of many continuing overlapping observations throughout the examination.

The Pre-Term Infant

Neurological examination
When carrying out a neurological examination of a pre-term infant one must take into account the fact that the normal muscle tone and power are relatively low, to make allowances for responses that at term would qualify as apathetic, weak or hypotonic.

In addition the pre-term infant is relatively unflexed because flexor tone is still underdeveloped and he has not experienced the flexural compressional effects of the final weeks *in utero*. The infant may, for instance, walk on tiptoe and have ankle clonus and this could be misinterpreted. The normal pre-term infant's gait is symmetrical and the foot goes flat when the body is supported in the vertical position and not tilted forward; ankle clonus is also symmetrical and is not sustained. Scissoring is not observed.

The infant should be re-examined at intervals to monitor neurological maturation and the final examination should be as near term as his discharge date allows. By then he should normally be free and full in the placing, extensor thrust and primary walking responses compared with the newborn term infant and within a few days past term there is little or no difference between them.

Assessment of maturity
In practice the use of gestational age assessment concentrates largely on whether low birth-weight infants (2500 g or less) are pre-term (less than 37 completed weeks of gestation) and physiologically immature but of appropriate weight for gestational age, or whether they are inappropriately small or light for gestational age, be this term or pre-term.

If the infant is in good fettle and performs up to the expected term level in neurological examination it can be assumed that this is his gestational age even if birth-weight is low. If on the other hand responses are poor, performance can either be physiologically appropriate to a pre-term gestational age or be due to neurological dysfunction characterized by 'apathy'.

The chart illustrated (Fig. 3.9), which combines selected items from Robinson

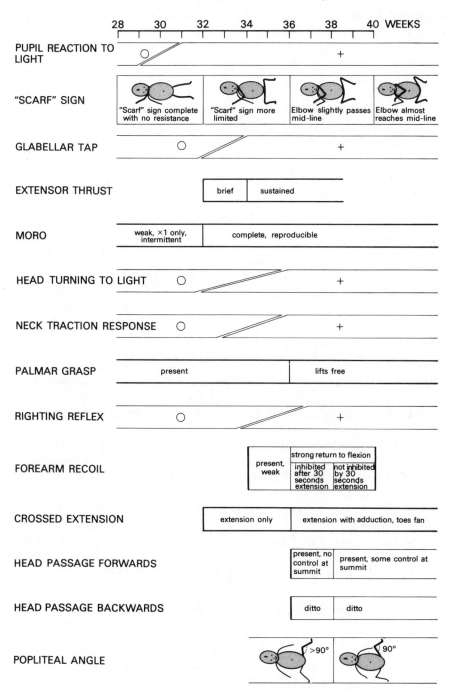

FIG. 3.9. Assessment of gestational age.

(1966) and Amiel-Tison (1968), has been found useful in assessing gestational age at roughly 2 week intervals (30–32 weeks, 32–34 weeks and so on). Certain physical characteristics are also noted. These were selected from the Farr score (Farr *et al.*, 1966) and chosen on the basis of easy objectivity. Four items are recorded; the condition of the pinnae, breasts and genitalia and the presence or absence of oedema. A similar modified Farr score for general use has recently been suggested by Parkin *et al.* (1976). The advantage of using some measures of external characteristics as an adjunct to neurological evaluation is that if immature performance is appropriate to gestational age suggested by these, all is probably well. However, if there is an obvious difference between the two measures then neurological dysfunction is significant.

Results of the Examination

The population divides into 4 categories:

(1) normal performance in all items;
(2) normal performance overall with some minor abnormalities or deviations, e.g. subconjunctival haemorrhage, isolated sixth nerve palsy or isolated high-threshold Moro response. What counts is the *cumulative overall* impression;
(3) minor neurological dysfunction;
(4) severe neurological dysfunction. In this category the baby presents with florid signs of convulsive, tonic, postural or motor disorders.

It is impossible to segregate these categories with absolute precision, no matter how experienced the examiner or how sophisticated his tests. One might say that the crucial group with significant minor neurological dysfunction is arrived at by subtraction: these infants would not be rated as showing gross signs of neurological abnormality and yet they show more than can be passed off as variations within the range of normal. The increased recognition of hemisyndromes has helped the primary care doctor in his evaluations and if in doubt a second opinion should be sought.

In a routine nursery service at West Middlesex Hospital and Chiswick Maternity Hospital (1968–72) minor neurological dysfunction was found in a little over 4 per cent of all infants, while the ascertainment in a partially overlapping survey of 2000 births at Chiswick (Hounslow Mother and Child Study) was 10 per cent in the hands of research fellows (Zinkin, 1976).

Management of Minor Neurological Dysfunction

Investigation
The question of immediate investigation depends to a large extent on whether there are additional high-risk factors in terms of inheritance and/or pre- and perinatal experience. One should be alerted, for instance, by a history of affected siblings or consanguinity, signs of intrauterine infection, light weight for gestational age or small head circumference. A history devoid of definable risk raises the possibility of congenital malformations or metabolic disorders. It should be

remembered that apparent overt risk factors such as breech birth or unexpected respiratory distress may themselves be indicators of underlying covert abnormality. In the event, much depends on the inclination of the individual clinician. It is found that very few infants exhibiting minor neurological dysfunction require investigation initially.

Explanation

Both parents are interviewed by the consultant, who explains that the baby shows a mild upset in the way he holds himself, moves or handles (experienced mothers generally confirm this) and it is expected that the baby will get over this of his own accord before long. This explanation is easily understood when seen to relate to factors such as difficulty in delivery, but even when there is no obvious cause parents usually accept these consequences of universal examinations at this level when the situation is suitably explained to them.

The family doctor is informed and a copy of that letter is sent to the appropriate community paediatrician.

Management

Babies who show minor neurological dysfunction in the newborn period may present with problems of behaviour and management in the early months at home. These are discussed elsewhere (p. 340). Some initial advice about posture may be helpful. The baby whose disorder is characterized by hypertonicity/ hyperactivity is suited best by the prone position and if there is strong lateral preference the mother is told how to position the baby so that he is induced to turn towards the opposite side.

The first follow-up visit is scheduled for age 4 weeks. If the neurological dysfunction is more obvious or if there is any suggestion of fits, no matter how mild or focal, then full investigation is mandatory. Even if there is no change investigation should be seriously considered, for the expected spontaneous improvement in these early weeks is quite rapid.

The counsel of perfection would be to follow these children until one is sure that they are developing normally up to the acquisition of normal speech. In practice those who improve most rapidly to perform within the normal range are often discharged from hospital follow-up at age 7–12 months. The local community child health doctor should be informed of the early findings to facilitate later identification of possible cerebral dysfunction in the preschool years or at latest on school entry. The remainder, who have a continuing problem, are managed according to the nature and dimensions of their needs.

Pro and Contra

The main arguments that are advanced by those who doubt the usefulness of routine neurological examination of the newborn are that the examination is time consuming, that it cannot test the higher functions of the brain, that minor neurological dysfunction does not call for intervention and will usually resolve spontaneously, that anything of importance would be revealed at examination later in the first year, that if abnormal signs are detected unnecessary worry is caused to parents by disclosing this, or alternatively that it may be misleading to tell a mother that her baby is normal on the basis of a brief examination, particularly if there is a background of risk factors. Similarly it is argued that the label of normal performance may be to the disadvantage of children whose problems are not discoverable in the newborn examination or arise postnatally.

The long-term outcome of infants exhibiting minor neurological dysfunction in the newborn period (p. 123, Francis-Williams, 1970, 1976) demonstrates that the lofty 'silent' areas of the brain can be well spoken for by responses definable at a more lowly level. Admittedly, early diagnosis and treatment is rare though not unknown. More importantly a plan for follow-up is arranged because neurological dysfunction is often the prelude to other developmental problems that become evident only after a 'normal' interval.

Parents are no more likely to be distressed by the need to watch the baby's neurodevelopmental progress than they are when the baby is kept under review because of a clicking hip or systolic murmur. If a high risk infant is found to be performing normally the mother is told so and if pressed about possible deleterious effects of high risk factors, she is told that he has performed in as normal a way as any baby in the unit with no such risk background. The generic validity of this statement is born out by the observed long-term results.

By 6 months many infants who had minor neurological dysfunction will pass as normal. Thus one cannot depend on significant dysfunction (in terms of later disability) being identified later in the first year. In any event only 70 per cent of infants in England and Wales visit clinics for routine surveillance.

Follow-up of some cases (Francis-Williams, 1970, 1976) has produced evidence that neonates with minor neurological dysfunction have, as a group, a significant liability to developmental disorders which may be capable of amelioration by early intervention.

Reliable neurological examination should be widely (and ultimately universally) available since it is illogical to offer routine physical examinations that virtually exclude an adequate assessment of the infant's most vulnerable system. There is no serious obstacle to proceeding with the widespread adoption of reliable neurological examination in the routine nursery service. However, it is imperative that the logistics and cost-effectiveness of any scheme operate as stringent determinants of the rate and extent to which it is put into operation (Holt, 1974). Furthermore, introduction of routine neurological examinations should proceed cautiously on a limited scale to allow adequate time for training and to have good quality work. This is not a system to introduce for all newborns at the same moment in time when there is a risk of ending up with a pile of paper work and little solid reward to show for it.

References

AMIEL-TISON C. (1968) Neurological evaluation of the maturity of newborn infants. *Archives of Disease in Childhood*, **43**, 89.

ANDRÉ-THOMAS S. and SAINT-ANNE DARGASSIES S. (1952) *Études Neurologiques sur le Nouveau-Né et le Jeune Nourrisson.* Paris: Masson et Cie.

ANDRÉ-THOMAS S., CHESNI Y. and SAINT-ANNE DARGASSIES S., (1955) *Examen Neurologique du Nourrisson.* Paris: Editions La Vie Médicale.

ANDRÉ-THOMAS S., CHESNI Y. and SAINT-ANNE DARGASSIES S. (1960) *The Neurological Examination of the Infant.* Little Club Clinics No. 1. London: Heinemann.

FARR V., MITCHELL R.G., NELIGAN G.A. and PARKIN J.M. (1966). The definition of some external characteristics used in the assessment of gestational age in the newborn infant. *Developmental Medicine and Child Neurology*, **8**, 507.

FRANCIS-WILLIAMS J. (1974) *Children with Specific Learning Difficulties.* 2nd Ed. Oxford: Pergamon Press.

FRANCIS-WILLIAMS J. (1976) Early identification of children likely to have specific learning difficulties: report of a follow-up. *Developmental Medicine and Child Neurology*, **18**, 71.

HOLT K.S. (1974) Screening for disease: infancy and childhood. *Lancet* **ii**, 1057.

PARKIN J.M., HEY E.N. and CLOWES J.S. (1976) Rapid assessment of gestational age at birth. *Archives of Disease in Childhood*, **51**, 259.

PRECHTL H. and BEINTEMA D. (1964) *The Neurological Examination of the Full-Term Newborn Infant. Clinics in Developmental Medicine No. 12.* London: Heinemann.

ROBINSON, R.J. (1966) Assessment of gestational age by neurological examination. *Archives of Disease in Childhood*, **41**, 437.

ZINKIN P.M. (1976) Personal communication.

CHAPTER 4

Developmental Assessment and Development Screening

Developmental assessment has been described as a systematized form of observation which allows some estimation to be made of the extent of activities of the brain.

The purpose of assessment is to identify, as early as possible, deviations from normal developmental behaviour, which may be the first indicators of mental, physical, neurological, behavioural or environmental impairment, so that appropriate measures can be taken to rectify or ameliorate the conditions identified.

Developmental screening is a brief examination, which might reasonably be applied to a total population of infants and young children, to detect those who appear to merit a more detailed assessment. The practicability and cost effectiveness of developmental screening on a large scale has not been established yet, nevertheless this method is widely used in clinical practice, a limited number of key questions and observations indicating whether or not developmental level appears to be appropriate for age.

The basic requirement for screening and assessment is understanding of how normal infants and young children behave when physically thriving and reared in environments which provide space and freedom to move, household materials and toys to handle and consistent adult attention giving physical contact, verbal stimulation and emotional satisfaction.

Predictive Value of Developmental Assessment

There is considerable controversy about the predictive value for later intelligence of developmental testing in infancy and early childhood. Those who maintain that infant tests have little predictive value are inclined to go further and suggest that without accurate prediction developmental assessment is valueless. Even the staunchest protagonists of the value of early developmental testing do not claim that the tests can do more than establish that, at the time of examination, the infant is, or is not, developing normally. Similarly an early physical examination can do no more than establish that the infant is healthy and adequately nourished at that time.

It is not always appreciated that the conclusions reached from developmental assessment are not synonymous with scored responses on a series of objective tests applied in isolation. In coming to a decision about current developmental functioning and probable mental potential, cognizance must be taken of pre- and perinatal events; postnatal environment; the child's developmental history as given by his mother; any physical, neurological or sensory impairments; the child's level of interest, alertness and concentration in the testing situation, the quality of his responses and possible reasons for failure to respond.

Rate of development gives a better indication of potential than status at one period in time and in many cases a second examination after an interval of 3–6 months is required before any opinion can be given. In other cases an estimate of likely potential cannot be given until an attempt has been made to modify adverse factors which may be affecting performance.

There is sufficient evidence from a number of studies (e.g. Drillien, 1964; Knobloch and Pasamanick, 1974; Illingworth, 1972, 1975) that given in-depth assessment as described below, most cases of mental retardation of a degree likely to preclude entry to normal school, can be diagnosed confidently before the age of 1 year and children who are mildly retarded by age 2 years. In addition, one can identify in the first 12–18 months of life (or have a strong suspicion about) most cases of congenital cerebral palsy, some neuromuscular disorders, moderate or severe defects of hearing and vision and some immediately treatable conditions such as squints and congenital disclocation of hip.

However, it is impossible to predict which children will suffer from later illness or injury. A larger number will be subjected to deprivation of experience, stimulation and emotional stability sufficient to seriously impair learning capability in school and children from backgrounds which are materially, culturally and emotionally impoverished are at high risk of later disability and merit regular developmental supervision on this account.

Conversely other children may catch up when adverse factors resolve or are removed, e.g. transient abnormal neurological signs in the first year of life, commonly seen in infants of very low birth-weight and others with evidence of hypoxic or traumatic damage in the perinatal period, are often associated with developmental delay; as the signs resolve there may be a spurt in development (Chapter 15); children removed from a depriving environment to a good foster home may show marked gains.

A more fundamental difficulty is that it is by no means sure how developing skills in infancy are related to the different skills required in the later learning situation in school (p. 111). Longitudinal studies relating early development to school performance, taking full account of intrinsic and extrinsic factors in the child's life history which might have a bearing on later learning ability, could throw light on this problem.

Although mental retardation and neurological abnormality can be diagnosed early, it is much more difficult to predict mental superiority, but this is of more academic than practical interest.

Prediction is a part of developmental assessment (and often parents press for prognoses before these can be given with any confidence), but assessment is more concerned with the causes of developmental lags as a preliminary to action and with the detection of physical, neurological and sensory defects and behaviour problems, which may be amenable to altered management or treatment. Assessment without consequent intervention is of little benefit to the child or to his family.

A full developmental assessment consists of:

(1) history,
(2) developmental testing,
(3) physical examination,
(4) neurological examination,
(5) tests of hearing and vision.

(1) and (2) are considered in this chapter, (3) and (4) in Chapter 7 and (5) in Chapter 8.

On Taking a History

The history given by the mother is probably the most important part of the developmental examination and adequate time must be allowed for this. If it appears likely that the child attending for assessment has a definite handicap, it is helpful if both parents are present at the first interview. However, unnecessary anxiety may be generated if the father is requested to attend with a child considered to be suspect only.

The two main areas of information to be elicited from history are:

(1) circumstances which place the child at increased risk (as compared with children in the general population) of suffering from brain dysfunction or damage, sensory defect and postnatal deprivation, and

(2) the child's health history and developmental and behavioural status, both past and present.

'At-risk' factors

The history should take note of the following:

(1) Family history: including socioeconomic circumstances, housing, patterns of child rearing and stressful domestic situations (the health visitor's knowledge is invaluable here); age, health (physical and mental), education and occupations of parents and some estimate of the parents' (or mother's) apparent level of intelligence; age and current status of siblings and the presence of particular developmental patterns in the family such as slow speech and sinistrality; history of handicapping conditions and sensory defects in near relatives.

(2) Reproductive history of mother: including outcome of all conceptions and if widely spaced or a long interval from marriage to first conception, whether intentional (contraception practised) or unintentional.

(3) Pregnancy history: with special note taken of infections, drug taking and threatened abortion in the first trimester and late pregnancy complications which carry risk to the fetus of malnutrition or hypoxia.

(4) Perinatal history: including gestational age at birth, complications of labour and delivery, immediate postnatal state of the infant and later neonatal complications. The behaviour of the prematurely delivered infant after discharge from maternity hospital must be considered in relation to expected performance

if he had been born at term. If gestational age is in doubt, a firm conclusion about developmental functioning is not possible in the early months of life. The effect of prematurity becomes relatively less important with increasing age.

Obstetric and baby records may provide most of the information specified under (2) to (4) above and whenever possible these records should be scrutinized in advance.

(5) Any circumstances in the child's postnatal life which might have an effect on current development: in particular any depriving situations such as poor maternal care, separation of mother and child due to hospitalisation of either, admission to residential or day nursery or foster home and specific physical or sensory defects which restrict opportunities for obtaining normal stimulations and experiences.

Developmental history

The mother is the best observer of her child and her account of his past progress and present skills is an essential part of the developmental assessment.

In a brief screening session the history may be all that can be elicited. The infant may be due for nap or feed or be frightened by strange surroundings and refuse to respond to friendly overtures or proffered toys. Older children may not demonstrate their abilities in the short time available for screening. In many such cases the history will allow the examiner to decide that the child appears to be functioning at or above the expected level for age, or that he should be seen again at an hour when he is likely to be awake and ready for play, or when more time can be allowed.

Past history. With skilful questioning even mothers of limited intelligence can give an accurate account of what their children are doing and how they are behaving here and now, but even perceptive mothers find it difficult to remember what their children were doing in the past. The further back, the more difficult; but whereas developmental minutiae may be important in the past history of the suspect infant or toddler, major milestones, rather than details, suffice at later ages.

It is helpful to relate past progress to particular dates such as Christmas, the summer holidays or the child's birthday, enabling mother to cast her mind back to events likely to be more vividly remembered.

Past history is of particular importance when it seems that development progressed normally up to a certain age and then the pattern of development or rate of progress altered noticeably. Some confirmation may be obtainable from health visitor, clinic doctor or family practitioner records.

Present functioning. The first essential in obtaining an accurate record is to ensure that what is meant by the examiner is correctly understood by the mother and *vice versa*. Vague terms such as 'sitting', 'walking', 'grasping' should not be used. Sufficient detail must be given in questioning to avoid any misinterpretation and to convey to mother a facsimile of the clear picture of performance in the examiner's mind. It follows that a useful developmental history can not be obtained if the questioner is not well experienced in the ways normal infants behave.

Questions should never be put in such a way that the mother gains the impression that her child *ought* to be doing something. The phrase 'can he . . . ?' should be avoided. The form of words 'tell me how he . . . ?', 'what happens when . . . ?' and 'I don't expect he can . . . yet?' are more likely to elicit accurate responses.

Pleasure should be shown in reported achievements and not too much concern about negative answers, unless mother herself is concerned. Positive responses are followed up with 'when did he start to do that?' and if appropriate 'how often?' or 'how well?', e.g. if mother reports that her 10-week infant has a social smile, it is important to know when he began to smile and whether he smiles readily and often or only occasionally after much coaxing.

Useful questions are those concerned with activities seldom regarded by parents as being associated with neurodevelopmental progress such as hand regard and finger play, discontent if left lying awake without entertainment, ability to deal with stodgy foods and chew a biscuit and persistent mouthing.

If there are siblings it is worth enquiring in general terms how this child compares with his siblings at like age (obviously quicker, obviously slower, much the same) in overall development and specific areas of functioning. Educational progress of school age siblings should be noted.

Time must be allowed for the mother to express her feelings about the child and his problems (if she admits that he has any) and discuss the reactions of father and other family members. Note should be taken of any aspects of mother–child interaction that are apparent.

Any mother who is concerned about any aspect of her child's development (that he is not seeing, hearing, taking notice, moving, using his hands or talking, like others of his age or siblings at like age) should be taken seriously, even if no obvious delay or deficit is found on examination. Such a child should be kept under review until both mother and doctor are satisfied that development is progressing normally.

The mother's account of current performance can be checked against findings on examination and some estimate made of reliability, which will influence the significance accorded to past history. Discrepancies in developmental history may throw doubt on reliability; alternatively they may suggest the presence of specific defects or deprivations.

Even with careful questioning answers may still be inaccurate. The mother may genuinely believe that facial grimaces imply a social smile, confuse reflex with voluntary grasping and sucking a biscuit with chewing, and interpret polysyllabic babbling as meaningful speech. Other mothers are unwilling to admit the possibility of developmental delay and make such comments as 'of course he's very intelligent', 'he doesn't say much but he is taking everything in', 'it's his shy nature, just like his Dad'. Such value judgements should be treated with reserve, particularly if examination fails to confirm the mother's optimism. In a few cases the mother's account of the child's abilities is so far removed from reality to suggest that she is in need of help herself.

Health history
Hospital attendances and admissions, other illnesses, particularly convulsions and middle ear infections and immunization record should be noted.

History of behaviour
In the first 6 months of life problems of management and behaviour may be the first indicators of mental or neurological impairment. Questions should be asked about feeding behaviour, sleep patterns, any difficulties encountered in the care-taking activities of nappy changing, bathing and dressing, reaction to loud sounds or sudden changes of posture and amount of spontaneous movement. The significance of these early behavioural characteristics is discussed in Chapter 15.

Temperamental traits and specific problems of behaviour of older infants and young children should also be recorded (Chapter 25).

Examination Environment and Equipment

The examination room must be warm enough for the child to be comfortable when undressed. Infants of 6 months or younger usually do not object to being stripped of clothes; mother is invited to undress the baby except for nappy towards the end of history taking, this remaining item will be removed before examination. The infant of 7–12 months is more wary of strangers and strange surroundings but in most cases will allow removal of shoes, socks, long-sleeved woollens and trousers without complaint; remaining garments are removed before assessment of locomotor function and physical examination. After the

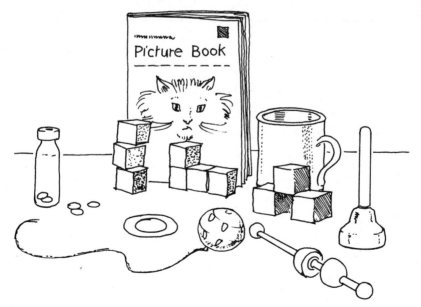

Fig. 4.1. Testing materials for the first 15 months of life.

age of 1 year it is diplomatic to avoid undressing until the developmental examination is completed apart from assessment of locomotion which necessitates removal of shoes, socks and long trousers.

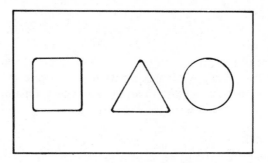

FIG. 4.2a. Three-hole formboard.

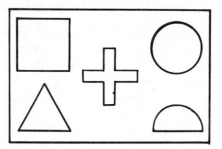

FIG. 4.2b. Five-shape colour forms.

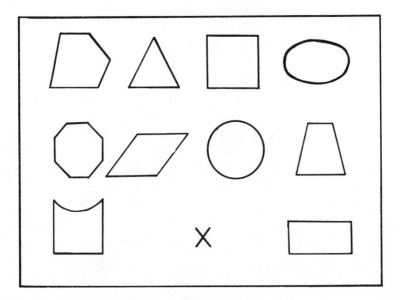

FIG. 4.2c. Ten-shape geometric forms.

TABLE 4.1. Equipment for developmental testing at different ages.

4–20 weeks

Dangling object; practice golf ball or 4 inch embroidery hoop on string 8 inches long and not thicker than 1/16th inch diameter

Teething ring; diameters, outer $2\frac{1}{2}$ inches, inner $1\frac{1}{2}$ inches

*1 inch cube, wooden or solid plastic, red colour recommended

20–40 weeks

Rattle

Pellets $\frac{1}{4}$–$\frac{1}{2}$ inch diameter, e.g. tiny ball of tissue paper or cotton wool or small sweet

*3 1-inch cubes

Bell; $2\frac{1}{2}$–3 inches high with wooden handle and metal bowl of $1\frac{1}{2}$ inch diameter

Ball or hoop on string

40 weeks–15 months

*6 1-inch cubes

Mug; aluminium, enamel or melamine, $2\frac{1}{4}$ inches high, 3 inches diameter

Ball or hoop on string

Pellets

Glass bottle; $2\frac{1}{2}$–3 inches high, neck 1 inch diameter, e.g. specimen bottle

Pencil and scribbling paper

Picture book with single common objects on each page, e.g. Ladybird First or Second Picture Book

Balls; small, $2\frac{1}{2}$ inches diameter, large, 5–6 inches diameter

15 months–3 years

*10 1-inch cubes

Mug

Pencil and paper

*Formboard; three-hole. Green board 8×5 inches, three equidistant holes, square $1\frac{1}{2}$ inches, triangle $1\frac{3}{4}$ inches, circle $1\frac{3}{4}$ inches. Red shapes slightly smaller than holes for easy fit

Colour forms, 5 shapes. White card 12×9 inches with five red forms; matching thick card cut-outs (3 inches) of square, circle, cross, triangle, half-circle

Balls

Books, one showing single familiar objects and one showing everyday activities

Picture cards, single pictures of common objects, e.g. using Ladybird First Picture Book: Card 1 flowers, cat, shoes, ball; Card 2 plate and spoon, dog, doll, bus, teddy, biscuits

Box of 10 miniature toys and other small objects, e.g. car, cup, spoon, plate, doll, aeroplane, pencil, key, coin, scissors

3–5 years

10 pellets and bottle

Blunt-ended scissors

12 1-inch cubes, 3 each of red, blue, yellow and green

Cards for copying: circle, cross, square and triangle, about $2\frac{3}{8}$ in diameter, length or sides, drawn in heavy black outline

Forms for tracing: double diamond outer diagonals $2\frac{3}{8}$ in, distance to inner lines $\frac{3}{8}$ in; double cross; height/width $3\frac{1}{2}$ in, outer arms height/width $1\frac{1}{4}$ in, distance to inner lines $\frac{3}{8}$ inch

Incomplete man; height 3 inches, head with eyebrows, trunk with buttons, one leg and foot

Geometric forms; white card 9×11 in., shapes width/height $1\frac{1}{2}$ in; matching set of shapes drawn on cards $2\frac{1}{2} \times 2\frac{1}{2}$ in

Card showing big/small circles (diameter $3\frac{1}{2}$ in/3 in); long/short lines $2\frac{1}{2}$ in/2 in

---

Basic furniture includes a low arm-chair for mother's comfort; a desk or table and two desk chairs, one of appropriate height for the infant or toddler, seated on mother's lap, to be able to play with table-top toys easily; an examination couch (if the couch is placed against a wall this should be free of distracting pictures); a foam rubber physiotherapy mat or washable rug of adequate size to allow rolling and crawling; a child-size table and chair without arms. Ideally the room should be large enough for demonstration of walking, trotting and throwing and kicking a ball.

Table 4.1 details equipment for developmental testing at different ages. Sizes of play materials are approximate except for items asterisked, when standard sizes are required. Test materials are illustrated in Figs 4.1., 4.2. and 4.3.

For a brief screening examination available ward or consulting-room equipment can be substituted for some items (e.g. stethoscope and tongue depressor for dangling object and rattle). Other items, such as 1-inch cubes, are indispensable.

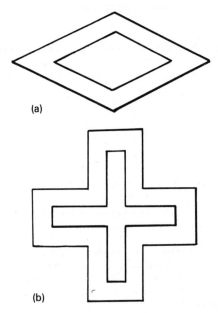

(a)

(b)

Fig. 4.3. Shapes for tracing: (a) double diamond; (b) double cross.

Apart from testing equipment it is useful to have a selection of other toys (e.g. doll, teddy bear, doll's cot with covers, wheeled toy on cord, squeaky bath toy, cars, string of wooden beads or plastic keys) to amuse the child during conversation with mother and demonstrate free play activities.

Sequences of Normal Development, 4 Weeks to 3 Years

Sequences of normal development from 4 weeks to 3 years are detailed in Table 4.2. Average age norms are given for guidance but it should be remembered that within the range of normal there is variation in the rate of development amounting to some weeks either way in the first 12–18 months, and some months thereafter. 'Stops and starts', which are later demonstrated to be of little long-term significance, are also seen. It is difficult to draw dividing lines between what would be considered acceptably normal, suspect or definitely abnormal, though it is obvious that the further the child deviates below average performance the more likely is it that he is abnormal.

Table 4.3 gives a rough guide to degrees of delay (in any area of development) at different ages which might be considered significant, in that the child appears to be functioning at four-fifths or less of what would be expected for age. Such children should be kept under review. As the child gets older it is easier to decide whether or not he is showing significant delay, e.g. 2 weeks delay at age 10 weeks has roughly the same significance as 10 months delay at 4 years, but is much more difficult to identify because items of objective testing are more limited.

Although rate of development varies in normal children, sequences of development vary less. Deviations in sequence within one area of functioning may be normal variants (e.g. the infant who shuffles on his buttocks instead of crawling), indicators of deprivation (e.g. the infant who bears little weight on his legs because he has not been allowed to stand) or indicators of pathological conditions (e.g. the infant with increased extensor tone whose performance in standing is 'better' than in sitting).

Similarly deviations in sequence between different areas of development may be normal variants (e.g. most children walk steadily before they have much useful speech, in a few talking comes first and walking is delayed) but more often discrepancies in level of functioning in different areas are due to deprivation or to pathological processes (e.g. the deprived child who is put down on the floor and is appropriate in motor function but is retarded in play behaviour because he has no play materials; the deaf child who has excessive delay in comprehension and speech; the cerebral palsied child of normal intelligence who shows excessive motor delay). Specific variations in sequence are discussed below in separate sections dealing with the four main areas of development. These are: posture and gross motor behaviour; vision, fine motor and adaptive behaviour; hearing, comprehension and communication; social development, play activities and self-help skills.

POSTURE AND GROSS MOTOR BEHAVIOUR

Gross motor function is the easiest area of development to assess both from history and observation. Because of this, undue stress may be placed on locomotor skills in a brief screening examination, particularly in the first 12–18 months of life. This is unfortunate as though, on average, retarded infants are late to reach motor milestones such as sitting and walking, a substantial minority (up to 20 per cent in some series) of children who are precluded from normal school on account of mental retardation were acceptably normal in early gross motor development. Conversely locomotor precocity is poorly correlated with

TABLE 4.2. Sequences of development 4 weeks–3 years

| | *Weeks* | |
	4	6
Posture and gross motor		
Supine (on firm surface)	Lies head to side; asymm. posture predominates; knees apart, soles of feet inturned; large jerky movements of limbs (especially arms); intermittently rolls part way to one side and other.	
Pull to sit from supine	Complete or marked head lag, head erect briefly when trunk at 90° to couch before falling forward.	Marked head lag, briefly holds head in line with trunk when trunk at 45–90° to couch.
Held sitting	Back rounded; head slumped forwards, chin on chest.	Back rounded; erects head momentarily.
Sitting supported with cushions		
Ventral suspension	Elbows flexed, hips partly extended, knees partly flexed; head intermittently held up in line with trunk.	
Placed prone (on firm surface)	Turns head to side, rests on cheek; elbows flexed away from or under chest, buttocks raised, knees under abdomen; intermittent crawling movements.	Head intermittently turned to midline, and briefly raised with chin just clear of couch; hips partly extended, knees intermittently under abdomen.
Standing, supported round chest under axillae	Reflex weight bearing.	Weight bearing disappearing.
Vision and fine motor		
Vision (see Chapter 8)	Head turns to light; regard of mother's face not sustained; 'picks up' briefly dangling object (not noise making) gently moved in line of vision at 6–10 inches to and from face (when supine); follows through less than 45°	Regard of mother's face sustained; follows dangling object brought in from side, 9–10 inches from face (when supine), follows up to midline.

8	12	16	20
Head to side; elbows flexed, hips and knees partly flexed; movements less jerky, more rhythmic; rolling reduced.	Head sometimes to side, sometimes midline; symmetric postures seen intermittently.	Symmetric postures predominate, head midline, both arms abducted or adducted with hands engaging in midline, both legs flexed or extended; smooth rhythmic movements of limbs.	
	Head lag lessening.	May or may not have slight head lag at beginning of pull up, quickly compensates and brings head up in line with trunk.	May lift head from supine at beginning of pull up, no head lag, head in line with trunk.
Back rounded, raises head frequently, maintains erect longer.	Back straighter, lumbar curve; head erect but thrust forward at angle to trunk, holds erect for several seconds then bobs forwards and downwards.	Back straight except for slight lumbar curve; head set forward but steadily erect, looks around; head bobs forward when trunk swayed.	Back straight; head erect in line with trunk, head control complete, no bobbing.
	Quickly wriggles down.	Sits 10 minutes+ with cushions at sides and back.	Sits 10 minutes+ with cushion at back.
Head held in line with trunk longer, keeps head in this position when lowered to prone.	Head held up beyond line of trunk; hips extended.		
Head maintained in midline, intermittently raised 1–2 inches above couch; buttocks lower, hips mainly extended, knees not under abdomen.	Head maintained with face at 45° to couch; buttocks flat, hips extended, rests on forearms, can get arms out from under chest; beginning to scratch at supporting surface.	Head and upper chest well up, face at 90° to couch, rests on forearms, beginning to push up on hands; 'swimming' (whole weight on abdomen), actively scratching at supporting surface.	Entire chest raised, arms extended, elbows straight, weight on hands; on verge of rolling.
Not weight-bearing on legs.	Bears small fraction of weight briefly, sags at knees.	Bears most of weight briefly, sags at hips and knees.	Weight bears for longer before sagging.
Follows dangling object beyond midline when supine.	Prompt regard of dangling object presented in mid-line when supine; follows from side to side through 180°. Sitting propped looks at faces rather than objects, turns head to watch elders moving. Hand regard.	Looks sustainedly at small toys in hand or within 12 inches on table top; may ignore very small still object (pellet) or look but not sustainedly. Hand regard lessening at 20 weeks.	

TABLE 4.2. Sequences of development 4 weeks–3 years.—*continued*

	Weeks	
	4	6
Hand posture	Hands firmly closed at rest, open during movement. Grasp reflex present.	Hands open more often. Grasp reflex present.
Teething ring, rattle, cube; approach and grasp		
Other play activities		
Hearing, comprehension and communication		
Hearing (see Chapter 8)	Startles to loud sounds, activity lessens momentarily when small bell rung about 4 inches from ear.	Activity lessens when mother speaks out of sight.
Vocalization (see Chapter 9)	Cries lustily when uncomfortable; small throaty sounds when comfortable.	
Comprehension	Watches friendly face speaking, opens and closes mouth, bobs head.	Smiles to friendly face.

	Weeks		
8	12	16	20
Hands loosely closed at rest. Grasp reflex disappearing.	Hands half open at rest. Grasp reflex absent but hands close on blankets, clothes, etc., with which they come in contact. Hands come together in supine and supported sitting.	Hands held mainly open.	Hands held open.
Teething ring placed in hand, retains briefly, does not regard.	Rattle placed in hand, grasps, retains, regards more than momentarily.	Rattle offered almost touching fingers, activation of arms without approach or two-handed approach, often overshoots but may secure; regards, retains, shakes, for 30 seconds or longer. Plays with fingers. Pulls dress over face.	Rattle offered 2–3 inches from fingers, two-handed accurate approach, secures, retains, may carry to mouth. Palmar grasp of cube. Plays with toys, crumples paper, splashes in bath with hands.
Stops whimpering when mother speaks out of sight, ignores voice if crying lustily.	Beginning to turn head to side to locate voice and other sounds.	Head and eyes turn in direction of sound.	
Definite vocal response to mother, short vowel sounds.	Coos (longer vowel sounds) in response, 'talks back', chuckles.	Excites, breathes heavily, laughs aloud. Makes sounds to himself and seems to listen to them.	More variety of sounds in vocal response, sing-song intonation, beginning to use consonants; high-pitched squeals.
Smiles and vocalizes in response.	Recognizes breast or bottle; when offered toy more interested in face; obvious pleasure on bathing, handling, tickling and other playful activities, especially when accompanied by voice.	Marked interest in toys, surroundings, people; wants to be propped when awake, fusses when left alone; needs entertainment; spontaneous social smile. Uses vocalization to attract attention.	Anticipates and excites on preparations for feeding, bathing. Recognizes, watches sibs. Still friendly to strangers.

TABLE 4.2. Sequences of development 4 weeks–3 years.—*continued*

	Weeks 24	28
Gross motor		
Supine and pull-to-sit	Supine, legs lifted high in extension, grasps feet. Lifts head at beginning of pull up, assists by flexing elbows and bracing shoulders.	Supine, raises head to look at feet. Raises head spontaneously in anticipation of pull up, head comes up in advance of trunk. Rolls supine to prone.
Sitting supported and unsupported (firm surface)	Sits erect in chair or pram, strapped for balance, leans forward to reach object, re-erects.	Sits on firm surface briefly unsupported, leans forwards, trunk at 45°, hands on on surface, arms extended; lifts arms, erects trunk momentarily.
Prone (firm surface)	Weight on hands, chest and upper abdomen raised. Rolls to supine.	Bears weight on one hand. Rolls over and over.
Standing, supported round chest; unsupported	Supported, bears almost all weight, hips extended, knees slightly flexed.	Supported, bears all weight, bounces actively.
Parachute (protective) reactions	Downwards present.	Sideways may or may not be present.
Fine motor and adaptive		
Reaching, type of grasp, release (cube)	Two-handed accurate approach. Whole hand palmar grasp to ulnar side. Holds one object only; if second placed in other hand drops first.	One-handed approach. Palmar grasp to radial side. Transfers object from hand to hand. Carries object to mouth. Two objects held more than momentarily if second object placed in hand.
Grasp of small object (pellet)	Looks intently at small object, still or moving. Tries to secure by raking into palm, all fingers and thumb flexing and extending in scratching movements, associated whole arm movements. May land on pellet with whole hand flat. May or may not be successful in securing.	
Exploitation of play materials Rattle	Secures when offered 6 inches from fingers; brings other hand across to touch; may achieve fumbling transfer or drop.	Leans forward to grasp when offered 10 inches from fingers; neat transfer; mouths.

32	36	40
Pulls up on two fingers needing little assistance.	Pulling self up to sit on pram or cot sides	
	just	easily

Sits on floor erect, hands up for 30–60 seconds, unsteady, easily topples or throws self backwards.	Sits steadily on floor, trunk erect 10 minutes +, leans forwards, recovers balance; topples when trunk rotated or stretching sideways; still throws self backwards; mother unwilling to leave sitting alone.	Sits as long as he wants; goes deliberately from sitting to prone and may go from prone to sitting; pivots using hands to assist; mother willing to leave unattended.
Pivots on abdomen through 45°, crossing one arm over other.	Beginning to pull self forward on abdomen ('sealing'); may get up on hands and knees and collapse forwards on to face or push self backwards.	Progresses forwards by mixture of hands/knees crawling and 'sealing'; may be 'hitching' (bottom shuffling).
On floor briefly, hands held, arms extended at shoulder height.	Placed standing at table or chair, holds on with 2 hands, chest not leaning against furniture; lets go and falls backwards or collapses on to buttocks. Attempting pull up, gets to knees.	Pulls up to stand in cot or on furniture; lets go and collapses on to buttocks.
Sideways present.	Forwards present	

One-handed accurate approach and grasp, first one object then another. Intermediate grasp, cube pressed against base of thumb by distal phalanges.

Digital grasp, cube grasped between volar pads of thumb and first 2 or 3 fingers; space between cube and palm. Presses down on firm surface to release.

Attempts to secure with thumb volar pad and side of curled or extended index finger; other fingers flex and extend in unison. Usually successful.	Succeeds in securing between volar pad of thumb and side of curled index finger, other fingers remain loosely curled (scissors grasp).	Succeeds in securing between volar pads of thumb and index or middle finger; forearm on surface for support. Extended index finger approach to pellet.

TABLE 4.2. Sequences of development 4 weeks–3 years.—*continued*

| | Weeks | |
	24	28
Cubes	Grasps one, approaches another; can only retain one.	Grasps one, grasps another placed in hand; retains more than momentarily.
Bell	Unselective grasp, as likely by bowl as handle; bangs, shakes but does not ring.	
Ring on string	Ignores string; may attempt to reach for ring, soon gives up.	Ignores string; reaches persistently for ring; fusses.
Comprehension and communication Vocalization (see Chapter 9)	Vocalizes tunefully to self and others; polysyllabic, distinct vowel sounds with some consonants, 'mm-mm-mm' when crying; low-pitched grunts and growls.	
Comprehension	Stretches hands to be lifted. Imitates actions (sticking out tongue) and noises, repeats when laughed at. Enjoys 'peep-bo'. Displeasure when toy removed. Ignores toy which falls outside visual field or searches around vaguely. Indicates does not want food by keeping lips shut. Smiles and vocalizes at mirror image.	
Feeding patterns	Accepts smooth 'solids' of consistency that does not run off tipped spoon. Hands round bottle.	Food mashed down but with tiny bits remaining.

| | Weeks | |
	44	48
Gross motor	When standing holding on, lifts and replaces one foot or one and then other. Crawls hands and knees or hitches.	Gets up to sit from supine without aid. Pivots on buttocks, using feet not hands. Side-stepping along furniture (cruising), sliding hands along. Walks 2 hands held, for balance.
Fine motor and adaptive Grasp and release, mouthing	Can remove object from container and thrust hand back in to replace, often does not release. Mouthing lessening.	Neat pincer grip of pellet, volar pads of thumb and index or middle finger from above, no forearm support.

	Weeks	
32	36	40

Grasps one, grasps second, retains prolonged period, ignores third cube offered.	Grasps two; when third offered drops one that he is holding to secure third.	Matches two cubes, bringing them together in mid-line, while watching them closely.

Everything to mouth.

Grasps by handle (low down) and bowl; shakes.

		Grasps by handle, shakes deliberately to produce sound, regards clapper and pokes with index finger.
Reaches for ring first; whole hand contact with string; may or may not secure ring via string.	Secures ring with effort; holds ring in one hand, string in other, manipulates both.	Secures ring easily by plucking string between thumb and index or middle finger.
Single consonant sounds, ('ba', 'da', 'ka'), sometimes preceded by vowel ('adah') but emphasis on consonant.	Two syllable consonant sounds ('dada') without meaning. Imitating sounds (cough, 'blowing raspberries').	Babbles loudly in extended, tuneful sequences, mainly for self amusement, less often for communication with familiars.

Clearly distinguishes strangers, may show marked anxiety. Responds to 'No-No' by temporary drawing back or change of expression. Recognizes own name. Imitates clapping hands. Looks after dropped toy.

		Wide variety of nursery games ('so big', 'round and round the garden'), responds to words and actions. Raises arms to be lifted. Uncovers toy hidden by cloth.

Household foods needing some chewing (minced meat, mashed down bits of fish with potato).

Chews biscuit, toast, piece of apple without choking.

	Weeks	Months
52	56	15

Lowers self deliberately from standing, looking down to floor. Holds on one hand, holds toy in other. May 'bear walk' (hands and feet). Cruises, lifting hands. Walks one hand held.	Stands alone briefly. May take 1–2 staggery steps forwards. May crawl up 2–3 steps. Crawls rather than walks.	Beginning to kneel unsupported. Gets up to stand from floor. Can walk across room; starts, stops after few steps, starts again; broad base, arms raised; steps uneven in length. Falls by collapse on to buttocks or forward on to outstretched hands. Walks rather than crawls.
Releases objects into container. Places cube on cube (to build) without release or tower falls when release attempted. Seldom mouths toys.	Grasps 2 cubes in one hand.	Repeatedly throws objects to floor or casts around. Sufficient control over release to build tower of 2 cubes. Can release pellet into bottle.

TABLE 4.2. Sequences of development 4 weeks–3 years.—*continued*

	Weeks	
	44	48
Exploitation of play materials		
Cubes and mug	Tips cubes out of mug, may lift out one.	Sequential play with cubes, moving about or picking up and dropping with concentration.
Ring on string	Goes immediately for string, watches ring approaching as he pulls.	Dangles ring with up and down movements of arm or sweeping side to side movements.
Pencil and paper		
Book	Treats picture book as object to be manipulated; tears.	
Ball play with adult		
Pellet and bottle	Points through glass at pellet in the bottle.	
Comprehension and communication	Extends toy in response to 'Give it to me' and gesture. May respond meaningfully to a few words ('Where's Daddy?')	'Dadda', 'Mamma' said with meaning.
Self-help-skills	Holds up arm for sleeve and foot for shoe. Drinks from cup, gets hands round but cannot control. Finger feeds biscuit, piece of apple.	

Releases 1–2 cubes into mug after several demonstrations. Attempts tower of 2, fails.	Releases 1–2 cubes into mug on request and gesture, without demonstration.	Places 5–6 cubes in mug with verbal encouragement. Builds tower of 2.
As for 48 weeks		

Pencil held in fist (palmar grasp), jabs at paper, may make faint marks.

Interested in book shown by adult.

Scribbles in imitation.

May scribble to and fro, spontaneously; attempts to copy stroke.

Helps turn pages. Pats pictures.

Pushes ball along floor from sitting.

Incipient throw, releases ball deliberately with slight forwards thrust from sitting.

Throws ball under or over hand from standing, may or may not go in intended direction; may topple over when throwing. Ignores request to kick, throws instead.

Tries unsuccessfully to drop pellet in bottle after demontion.

Drops pellet in, cannot get out after demonstration of 'dumping'; shakes bottle, pokes index finger in neck.

Jargons loudly and persistently, using vowels and many consonant sounds. Responds to words only of nursery games. Understands more words ('Where's teddy, the tick-tock, the car?').

May hand a few named objects. May demonstrate understanding of use ('drinking' from cup, brush to hair). Responds to some simple commands and gestures.

3–6 intelligible words apart from Mamma, Dadda. 'Understands a lot', demonstrates by responding to some simple commands without gesture. Makes wants known by pointing, saying 'uh-uh'.

Lifts cup or feeder beaker and drinks, then drops or turns upside down. Likes to hold spoon but cannot use.

Takes off shoes. Picks up cup, drinks, replaces with little spillage. Tips spoon. May indicate by gestures when soiled or wet.

TABLE 4.2. Sequences of development 4 weeks–3 years.—*continued*

	Months	
	18	21
Gross motor	Walks well, feet slightly apart, arms down; seldom falls; can carry large toy while walking. Runs stiffly and carefully, trunk and head erect; stops at obstacles. Kneels upright on floor. Squats to pick up toy, rises with aid of own hand to floor. Crawls upstairs to the top, backwards down stairs; walks up one hand held. Climbs forward into adult chair, turns to sit. Seats self on child size chair, sliding in sideways or edging backwards.	Running more smoothly, negotiates obstacles. Walks backwards in imitation. Stoops forward to pick up toy from floor. Squats for 5 minutes+ in play. Walks upstairs holding rail or hand against wall; walks down hand held.
Fine motor and adaptive, exploitation of play materials		
Cubes and mug	10 cubes in and out of mug spontaneously. Tower of 3–4 after demonstration.	Tower of 5–6 with demonstration and encouragement. Cannot align cubes (continues to build) but will imitate pushing 'train'.
Pellets and bottle	Inserts pellet spontaneously or on request. When asked to get it out, pokes finger in, shakes and finally turns bottle upside down on table ('dumping'). May or may not need demonstration.	
Pencil and paper	Pencil held in fist, mid shaft or near point. Spontaneous scribble. Makes single stroke after demonstration, without regard to direction.	Holds mid shaft or near point between volar pad of thumb and distal interphalangeal joints of first 3 fingers. Vigorous spontaneous scribble with preferred hand. Imitates single vertical stroke, roughly in the right direction.
Three-hole formboard, five colour forms	Piles blocks on board indiscriminately. May succeed in inserting round block after several demonstrations.	Piles blocks on board. After demonstrations inserts 2–3.
Book	Sustained interest in picture book. Places index finger on familiar objects, if largely and clearly depicted, with obvious recognition. Turns 2–3 pages at a time to find other pictures.	
Ball	Throws from standing, tends to take a few steps in the intended direction before and after throwing.	
	After demonstration kick, steps against, walks into or on to ball, does not lift foot to kick unless hand supported.	After demonstration lifts foot and pushes ball forward short distance, may miss it.

Runs, still on whole soles of feet, knees flex and arms alternate; seldom falls; may prefer running to walking. Squats for long periods to play, rises to feet without aid of own hands. Walks up and down stairs holding rail, two feet to one tread.	Runs well but still has difficulty in stopping suddenly and running round corners. Jumps 2 feet together on floor. Walks tip-toes, may need hand to start.	Runs like older children on forefeet; as one foot goes forward, other lifted well up behind; arms alternate. Can decelerate suddenly and run round corners. Jumps 2 feet together off bottom step. Walks tip-toes. Balances momentarily on preferred foot. Walks up stairs, hand to rail, one foot to tread; down two feet to tread; can carry large toy up and down stairs.
Unscrews lids, turns handles. Tower of 6–7, may construct on request and gesture without demonstration; aligns 2 or more to make train.	Tower of 8 on request; aligns 3 to make train, adds chimney after demonstration.	Tower of 9–10. Constructs bridge (door) after demonstration, model left standing. On request to insert pellets singly and as fast as possible, inserts 10 in 30 seconds.
Holds well down shaft near the point between volar pads of thumb and first 2 fingers, shaft still in palm. Imitates vertical stroke and circular scribble.	Holds pencil adult fashion but low down near point. Imitates circle, vertical and horizontal strokes. Makes two strokes for cross.	Copies circle when shown one previously drawn. Imitates cross. Names own scribbles as being man, house, car, etc.
Inserts 3 blocks after demonstration or verbal assistance. After repeated demonstrations may adapt to rotation of board through 180°.	Inserts blocks on request. Adapts to rotation with errors, corrects with verbal assistance, but repeats errors. Places one colour form, may need demonstration of circle first.	Adapts to rotation without error or immediate correction without verbal comment. Places 3 + colour forms.
Identifies fine details in familiar books. Turns single pages, forward and back-wards. Enjoys being shown pictures.	Turns single pages forwards, names some objects spontaneously. Enjoys being read a favourite story.	Describes actions in response to 'What is . . . doing?' Demands to be read to.
Stands still to throw.	Throws ball in correct direction	Catches large ball with extended arms.
Kicks on command, more swing of the kicking leg. Does not overbalance. Kicks better with preferred foot.	Forcible swinging kick. May run up to ball but stops before kicking.	Running kick at ball, may miss it.

TABLE 4.2. Sequences of development 4 weeks–3 years.—*continued*

	Months	
	18	21
Play activities	Plays happily alone but needs familiars within eye or earshot.	
	Box of junk, taking out, manipulating, arranging, putting back. Casting reduced. Lids on and off containers (e.g. saucepans). Carries, hugs doll, teddy. Pulls wheeled toy on string when walking. Pushes pram or trolley. Domestic mimicry beginning.	Imitates domestic activities (putting doll to sleep, reading newspaper, domestic play with duster, brush, in the sink). Meaningful floor play with cars, trains. Casting absent.
Comprehension and speech	Still jargoning particularly when playing. 5–20 words used with meaning, including family names. Understands much more and demonstrates by response to a variety of simple commands. Attends to speech addressed to himself and echoes words. Enjoys rhymes and TV jingles, echoes last word/s of lines. May only be understandable to family. Identifies 1 of 4 pictures by pointing. Points to 2+ body parts. Carries out 2 directional commands.	Jargoning lessening. Combining 2 words spontaneously to express two ideas, as opposed to learnt phrases. Uses single words for some needs (food, drink, toilet). Pulls adult, by hand or clothes to show. Identifies 1 by naming, 2 by pointing of 4 pictures. Carries out 3 directional commands.
Self-help skills		
Undressing, dressing	Takes off shoes, socks, hat.	Gets feet into loose slippers, no regard to which foot. Pulls up pants to curve of buttocks. Unzips.
Toileting	Bowel control attained. Fairly dry with regular potting. Can indicate (word or gesture) when about to urinate, often too late to catch on account of urgency.	'Accidents' less frequent but occur particularly when engrossed in play. Using word to ask for pottie. Wet at night.
Self-feeding	Lifts cup 2 hands, drinks, replaces. Can get spoon to mouth without tipping but tends to bring spoon to mouth sideways; uses preferred hand: still very messy, still prefers to finger	Lifts cup by handle. Gets most stodgy food off plate into mouth without too much mess using spoon.

	Years	
2	**2½**	**3**

Enjoys play beside other children with adult in vicinity. Will not share toys. Pretending games with verbal accompaniment (scolding doll); dressing up (hats, shoes); uses miniature toys appropriately (tea set).

Vigorous outdoor activities (and in house), running, climbing, jumping. Beginning to pedal tricycle at 2½, can pedal and steer round wide corners at 3. Painting; cutting out at 3. Increasingly inventive make believe in solitary and co-operative play with other children.

Not jargoning although sustained monologue (with marked echolalia) while playing maybe difficult to understand. 50+ words; many 2–3 word combinations. Uses speech instead of gesture for needs. Constantly echoes speech addressed to him. Asks 'What's that?' and repeats after being told. Refers to self by name. May use pronouns (I, me, you). Understandable to strangers. Names 3 of 10 pictures of common objects, identifies by pointing to 5 or more. Points to 3–4 body parts, and repeats names. Carries out 4 directional commands.

Expresses immediate experiences. Still leaves out many inessential words. Sentence length 3–5 words. Listens with interest to general talk, not specifically addressed to him. Refers to self as 'I' or 'me'. Gives full name. Picture cards, identifies 7 of 10 (5 named). Gives uses of objects at simple level (penny/'sweeties', cup/'juice'). May give actions at simple level ('running', 'dinner').

Can carry on conversation. Still some mispronunciations. Echolalia infrequent. Constantly asking 'Who?' 'What?' 'Where?' 'Why?' Uses plurals, understands prepositions (under, behind). Picture cards 8–10 of 10. Uses at more advanced level ('Buying sweeties', 'That's for my juice'). Actions at more advanced level ('The boys are running', 'She's having her dinner').

Given time can remove most clothes excepting those going over head. Tugs at buttons. Takes pants down and up for toileting. Tries to put on socks (often toes into sock heels), shoes (often wrong feet), pants (may put both legs through one hole), hat.

Puts on simple garments efficiently. Needs help with second sleeve and arms into sleeves after putting garment over head. Puts clothes on back to front.

Undoes front buttons, does up big buttons. Can dress completely with advice about back and front, which shoe for which foot and help with small buttons and back fastenings.

Toilet needs verbalized fairly consistently and in time. May or may not be dry at night if lifted. Washes hands.

May use pottie himself, needs help with wiping. May climb on to lavatory seat.

Uses lavatory. Goes without asking, may tell he is going and shout for help with wiping.

Complete self-feeding with cup and spoon. Sits up to table.

Uses fork efficiently.

Uses spoon and fork.

mental superiority. In non-specific mental retardation, development is usually delayed in all areas but less so in motor function than in adaptive behaviour and speech.

TABLE 4.3. Degree of developmental delay at different ages which might be considered significant.

Chronological age	Developmental age	Developmental delay
Weeks		
8	6	} 2
12	10	
16	12	
20	16	} 4
24	20	
28	22	} 6
32	26	
36	28	
40	32	} 8
44	36	
48	38	
52	42	} 10
56	46	
Months		
15	12	} 3
18	15	
21	17	} 4
24	20	
30	24	6
36	28	} 8
42	34	
48	38	10
54	42	} 12
60	48	

Examination procedures

From birth to 28 weeks the infant's posture and motor performance is observed on lap and couch in four positions: sitting on mother's lap and supported on a firm surface, supine and pulled up to sitting, ventral suspension (in the first 12 weeks) and prone on a firm surface, and held standing on lap and on a firm surface.

After 28 weeks sitting and standing balance are observed on the floor and spontaneous movement encouraged by the use of a lure such as a small shining bell, brightly coloured rattle or squeaky toy.

Birth to 20 weeks. How mother carries the infant into the examination room and how she holds him on her lap gives the first indication of motor level. As long as head control is incomplete, mother will support the head in the crook of her arm.

After the history has been elicited and the infant undressed the examiner takes him from mother, tests standing balance on lap before carrying to the couch.

The young infant does not object to being lain supine and observations of posture and spontaneous movement are made first. In the pull to sit manoeuvre the infant's forearms are grasped above the wrists, he is encouraged to keep his head centred by talking to him (before 8–10 weeks the infant's head is positioned centrally) and he is gently pulled up to sitting. The position of the head in relation to the trunk is observed. Position of the head and curvature of the back in supported sitting is noted.

With the infant supported under the axillae, weight bearing when standing on a firm surface is elicited. Placing and walking reflexes are tested (pp. 35, 36).

If the infant is 12 weeks or younger, positions of head and limbs are observed in ventral suspension (the infant held in the prone position, examiner's hands under lower chest and upper abdomen) and on lowering to prone lie on the couch. The infant of 8 weeks or younger may fail to demonstrate abilities in prone spontaneously. If he continues to lie with head to one side and cheek resting on the couch, his head is gently turned to mid-line while mother speaks to the infant at front to encourage optimal head-raising. The presence of crawling reflex is observed, either spontaneous crawling movements or induced by pressure with thumbs on the soles of the feet.

Before handing back to mother the Moro reflex is tested (p. 36).

20–28 weeks. Order of examination is as above except that if the infant protests at being lain supine, this position is deferred to the end of the motor assessment. In the pull-to-sit manoeuvre the infant is held by his hands.

Progression reflexes and full Moro response cannot normally be elicited at this age.

28–36 weeks. After 28 weeks examination is more conveniently carried out with examiner, mother and child on the floor.

Supported and unsupported sitting balance is tested first and sideways protective reactions (p. 185). If the infant appears to be on the verge of unsupported sitting he is positioned with legs in abduction at hips and semi-flexion at knees and hands in a propping position alongside his feet. If balance is maintained a lure is offered at shoulder height front, to test ability to erect the trunk and lift one hand. The lure is presented by mother or examiner, the other being strategically placed to protect the infant from toppling over. With more secure sitting balance the lure is placed on the floor at front (to demonstrate ability to lean forward and re-erect) and to either side (to demonstrate extent to which the trunk can be twisted before balance is lost).

Next the infant is placed prone and observations made on rolling, pivoting and forward progression by any means, again using a lure to stimulate movement. These manoeuvres should be carried out rapidly and if the infant shows signs of frustration at any stage he should be rewarded with the lure and another provided for later testing after a few moments play with the first.

Standing is tested with the infant's hands held at shoulder height and with the infant placed standing at the low table.

Ability to pull up from supine with the infant grasping examiner's two fingers is elicited and finally forwards protective reaction (p. 185).

36 weeks to independent walking. Sitting balance is again tested first and the child's ability to pivot in sitting to reach a lure, with or without use of hands for stability. The lure is then placed out of reach in front to demonstrate ability to go deliberately to prone and method of forward progression, or hitching.

The lure is placed on the low table to demonstrate pulling up to stand and behaviour when standing, moved along the table to stimulate cruising and removed from table to floor to show how the child gets back to the floor from standing.

Walking with one or two hands held by mother is demonstrated.

After independent walking. After the child has attained independent walking, locomotor performance is observed incidentally in free play and ball activities.

Kicking a ball and standing on one leg can be encouraged by allowing mother to hold the child's hand initially and then gently let go.

If mother has any concern about gait some free space, such as an adjacent corridor, must be found for demonstration of running. Ball play with mother is the best way to encourage running, decelerating, turning and kicking.

Motor variations and delays

Motor variations and delays may be of no significance, due to lack of opportunity or due to pathological conditions.

The amount of spontaneous movement of the young infant placed supine shows considerable normal variation. Excessive rolling from side to side, with persistence of jerky rather than smooth rhythmic movements and prolongation of the ATNR posture (p. 29) may indicate neurological abnormality.

Slow motor development, more noticeable in age of walking than age of attaining head control and sitting balance, may be a familial feature and of no significance. Conversely, precocious motor development may run in families.

A number of studies suggest that negro infants are advanced in motor skills in the early months, compared with Caucasian infants.

Infants who hitch (bottom shuffle) are later by a few weeks to pull up to stand and walk than crawlers.

Age of independent walking is affected by temperament. Cautious toddlers may prolong the period of needing minimal support. When such a child eventually lets go and walks alone it is obvious that gait is relatively mature and that he could have walked at an earlier age if confidence had permitted. Conversely some adventurous toddlers will step out as soon as independent standing is achieved and then go through a longer period of taking one or two steps, collapsing on to buttocks or outstretched arms, crawling to pull up on furniture before stepping out again. Because of these temperamental differences questions about walking alone should specify distance walked.

Infants who are seldom placed prone show some delay in this position. Conversely infants who are traditionally placed prone for sleeping (as in North America) tend to show superior performance in prone in the first 6 months.

Infants who are given little opportunity to stand can be markedly delayed and show discrepancy between sitting balance and weight bearing on legs to the extent that, e.g. a 6-month infant who can sit erect with minimal support, immediately sags at hips and knees when assisted standing is attempted, or flexes at hips and extends at knees assuming a sitting position in mid-air. The latter posture suggests that the infant is spending most of his time strapped into a pram.

Over-use of baby walkers and bouncers can delay mobility by crawling or hitching to the extent that some who have spent most of their waking hours in these devices from 6–12 months may sit unsupported at the usual age but 3 months later are still immobile when placed sitting on the floor, while able to cruise when placed standing at a low table. Scrutton and Gilbertson (1975) suggest that walkers and bouncers show a child how not to stand, since standing means taking weight through the feet, the body being supported by them and balanced over them. In a walker or bouncer the trunk becomes the base and the feet can be drawn up without disturbing balance.

Increase in extensor tone produces discrepancies in motor performance in different positions, the infant appearing 'mature' in standing and prone compared with immaturity in supine pull to sit and supported sitting.

Retarded motor development
Motor development would be considered very slow if the child had not achieved:

complete head control by age 24–28 weeks,
sitting erect on the floor (5–10 minutes) by age 44–48 weeks,
mobility by crawling or hitching and pulling to stand by age 52–56 weeks,
walking alone or with minimal support by age 18–21 months.

The main causes of retarded motor development are as follows.

Mental retardation. In spite of the provisos given above, in numerical terms mental retardation is still the commonest cause of slow locomotion. Nevertheless, a disproportionate delay in motor development is unlikely to be due solely to mental retardation.

Cerebral palsy. In cerebral palsy the extent and pattern of locomotor retardation depends on the type, severity and distribution of the cerebral palsy and on the child's intelligence (Chapter 14). Tone can be hypertonic, hypotonic or variable. A marked and disproportionate delay in motor development, even if overt abnormal neurological signs are few, is most likely to be due to a developing cerebral palsy and the child should be closely followed up with this in mind. At a later stage, delayed motor development in cerebral palsy is associated with abnormal patterns of posture and movement.

Hypotonia. Apart from cerebral palsy, hypotonia can also result from lesions of spinal cord or lower motor neurone, intrinsic muscle pathology, deprivation or from general physical disorders such as rickets or any severe illness (Chapter 19). Children with non-specific mild retardation are often somewhat hypotonic but not to an extent that leads to relative motor delay.

Deprivation. Restriction of opportunity ranges from the infant left too long in cot or pram by the harassed mother of a large family, to the blind child whose mother is fearful that he will bump himself if he is allowed the freedom of the floor. Blind children may also have to be taught to walk in a way that is unnecessary with sighted children. Blind infants often omit the crawling stage.

There is little evidence that overweight children are later to walk, given normal opportunities to do so, though it is certain that some mothers of overweight infants discourage weight bearing for fear of inducing postural deformities of the legs.

Congenital dislocation of hip. Opinions differ as to whether congenital dislocation of hip delays age of walking. Illingworth (1975) states that it does not even when bilateral. This is not the opinion of some orthopaedic surgeons.

VISION, FINE MOTOR AND ADAPTIVE BEHAVIOUR

Assessment of vision is considered in Chapter 8.

Adaptive behaviour has been defined as the effectiveness with which the individual copes with the natural and social demands of his environment and the ability to utilize previous experience in the solutions of new problems.

In infancy and early childhood adaptive behaviour is demonstrated by the way the child utilizes his developing motor skills in purposeful and increasingly complex exploitation of play materials, the extent to which he perceives relationships and how he initiates new adjustments to solving simple problems.

Adaptive behaviour is affected by visual competence, hand–eye co-ordination and manipulative skills, e.g. the ability to secure a ring by pulling on a thin string demonstrates that the infant can see ring and string, reach accurately, is capable of plucking the string and also appreciates that the ring can be secured by this strategy.

Adaptive behaviour gives a better indication of intellectual potential than does gross motor function, but optimal performance is more difficult to elicit, as this depends to a greater extent on rapport between examiner and child, the child's temperament (friendly or shy) and his mood at the time of examination. Therefore it is the more important that the child be relaxed and aware that a friendly relationship exists between his mother and the examiner, comfortably and securely seated and that the testing materials presented have an inherent interest appropriate for age.

Up to age 20 weeks, hand function, interest in and exploitation of play materials are assessed with the infant on mother's lap. At later ages fine motor skills and adaptive behaviour are demonstrated with play materials on table or desk top. After 15 months the child may accept the child-size chair and table but may prefer to stand at the table or be seated on the floor.

Tests should be presented quickly to sustain interest.

If the child shows initial anxiety and suspicion the examiner should withdraw to increase the distance between himself and the child; with continuing inhibition mother can offer the first test objects or they can be placed within reach on the table top while the examiner continues a friendly conversation with mother, apparently ignoring the child.

In the first 3 months degree of hand closure is noted, any difference between right and left and presence or absence of grasp reflex (p. 34).

Voluntary grasping is observed from 12 weeks, ability to reach and secure a proffered rattle from 20 weeks, evolving grasp of cube (palmar to digital) from 20 weeks, attempts to secure a tiny object from 24 weeks and method of securing from 32 weeks, ability to release voluntarily from 40 weeks and increasing skill in fine motor control as demonstrated by cube play, pellet in bottle test and use of pencil from 52 weeks.

Examination procedures

Birth to 20 weeks. Vision testing in the early months is described in Chapter 8.

At 12 weeks, when hands are held loosely closed or half open, a teething ring is placed in each hand in turn and note taken of voluntary grasp and regard.

At 16 weeks the rattle is presented almost touching the infant's fingers. Excitation, activation of arms and two-handed attempts to reach are noted. If the infant fails to secure, the rattle is placed in one hand and in the other.

20–28 weeks. The rattle is offered first and method of reach and grasp observed, and also whether or not the rattle is transferred to the other hand and carried to the mouth. Similar observations are made on reach, grasp and transfer of a cube. If one cube is handled dextrously, a second is placed in the free hand and the infant's ability to retain two objects noted.

Presentation of the pellet on desk top demonstrates the infant's ability to see a small object placed to either side and whether he will follow this with his eyes if it is gently flicked across the desk. From 24 weeks he may try to secure, usually without success.

Manipulation of bell and reaction to the ring on string problem are noted from 24 weeks. These items are also presented on desk top.

28–40 weeks. The following test items are presented on desk top:

Three cubes; the first cube is tapped on desk top to attract attention and when the infant is looking at the cube it is slid smoothly within reach. This is repeated with the second and third cubes. Observations are made on type of grasp, number grasped and retained and matching of two cubes (i.e. bringing the cubes together in the mid-line while watching them intently). From 32 weeks cube play is concluded by noting following of dropped object (cube pushed off the edge of the desk while the child is looking at it).

Ring on string; the string is placed within and ring out of reach. If the infant ignores the string but reaches persistently for the ring, the examiner demonstrates how this may be secured by pulling on the string.

Bell; this is placed centrally within easy reach after demonstration of how to obtain a ringing tone. Method of grasping, banging or shaking is noted, also if the infant searches for the source of sound and pokes the clapper.

Pellet; index finger approach and method of securing is observed.

40 weeks–15 months. At this and older ages a wider variety of test items is available. It may not be possible or necessary to apply all these tests, but the method of doing so is described for all.

Cup and six cubes; the cubes are presented in a cluster centrally and the cup to the child's left; spontaneous play is observed. At age 44–52 weeks two cubes are dropped into the cup and method of re-securing noted. After 52 weeks the child is encouraged by demonstration, gesture or verbally to release one or more cubes into the cup.

Before the cup is removed the 'hidden toy' test can be carried out with infants of 48–56 weeks. All cubes but one are removed, the child's attention is drawn to the remaining cube before the cup is placed upside down over it. The child is asked to find the cube; gesture or eye-pointing should be avoided.

Following discovery of the cube the cup is removed and the examiner tests for 'offers toy and releases' by holding out his hand and asking the child to give the cube. If there is no response the child is offered another cube and after he has taken it, the examiner again holds out his hand with the words 'now you give me one'. If he still refuses mother is instructed to ask for the cube.

From 52 weeks tower building can be attempted. With four cubes on the desk the examiner slides two close to the child and with the other two demonstrates building a tower. If the child makes no response to 'now you do it with your blocks', a second demonstration is given using the child's cubes; that tower is dismantled and the child again encouraged with 'now you do it'.

Pellet and specimen bottle; method of securing a tiny sweet is observed, both hands being tested. The sweet (or another one if the first has been eaten) is then dropped into the bottle which is shaken and placed in front of the child. Attempts to retrieve the sweet are noted.

From 15 months retrieving by 'dumping' (turning the bottle upside down) is demonstrated by the examiner. If the temptation to eat the sweet is too strong a paper clip can be used instead, taking good care that the child does not put that in his mouth.

Pencil and paper; from 52 weeks paper and pencil tests can be attempted. A sheet of paper is placed centrally, the examiner demonstrates a scribble, places the pencil in the middle of the paper pointing away from the child and encourages with 'now you do that'. One pencil only should be used; with two the child may be more interested in swapping pencils than in demonstrating use. However, sometimes the child shows signs of distress if his pencil is removed and the examiner is obliged to use another one. This should be concealed after strokes are demonstrated. Observations are made on method of holding the pencil and progress from jabbing at the paper making a faint mark, scribble in imitation or spontaneously to first attempts to copy strokes.

Book; ability to turn pages is elicited when testing reaction to pictures in language assessment.

15 months–2 years. By this age it is to be hoped that the child-size chair and table will be acceptable. The tests described below (and *2–3 years*) throw light on a wide range of abilities; increasing control over fine motor function, perception of shapes and relationships of increasing complexity and problems of increasing difficulty. How much can be accomplished depends on the child's continuing interest and co-operation. Some tests may appeal to him more than others. The examiner should be prepared to move on to fresh material if the child shows signs of frustration, waning interest or resistance and in any event move on quickly to another activity when the child has reached his ceiling in one.

Cubes and cup; a cluster of 10 cubes and a cup are presented. The child is asked to place the cubes in the cup. If there is no response gesture or demonstration is permitted. Tower building is attempted without or with demonstration. The child may need urging and encouragement (e.g. by counting) to produce his optimal performance. Some children cannot be prevented from deliberate knocking down and one suspects that the maximum number of cubes that could have been built is not demonstrated. Aligning cubes to make a train is more difficult. The child will imitate pushing a train, constructed by the examiner, before he can make one himself.

Pellet and bottle; the problem of insertion is solved before that of retrieval.

Paper and pencil; responses depend in part on practice at home. This information must be elicited. Paper and pencil are presented as before. Method of holding the pencil is recorded. It may be helpful if the examiner steadies the paper but some children object. After spontaneous scribble has been observed the child is asked to copy a firm line drawn down the margin (to the child's left) and a firm circular scribble (going round and round) at the top of the paper. Two attempts at each are allowed. A fresh side or sheet of paper is used for each demonstration.

Three-hole formboard; this is placed empty on the table, round hole to the child's right. The shapes are placed between child and board, each one opposite its appropriate hole, and he is asked to put the blocks in their right holes. If he looks puzzled it is permissible for the examiner to run his index finger back and forth across the top edge of the board while repeating 'you put them in the right holes'. If the child piles the shapes on the board indiscriminately or starts playing with them, insertion is demonstrated. The younger child may be assisted in adjusting corners of square and triangle at first attempt. Three attempts are allowed. The 2-year-old may adapt to rotation of the board (see below) after repeated demonstrations.

2–3 years. The child is seated at the table as above.

Cubes; ten cubes are presented and the child requested to build a tower (or house). Then all but three cubes are removed from the child's reach and the examiner demonstrates constructing a train, which the child is asked to copy. If successful the remaining four cubes are placed within reach, the examiner adds a chimney to his own train and exhorts the child to do likewise. At 3 years the examiner constructs a bridge (or door) of three cubes, leaves the model standing and asks the child to make another.

Pencil and paper; these are presented as before. Spontaneous scribble is permitted first. The 3-year-old may describe his scribble (if asked) as being a man, car, house and so on.

Demonstration strokes (for the child to copy) in increasing order of difficulty are vertical line and circular scribble as above, a horizontal line across the top of the paper, a cross at the top of the paper (vertical stroke first) and finally a card is presented on which a circle has been drawn. After each demonstration the child is urged to 'do one just like that'. A second demonstration stroke is made if the child fails to copy the first. The words 'circle', 'round' or 'cross' should not be used. When demonstrating the cross it is permissible to say 'one like that and one like that' as each stroke is drawn.

Pellets and bottle; at 3 years ten pellets and the bottle are placed before the child, pellets to the side of his preferred hand (demonstrated in drawing) and he is asked to drop the pellets into the bottle one by one, and 'as fast as you can'. If he enjoys this activity and will permit restraint of the preferred hand, he is asked to complete the task using the other hand.

Three-hole formboard; this is presented as before and the child asked, without gesture, to replace the blocks in their right holes. The shapes are removed and the child told to 'watch what I am going to do now'. When his attention is fixed on the board, this is rotated through an arc of 180°. The shapes are replaced in their initial order (round block now opposite the square hole) and once more the child is requested to replace them. Three or four attempts are allowed. If the child succeeds after one or two abortive attempts, he is invited to do it just once more, in order to demonstrate whether or not he has learnt from his previous errors and can now complete the task without error.

Five colour forms; at 2½–3 years the more complicated colour form board is presented. First the child is given the round form and asked 'where does that one go? You put it on'. If he is unsuccessful the round form is placed appropriately, before presenting the other four shapes.

Delay in adaptive behaviour and poor hand function
Ability to grasp, reach, secure and release would be considered very slow if the infant was not demonstrating:

voluntary grasp of rattle placed in hand, retention and regard	by 16 weeks;
accurate reach and grasp of rattle and transfer to other hand	by 40 weeks;
pincer grip to secure pellet	by 52 weeks;
voluntary release (cubes into cup)	by 18 months.

Hand regard and finger play (a normal activity between 12 and 20 weeks) persisting beyond 24–28 weeks, and mouthing (i.e. all toys going to the mouth, often with excessive drooling) well into the second year of life would also be cause for concern. Mouthing is not due to dental eruption.

Infants who are left lying in their cots with no playthings may continue to play with their fingers, simply because they have nothing else to do.

Poor hand control is seen in retarded children and is a more reliable indicator of low intelligence than late age of walking. However, after the child has passed the stages of voluntary grasp, reaching to secure, use of the fingers in grasp and deliberate release, ability with the hands depends to some extent on special aptitude. Some children are good with their hands, some are not. Among the latter will be some who are considered normal and some who are clumsy children with special problems (see Chapter 16).

A more important indication of retardation is lack of interest in play materials, the infant failing to exploit the fine motor skills which he possesses. Interest and ingenuity are difficult to quantify. It is also difficult to separate 'can not' from 'will not' and with shy reserved infants and unforthcoming or negative toddlers more than one session may be necessary before one is confident that the child has displayed the full range of his abilities.

Children reared in a depriving environment may be inhibited by the unfamiliarity of the test situations presented.

Hand preference. In the first year of life the infant is ambidextrous using which ever hand is nearest to the object he wishes to secure. If there is noticeable hand preference one should not accept the explanation that 'he is left/right handed just like his Dad'. Some evidence of hand preference may become apparent between 12 and 18 months, the child more frequently using the preferred hand for spoon and pencil. However, more often a clear preference is not obvious until 2 years. Even then many children still use either hand indiscriminately. Dominance is usually well established by age 5 years.

Abnormal hand posture, movement and function. In the neonatal period the hands are held firmly closed at rest, though they open on movement; grasp reflex is easily elicited. By 12 weeks the hands are held half open and the grasp reflex is weakly present or absent. It is unusual at any age for the hands to be so tightly clenched that difficulty is experienced in washing and drying the palms. It is also unusual for thumbs to be held across the palms although sometimes this isolated finding is seen in infants who appear entirely normal on neurological examination.

Differences in degree of fisting on right and left, prolongation of grasp reflex on one side and differences in amount of upper limb movement may be first indications of a developing hemiplegia, as may differences in arm movement or hand opening between right and left in sideways and forwards parachute reactions and during crawling.

By 36 weeks one would expect an accurate, rapid one-handed approach and grasp of a rattle or cube. Inco-ordinate, ataxic reach, which is normal at earlier ages is abnormal at this age. With increased tone in the arms the reaching movement is slower and there is a characteristic dorsiflexion at wrist and spreading of fingers.

In the second year of life cube building and the pellets in bottle test show up clumsy or ataxic hand function and intention tremor (p. 148).

HEARING, COMPREHENSION AND COMMUNICATION

Hearing
Assessment of hearing is considered in Chapter 8.

Comprehension and communication
Assessment of comprehension and communication skills is the most difficult to make in an outpatient clinic and to the greatest extent depends on the mother's account. Unfortunately this area of development is also the hardest to describe and to interpret from mother's history.

Comprehension includes recognition of and response to persons, understanding the significance of domestic equipment and events, understanding the meaning of gesture and tone of voice and finally understanding the spoken word. Communication includes preverbal vocalization, either spontaneous or evoked; communication by facial expression, total body movements and finer forms of gesture; mimicry and finally spontaneous speech in words, phrases and sentences. More than in other areas of early development comprehension and speech level appear to be related to later intelligence.

The development of speech is considered in more detail in Chapter 9.

Examination procedures
Birth to 28 weeks. The young infant's recognition of and response to a friendly face by looking, smiling and vocalization ('talking back') should be demonstrable. It is not enough to accept the mother's account, especially if this is her first child.

Some estimate of interest in surroundings, toys and people can be made from observation of the infant in the examination room. Interest in and anticipation of domestic activities; recognition of father, siblings and other familiars may be reported in mother's history. The normal infant of 3–5 months is unlikely to be content to lie in cot or pram for long periods when awake (usually he demands attention and entertainment), although the mother of an infant who does is more likely to think of him as particularly good rather than possibly slow.

The infant may be silent in the examination room and again one may be dependent on the mother for an account of vocalization and increasing maturity of babble.

28 weeks–15 months. In the second half of the first year the chances of hearing the infant's range of babble are even less, as at this age there is an increasing awareness of strange persons and strange places with concomitant reserve. Mother may be able to do no more than confirm that the infant does babble, that this is mono- or polysyllabic, and that he has a range of sound with tuneful intonation. However, at this age there are more ways in which the infant clearly demonstrates understanding and mother's history is more positive. He is also beginning to imitate actions, noises and later nursery games and shows that he understands some words addressed to him by appropriate responses, though none of this may be demonstrated in the clinic.

At 1 year the child may have a few sounds used consistently with meaning but even if he does not, one would expect recognition of family names and the names of a few objects. He may demonstrate this by looking at objects (e.g. light, teddy, car) named by his mother.

The significance of vocalization and the indications of comprehension, as seen by mother, are particularly open to wishful thinking. In this area, more than in others, mothers tend to give those answers which they judge (from tone of voice or form of question) are expected. For this reason it is very important that no suggestion should be made that the child ought to be understanding, vocalizing or speaking at any preconceived level. Questioning should start at a level well below that expected for age.

15 months–2 years. It is to be hoped that some spontaneous speech will be heard during the examination, but in any event mother should be asked about level of understanding, how wants are indicated and how much speech the child uses at home, single words, types of words and word combinations. It is important to differentiate learnt phrases such as 'all gone', 'night-night' and 'oh dear' from spontaneous word combinations.

Jargoning is the largely unintelligible but expressive sounding 'conversation' of the 15–18 month child, described by mother as 'talking in a foreign language'.

At this age it is possible to include objective items to test comprehension and expressive speech.

Picture book; this is a useful introduction, demonstrating interest in pictures in the younger child and at older ages providing an opportunity for spontaneous speech of both child and examiner in a familiar setting, if the child is used to books at home. As this is not a formal testing situation the examiner can both ask a question and answer it for the child reluctant to speak, which may put the child at ease for the tests to follow. If the older child of 21 months–2 years shows facility in naming the pictures, he can be taken through the first 10 pages and the picture cards test below omitted.

Picture cards; at 18 months the first picture card with four common objects is presented. Mother is warned not to help the child. The child is asked to show one of the objects by pointing. If he is unable (or unwilling) the examiner points to one picture and says, e.g., 'look there's the teddy bear, now you show mummy the teddy'. If the child then points to that picture, he is asked to 'show mummy' the others. If he does not and mother thinks the child should be capable of this task, she can be asked to give the instructions. Some younger children, who will not point, do indicate recognition by eye movement. The child of 21 months or older is first asked to name each object. If he fails to respond he is asked to show by pointing. At 2 years the second card of six pictures is added.

Many mothers become tense and anxious when their children refuse to respond to this sort of test and if this is so it may be diplomatic to move on to the next test with a word of reassurance. In any event the test is abandoned if the child fails to respond to three pictures.

Miniature toys; the shy child who will not respond to pictures may show understanding by identification of small toys and other familiar objects. Four of these are laid out on the table, the examiner withdraws, asking mother to request each item in turn. At 2 years a further set of six objects is presented.

Directional commands; at some convenient time (or times) during the examination the small ball or some other toy which has taken the child's fancy, can be used for demonstration of ability to follow directions. The child is directed to 'give it to mummy', 'put it on the table', 'give it to me', 'put it on the chair'. No gesture is permitted and eye-pointing should be avoided.

2–3 years. In the third year of life more children are prepared to talk with a friendly stranger, if they are given time to settle down before a direct approach is made. The child is invited to look at, or play with, the toys provided for free play activities during preliminary conversation with mother. These toys provide subject matter for subsequent talk with the child, which may demonstrate intelligibility, sentence length and grammatical construction.

If the child is chatty, language tests are best given before adaptive tests. With shy children the latter should be given first.

Picture books; the book showing single objects is presented first and the child asked to name the first ten pictures. The second book showing everyday activities is presented next and the child asked to describe the pictures. The younger child is likely to name people or objects first.

He is then asked e.g. 'what is the boy doing?' Single word indications of action (e.g. 'running', 'dinner') are expected at $2\frac{1}{2}$ years. The 3-year-old is more likely to describe actions spontaneously or respond to question with phrase or sentence (e.g. 'he's chasing that dog', 'eating his dinner').

Picture cards; if the child has not named pictures in the first book the two picture cards are presented.

Miniature toys; five are laid on the table (e.g. cup, pencil, key, coin, spoon). The child is asked to name each object and if successful is asked 'and what do you do with that?' Again at $2\frac{1}{2}$ years the child would be expected to give a single word indication of use (e.g. 'juice', 'draw') and at 3 years a word combination ('that's for juice', 'draw a man').

Giving full name; at some convenient time during the interview the child is asked what is his name and if first name only is given the examiner follows up with e.g. 'Johnny who?'

Prepositions; understanding of prepositions is tested at 3 years in table-top play or floor play with ball or other toy. The following prepositions are used (in ascending order of difficulty): on, under, behind (at the back of), in front of, beside.

Delay in comprehension and communication

There are wide variations in the ages at which normal children acquire useful speech and not uncommonly there are lulls and spurts in speech development. However an infant or young child would be considered very slow if he had not achieved:

a ready social smile	by 10 weeks
social-vocal response	by 12 weeks
polysyllabic tuneful vocalization and sustained interest in people, surroundings and toys	by 32 weeks
variety of nursery games and understanding some words	by 15 months
understanding a lot of what is said to him with 3–4 useful words	by 21 months
20 + words, using speech for some needs	by $2\frac{1}{2}$ years
50 + words and many 2–3 word combinations, words for all needs	by 3 years

Disorders of articulation are discussed in Chapter 24. Here it is sufficient to say that although the 18-month child may be understandable only to his family, the 2-year-old is largely intelligible to strangers in spite of many mispronunciations, such as substitutions and omissions. Intelligibility to the examiner may depend on his understanding of the local accent. Mothers resent the suggestion that their children are not talking properly, when in fact they are talking just like their parents and siblings. Elocution is not necessarily equated with language development.

Children of bilingual parents are rather later to acquire intelligible speech in either language. Up to age 3 or 4 years they tend to speak in a mixture of the two languages, but by the age of 5 years are speaking fluently in both without admixture.

Twins are often later to talk than single children, particularly if they have a close relationship, which makes communication with other members of the family less important. Jargoning may be prolonged and appear to be mutually understandable. Slower speech development in twins may also be due to their rather lower intelligence on average and the fact that mothers have less time to devote to two children than to one. In addition some mothers think it less necessary to talk to and play with twins as they have each other for companionship. That speech development is more dependent on adult attention and adult speech patterns than on the verbal stimulation of siblings is indicated by the well-documented advantage of first-born over later-born children.

Children are not slow to acquire useful speech because of tongue-tie, 'laziness' or because their siblings 'do everything' for them. The tactic of refusing to respond to needs unless the child uses speech to ask may lead to a variety of behaviour disturbances if in fact the child is not speaking because he can not do so, which is the usual situation.

The causes of slow language development are as follows.

Mental retardation. In numerical terms, mental retardation is by far the commonest cause of slow language development. The retarded infant is slow to smile, slow to vocalize, slow to show interest in surroundings, people and toys, slow to imitate and mimic and slow to speak. Poor articulation is more common in retarded than in normal children, but the more important problems are poor comprehension and delay in the acquisition of useful speech. Immature patterns such as echolalia (the child repeating a question instead of answering it and repetition of phrases or the last few words of sentences addressed to the child) are prolonged in retarded children.

Defective hearing. It is obvious that normal speech will not be acquired if the child has a hearing defect, though with partial deafness the earlier indicators of comprehension may not be much delayed and vocalization in the first 6 months may approach normal.

From a practical point of view (i.e. what can be done) deafness is the most important cause of slow speech development requiring early diagnosis. This subject is discussed in detail in Chapter 22.

Delayed auditory maturation. Occasionally one comes across an infant who gives little indication of responding to sound in the first 4–6 months of life but later is found to have normal hearing. One assumes that here there has been delay in auditory maturation or in the ability to localize sound.

Developmental speech disorders. Some children who respond up to age on non-verbal tests of intelligence and are not deaf, deprived or disturbed show slow speech development, ranging from a mild delay in the production of intelligible speech, to a more obvious delay in the development of expressive speech (with comprehension remaining near age). In the severest forms of developmental speech retardation there is impairment of both expression and comprehension (Chapter 24).

Cerebral palsy. Delayed speech and defective articulation are common in cerebral palsied children and may be due to low intelligence, spasticity of the muscles involved in speech and respiration or to inco-ordination and involuntary movements of these muscles. Defective hearing is more common in cerebral palsied children (especially dyskinetics) than in the general population.

The common discrepancy between comprehension and expression in cerebral palsied children of normal intelligence at 2–3 years may be due in part to the concentration that still needs to be devoted to movement. In normal children a spurt in expressive speech comes at 21–24 months when they no longer need to concentrate on balance, starting and stopping and changing direction.

Speech problems due to neurological abnormality are often preceded by early feeding and chewing difficulties. Persistent drooling, due to inability to swallow saliva, is also reported commonly.

Emotional disturbance. In the extreme case of infantile autism (p. 487) the child shows no response to speech or to other forms of communication and exhibits gross retardation in speech development. In lesser degrees of disturbance the child may be described as unforthcoming, shy, not cuddly or affectionate and more interested in things than people. It may be that other behaviour disorders (such as the reactions of the child with rigid or rejecting parents) can affect speech development, but this is less well documented.

Deprivation. Deprivation of consistent adult attention and verbal stimulation can affect all areas of development but particularly speech. Children cared for from birth in day nurseries or reared in residential institutions and children of non-speaking deaf parents will be retarded in speech unless special attention is given to providing them with the same sort of verbal stimulation that is available in a normal home environment.

To a lesser extent children from poor homes who spend much time playing outside from the second or third year of life fall behind in speech development as compared with children who are shown pictures, read stories and are the recipients of speech stimulation from their parents which is consciously geared to the correct developmental level.

SOCIAL DEVELOPMENT, PLAY ACTIVITIES AND SELF-HELP SKILLS

Social development includes the development of personal relationships, growing awareness of self and others, reactions to the social culture in which the child is reared, self-occupation and play with others and response to training in self-help skills.

Social development is influenced greatly by temperament, patterns of child rearing, social expectations of the family and opportunities given to the child. Individual variation is considerable and one can only relate social behaviour to developmental status in the broadest terms. Nevertheless, consideration of social development may provide clues to developmental and behavioural functioning and to environmental influences.

Responses to persons

Social interaction between the child and other people is indicated by physical contacts and language, both non-verbal and verbal. The development of comprehension and communication, which are major components of social behaviour, is discussed above.

In the first 4 weeks of life the infant who is adequately nourished and physically thriving sleeps most of the time except when being handled or fed. He stops whimpering when lifted or spoken to but does not quieten if crying with hunger. He stares vaguely at his surroundings but from 3–4 weeks looks at his mother's face, when she is feeding or talking to him, with an increasingly alert expression, progressing to a social smile at 4–8 weeks and a definite vocal response shortly afterwards. The 3 month infant shows obvious pleasure in bathing and playful handling especially when accompanied by voice.

By 4 months the infant is initiating social contact by smiling and by vocalizing to attract attention and enjoys this contact to the extent that he fusses when put down or left alone. He recognizes and responds to father, siblings and other close family members.

At this age and until 5–6 months most infants will respond readily to any friendly adult. Thereafter the infant begins to discriminate between familiars and strangers, at first with a slight reserve but by 9 months clearly distinguishing strangers and resisting attention from them or needing reassurance from mother before a stranger is accepted. At 9 months he may show a distinct preference for one parent or the other and identify with siblings to the extent that he cries in concert with a crying sib.

Likes and dislikes of people, objects and events become more specifically expressed at 9–12 months, the infant actively pushing away the unwanted person, toy or hand attempting to feed him and going to another (usually a parent) for support and comfort. Affection is clearly demonstrated as is distress or withdrawal on disapproval.

The child of 12–18 months can entertain himself with toys but needs to be within eye or earshot of a familiar adult. He is increasingly exhibiting his urge towards independence by resistant or negative behaviour, alternating with clinging and the need for comfort. He is still very demanding and dependent on his mother or principal caretaker.

With increasing understanding and the acquisition of a useful vocabulary between 18 months and 2 years there is more social contact with adults and children outwith the immediate family circle. Given the opportunity the 2-year-old is happy to play beside other children (parallel play) so long as they do not touch his possessions or too obviously claim the attention of his mother. Behaviour is still demanding and labile. Mood swings rapidly from cheerful contentment to temper tantrums, if the child is frustrated or thwarted (particularly if instant gratification is not forthcoming), and as rapidly return to smiling (since the 2-year-old can usually be distracted readily).

During the third year most children become more amenable with a growing desire to please. Because now he understands the rights and wishes of other people it is possible to reason with the 3-year-old. By this age co-operative play with other children is possible, including a degree of give and take. Now the child is old enough for brief separations from family and home in a play group.

Play activities

Sheridan (1975) defined play as 'eager engagement in pleasurable physical or mental effort to obtain emotional satisfaction'.

In the first 18 months of life enjoyment comes from the practice of developing locomotor and manipulative skills together with adult initiated playful handling and imitative and verbal nursery games. Concentration span is short and constructive play initiated by the child is limited. Toys are no more appreciated than common household objects such as packets and boxes, clothes pegs, saucepans and spoons.

By 18 months the child will play contentedly on the floor with a box of junk, taking out, putting in and arranging in clusters. He is becoming attached to teddy-bear or doll (and carries this around with him) and showing interest in push and pull wheeled toys.

By age 2 years conventional toys are used with meaning and initiative (dolls, pram and cot, cars, train, building blocks). Domestic mimicry (with or without mother) is sustained, the child following mother round the house and 'helping' or engaging in simple make-believe with dolls, tea-set and dressing up games.

Table-top activities such as drawing, painting, play dough, cutting out, puzzles and simple constructional toys, are appreciated at $2\frac{1}{2}$–3 years.

Given the opportunity, books are enjoyed from age 12–15 months. At first pictures are patted and familiar, clearly depicted objects are pointed out. Later a short jingle or nursery rhyme associated with a picture is recognized, with the child joining in on final words. By $2\frac{1}{2}$ years the child enjoys stories and these are demanded frequently by the 3-year-old.

At all ages motor activities provide enjoyment. As locomotor skills develop, running, climbing, jumping, chasing games, riding a tricycle and ball play provide pointers to motor competence.

Self-help skills

Self-help skills of undressing, dressing and feeding give some indication of manual dexterity and adaptive behaviour. There is a strong practice effect and only if given ample time and opportunity would the child be expected to achieve the average norms given in Table 4.2.

Age of achieving bowel and bladder control is little related to overall developmental status. The intelligent 2-year-old left in nappies is unlikely to have achieved continence whereas with patient training the mentally retarded 2-year-old may be reliably dry. There also appear to be constitutional differences, sometimes familial and unrelated to intelligence, which determine the age at which sphincter control is achieved (p. 477).

Sequences of Normal Development, $3\frac{1}{2}$–5 Years

Developmental assessment, as carried out by the paediatrician, has less value in the immediate pre-school years than at earlier ages. In districts where checks are maintained on developmental progress it is to be hoped that significant mental, neurological and sensory defects will be identified before 3 years. With

TABLE 4.4. Sequences of development 3½–5 years.

	3½	4
Gross motor	Runs smoothly and well, keeping up with his peers. Stands on 1 foot 2 secs. Running kick at ball, accurate.	Runs tip-toes. Down stairs 1 foot/tread. Broad jump from standing or running. Overhand throw of and catches bounced ball. Stands 1 foot 4–8 secs. Skips 1 foot.
Fine motor		
Pellets in bottle		10 in 25 secs.
Scissors	Controlled cutting along line.	
Tracing	Double diamond.	
Adaptive		
Cubes	Tower 10, copies bridge.	Imitates gate.
Pencil/paper	Copies circle, imitates cross.	Copies cross.
Draw-a-man	Head+1 other part.	3–4 parts.
Incomplete man	Adds 2 parts.	Adds 3 parts.
Geometric forms	Points to 6	8
Language	Speaks in well-constructed sentences, still some mispronunciations and confusions of grammar. Can give a coherent connected account of what has been happening to himself, family and friends. Questioning at its height. Repeats rhymes, sings jingles. Gives full name, address. Differentiates big/small, long/short. Matches 3–4 colours, names 1–2. Counts by rote to 10; by pointing, 2–3 objects. Repeats 3 digits (2 or 3 of 3 trials).	
Self-help skills		
Undressing, dressing		Completely with supervision, some advice and help with back fastenings and laces.
Washing	Hands and face, reminder to dry. Brushes teeth.	
Feeding	Spoon and fork. Pours from jug to cup, no spilling.	
Toilet	Attends to own needs, help with wiping.	

mild to moderate degrees of intellectual impairment and minor neurological dysfunction likely to cause problems in school, full assessment by a clinical or educational psychologist is indicated, particularly when the question of school assignment must be considered or prior placement in a nursery class may be recommended. At this age problems are more often concerned with educational planning than with developmental diagnosis.

Nevertheless the community paediatrician or family doctor is not infrequently presented with a child whose parents have become concerned about developmental progress (particularly on account of poor speech, clumsy motor performance and behaviour problems) as the age for school entrance comes nearer. Although the paediatrician should not usurp the role of the psychologist, he should be capable of identifying those children who merit referral for psychological assessment or other expert examination.

4½	5
Hops forwards on preferred foot. Plays safely on 'jungle gym.' equipment.	Stands on either foot 8 secs., and on preferred foot with arms folded. Hops forward with either foot. Skips alternate feet. Walks along chalked line.
	10 in 20 secs.
Controlled cutting round circle. Double cross.	
Copies gate. Imitates square. 5–6 parts. Adds 5–6 parts. 9	May imitate 3 steps. Copies square. 7 parts. Adds 7 parts. 10

Correct grammatical usage and pronunciation. Enjoys jokes, riddles. Uses abstract words. Knows age and birthday. Matches 6–10 colours, names 3–4. Counts by rote to 20; by pointing, 4–6 objects. Repeats 4 digits (1–2 of 3 trials).

Completely without supervision. May tie laces loosely.

Washes and dries face, hands. Baths with supervision, needs to be dried. Knife and fork. Independent.

Table 4.4 gives some broad categories of performance in different areas of behaviour at ages 3½–5 years and some simple tests of gross and fine motor control, perceptual ability and cognitive development, which have proved useful in deciding whether the child is acceptably normal and likely to maintain reasonable progress in primary school or whether additional examination and assessment is needed.

GROSS MOTOR BEHAVIOUR

By age 3½ years virtually all healthy children have opportunities for outdoor play and most play with other children. A mother's concern that her child does not keep up with his contemporaries in physical activities would be an indication for a more detailed assessment of gross motor function and examination for the detection (or exclusion) of signs of minor neurological dysfunction.

Conversely if mother confirms that her child runs, jumps, climbs, hops, skips and plays ball games with an agility comparable to that of his peers, it is likely that gross motor behaviour is acceptably normal.

FINE MOTOR AND ADAPTIVE BEHAVIOUR

Fine motor function is demonstrated in cube building and control of a pencil. The cube tower is a useful test with which to start table top tasks, as the child is guaranteed a degree of success in an activity which most enjoy.

If hand function appears to be clumsy or if, in answer to the question 'how good is he with his hands?' mother reports that the child is awkward, 'fumble-fisted', 'all thumbs', additional tests of fine manipulative ability provide confirmation:

Pellets in bottle test is carried out as above.

Cutting with scissors; the child is instructed to cut along a 6-inch line, drawn with a wide-tipped ($\frac{1}{8}$ inch) felt pen. If successful he is asked to cut round a circle of diameter approximately 3 inches.

Tracing; the child is instructed to draw a line right around the inside diamond without crossing either of the double lines. The examiner may demonstrate by moving a pencil along the path to be traced without marking the paper. If the child is successful the double cross is presented.

Perceptual abilities are demonstrated by the child's skills in drawing shapes, either after demonstrations or from models and by his success in matching shapes on the uncoloured geometric formboard.

In the latter test the card, on which are drawn ten geometric forms, is placed before the child and the matching circle is laid in the space provided (middle bottom row). The child is asked to show 'the other one just like that'. If he fails to respond or incorrectly indicates, the examiner points to both circles and then presents the next matching card. No other demonstrations are permitted. On no occasion is the child told that he is wrong. The matching cards are presented in the following order: circle, square, triangle, oval, rectangle, octagon, rhomboid, square with indented arc, trapezoid and irregular.

Recognition of body image is demonstrated in the draw-a-man and incomplete man tests. Technical ability in drawing is not measured in these tests. It is inadvisable to present these two tests in sequence because of possible practice effect.

The child is asked to draw a man (or a picture of Daddy) when paper and pencil are first presented, drawing shapes follows and finally the examiner produces the incomplete man and asks the child 'what is this?' If the child recognizes the drawing (or if he does not) the examiner comments 'yes, it's a man' (or 'it's a man isn't it?') and adds 'see he only has one leg, you finish the drawing, you draw all the rest of him'. If the child's additions are unrecognizable as body parts, he should be asked to tell what he has drawn.

LANGUAGE

By age $3\frac{1}{2}$ years one would expect the child's speech to be fully understandable and by 4½ years for mispronunciations to be few and grammatical usage to be largely correct. Soliloquy during solitary play, which is common up to 3 years decreases thereafter. Now the child wants to talk to others about his games. Between 3 and 4 years questioning is at its height; reasoning (or arguing) with adults and playmates is characteristic of the 4–5 year-old.

Some indications of expected levels of spontaneous conversation and some simple tests of cognition and memory are given in Table 4.4. Cubes are used for colour matching, colour naming and for counting.

The causes of slow speech development at this age are as discussed above. Identification of disorders of articulation becomes relatively more important after the age of 3½ years since the child is now old enough to respond to formal speech therapy (Chapter 24).

Development Screening

Screening in medical care has been defined as the presumptive identification of unrecognized disease or defect by the application of tests, examinations or other procedures which can be applied rapidly. It is suggested that for effective screening, tests should be relatively simple, reliable, with few false-positive or false-negative results, economic in terms of manpower and materials and cause no anxiety to subjects or their relatives. Furthermore, confirmatory tests should be available and the confirmed abnormality should be amenable to readily accessible effective treatment (Nuffield Provincial Hospitals Trust, 1968).

A Scottish Home and Health Department working party report (1973) on integration of the child health services considered that one of the major responsibilities of an integrated service would be to detect children with developmental abnormalities at as early an age as possible. Early detection was regarded as important for two main reasons: 'First, the most rapid period of growth takes place during the pre-school years so that undetected and untreated defects in this period can adversely affect both the child's present functioning and his later educational progress and social adjustment. Secondly, emotional development depends on a number of social and cultural factors and if faulty patterns of child rearing are identified early enough and modified, harm to the child may be prevented'. It was concluded that development screening (defined as the simple determination of developmental status) had a valuable part to play in the early detection of handicap and recommended that this service should be available to all children nationwide.

It is evident that screening for the detection of neurodevelopmental disabilities, as envisaged in the SHHD report, does not fulfil the criteria for effective screening given above. Simple tests with few false-positive or false-negative results have not been validated. The procedure is time-consuming and requires application by skilled personnel. Unlike some screening tests a series of examinations is needed.

Facilities for confirmatory assessment of suspect or abnormal subjects are now available in most areas but in general these facilities are better developed than are those for management and treatment of the conditions identified. In many areas there is a shortage of therapists, psychologists and remedial teachers, a lack of play groups, day nurseries and nursery classes able to accommodate young children with neurodevelopmental disabilities and inadequate social work, home help and baby-minding supportive services.

Detection without intervention is a largely academic exercise. If facilities for referral and thereafter for management are not available, detection by means of development screening is of little value to children or their families.

Unnecessary anxiety may be caused to parents when children, who are later shown to be normal, are referred for further assessment. However, most parents can appreciate that some children do not respond appropriately in the limited time available for a screening examination and that reported problems also require additional time for full discussion. Handled wisely anxiety can be minimized or avoided until a more detailed assessment is arranged. Certainly no parents should be told for the first time in a screening clinic that their child is abnormal. Referral to a hospital outpatient department is often a cause for anxiety and unless there is strong suspicion of definite abnormality (and in many of these cases parents are already aware that all is not well) there is some advantage in 'second tier' clinics being sited in local health centres or in assessment centres not located in hospital premises.

The value of screening for phenylketonuria and congenital dislocation of hips in the neonatal period and for hearing defects in the second 6 months of life is not questioned. Routine screening for squints is also of obvious value.

Moderate and severe mental and neurological handicaps are likely to be detected at earlier ages when infants are enrolled in screening programmes and relatively simple tests suffice to provide a high index of suspicion. However, unlike the conditions just mentioned, firm evidence that early intervention is of definite benefit to child patients with these handicaps is not yet available, although there is no doubt that parents and families benefit from early advice and support.

The detection of less obvious and less serious disabilities requires more skill on the part of screening personnel. Nevertheless it may well be shown that, in terms of practical benefit, the main value of development screening of total populations is in identification of developmental lags, mild neurological impairment, minor defects of vision and hearing, speech delay, behaviour disorders (including disturbances of mother–child interaction) and environmental disadvantage. These problems may be amenable to altered management, added stimulation and specific therapy.

Little evidence is available yet about the most effective and economic methods of screening, at what ages this should be carried out and by whom and the prognostic significance of different observations and procedures. The usefulness of development screening cannot be fully estimated with confidence until children included in screening programmes have reached a minimal age of 7 years. Information about the numbers of problems identified for the first time after school entry, the numbers identified and treated in the preschool period, together with evaluation of the effects of earlier intervention would provide the firm data needed before development screening of all infants and young children should or should not be recommended and, if the former is decided, furnish convincing evidence of the value of screening for those who would be called upon to implement that recommendation. Those who are not convinced of its usefulness are unlikely to become skilled in the techniques of screening.

At the present time different types of programmes are being used in different areas. These collective experiences could provide the important information about effective methods that is so much needed.

DEVELOPMENT SCREENING SCHEDULES

It has been suggested that an agreed schedule of what constitutes a basic screening examination should be worked out for universal use, but until such time as different methods can be compared there is much to be said for local communities developing programmes which seem best suited to local conditions. For this reason broad guide lines only are given here.

If development screening is to be carried out with all infants, the schedules employed must be brief but must scan all areas of development, include tests of vision and hearing and some items about behaviour. To avoid frequent recalls the one examination should identify those who appear to be definitely retarded in one or all areas of development and merit immediate referral, those who are suspect and should be seen again before the next routine screening examination and those who appear to be within the normal range for age.

Most schedules in current use carry a number of developmental items covering different areas of behaviour appropriate for the ages of screening and with Yes/No options for response. There are two disadvantages in this type of schedule. In practice many children are not brought for screening at the exact ages specified. If because of absence on holiday, illness, climatic inclemency or the need to use persuasion before mother will attend, the child has passed the age for examination the schedule may no longer be appropriate. In the event of failures on developmental tests, the Yes/No option gives no indication of degree of delay or the level at which the child is functioning. A schedule covering an age span is more informative and with less experienced screening personnel reduces the number of unnecessary referrals.

The number of examinations depends on availability of staff and their other commitments but the basic minimum for effective screening should not be less than 3 examinations at ages 9–10 months, 2 years and 3 years.

Methods of screening range from a simple developmental check list completed by health visitors to a structured interview and examination carried out by doctors with special training and including physical and neurological examination, developmental items and tests of vision and hearing. A National Children's Bureau project (Evans and Sparrow, 1975) is experimenting with a developmental guide for parents.

However simple or complex the schedules a detailed manual of instructions, geared to the least experienced of the many who will be involved in a total screening programme, will facilitate standardization of procedures and recording.

A number of publications about development screening exist (e.g. Egan *et al.*, 1969; Illingworth, 1973; Sheridan, 1973) which are invaluable in general training, but may not provide the exact details needed for implementing programmes designed to suit local needs.

Schedule items

Minimal requirements are some items covering gross motor function, hand manipulation and adaptive behaviour, language, social skills and observations on vision, hearing and behaviour.

The most useful developmental items are those in which the same test procedure elicits increasing maturity of response with age and those which are least affected by opportunity and practice. The recording form should enable observed responses to be differentiated from information supplied by mother. Warning signs of abnormality should be detailed in the manual and there may be some advantage in having such signs itemized on the schedule.

Gross motor function. The following items give the best simple indications of motor maturity at different ages.

4–12 weeks, posture in ventral suspension, particularly noting the position of the head relative to the trunk.

16–24 weeks, position of the head in the pull up from supine manoeuvre and head control in supported sitting.

28–40 weeks, balance in unsupported sitting and ability in standing.

44 weeks–15 months, method of moving by 'sealing', crawling, hitching, cruising, supported or unsupported walking. History will suffice if the child is reluctant to demonstrate his abilities.

18 months–3 years, stability, ease and grace in walking, trotting and running should be observed.

Hand manipulation and adaptive behaviour. The following observations and procedures are recommended.

4–12 weeks, observation of degree of hand closure.

16–24 weeks, grasp of and approach to a proffered rattle noting gradations of maturity from grasping and retention when rattle is placed in hand to accurate one-handed approach, grasp and transfer.

28–40 weeks, ability to grasp and retain two 1-inch cubes and method of grasp.

32–52 weeks, method of securing a pellet. Ring on string test demonstrates hand control and problem solving ability.

52 weeks–18 months, cup and cubes test demonstrates voluntary release and maturity in putting in/taking out games.

15 months–3 years, tower building provides information about fine motor control and construction of train and bridge pointers to problem solving and perceptual abilities. Similarly, pencil and paper tests demonstrate manual dexterity and perception of shape.

Comprehension and communication. Observations in this area of behaviour are the most difficult to quantify. There are few simple tests or substitutions for skill in history taking and experience in the ways that infants demonstrate understanding. The following observations should be recorded.

4–12 weeks, social smile and social vocal response should be clearly demonstrated, mother's history is insufficient.

16–24 weeks, interest in surroundings, toys, people may be evident in the screening situation or elicited from history. Vocalization may not be demonstrated but information should be sought from mother.

28–52 weeks, response to nursery games (actions, words and actions, words only) indicates increasing comprehension. Again, mother's account of maturity of vocalization is noted.

15 months–3 years. Questions are asked about number of words, word combinations, use of words and intelligibility. Response to pictures is included from 18 months.

Social skills. The acquisiton of social skills is much affected by child-rearing practices and the child's achievements are poorly correlated with overall developmental status. However, it is worth noting difficulties or delays in feeding behaviour (see below) and a history of ability in self-feeding at age 2–3 years provides some indication of fine motor control in children who refuse to respond to test items.

Vision. In the first 3 months fixing on mother's face and following a moving object are indicators of developmental status and visual competence. Thereafter the infant gives many indications of ability to see, immediately fixing on a rattle placed in hand at 16 weeks, fixing on play materials on table top within 6–12 inches at 20–24 weeks and 'picking up' with eyes a tiny object still or moving on table top at 24–28 weeks. In the 2nd and 3rd years of life peering at pictures may suggest myopia. If there is any doubt about visual acuity formal testing should be carried out (p. 151).

Hearing. Mother should have no doubt about response to unseen voice by 12–16 weeks. If any doubt exists formal testing should be carried out (p. 161). In any case routine hearing screening in the second 6 months of life is mandatory.

Behaviour. There is little time in a brief screening session for full discussion of behaviour. Some note should be taken of initial difficulties of management. If in answer to the question 'Is he an easy child to manage?' mother reports marked problems of feeding, toilet training or sleeping, frequent temper tantrums, excessive timidity, overactivity, aggression or negativism, or specific problems such as head banging, breath holding, enuresis and so on, these should be recorded but discussed in detail at a later session.

Warning signs
The following should be recorded if observed or reported.

Convulsions; major fits or 'blank spells', odd mannerisms or other episodes suggestive of minor fits.

Abnormal head size; too big (could be familial) or too small for weight, abnormal rate of growth, i.e. crossing percentile lines on OFC chart.

Abnormal eye movements; nystagmus and squint, apart from occasional horizontal squint noticed in the first 3–4 months of life.

Abnormal feeding patterns; difficulties in sucking, inability to take smooth stodgy foods at 24–28 weeks, foods containing bits at 32–36 weeks or to chew a biscuit from 40 weeks.

Other problems of management in the first 3 months; difficulties in handling and bathing, irritability, excessive response to loud noise and changes of posture, described as 'jumpy', 'jittery' or 'very easily startled'.

Abnormalities of tone; on handling, feels stiff ('doesn't cuddle up') or floppy ('like a rag doll').

Poverty and asymmetry of movement; lies still and extended, tight clenching of hands with thumbs across palms, persistence of ATNR attitude in supine beyond 16 weeks.

Tendency to come right up to standing on pull to sit manoeuvre and weight bearing on tip-toes.

Clumsy ataxic gait beyond 18 months. Ataxic reach beyond 28 weeks, intention tremor.

Persistence of hand regard beyond 24 weeks and mouthing of toys (often with excessive drooling) beyond 52 weeks.

Disinterest in surroundings at 16–20 weeks (the infant content to lie when awake); disinterest in toys beyond 28 weeks, persistent casting of toys beyond 18 months; aimless overactivity with little constructive play from 2 years.

Persistent jargoning beyond 2 years and echolalia beyond 3 years.

Children exhibiting any of these forms of behaviour should be referred for further assessment and neurological examination.

References

DRILLIEN C.M. (1964) Correlation between pre-school testing and intelligence testing in school. In *Growth and Development of the Prematurely Born Infant*, p. 202. Edinburgh: Livingstone.

EGAN D., ILLINGWORTH R.S. and MAC KEITH R.C. (1969) Developmental Screening 0–5 years. *Clinics in Developmental Medicine*. No. 30 London: Heinemann.

EVANS R. and SPARROW M. (1975) Trends in the assessment of early childhood development. *Child care, health and development*, 1, 127.

ILLINGWORTH R.S. (1972) Predictive value of developmental assessment in infancy. In *Mental Retardation: Prenatal Diagnosis and Infant Assessment*, eds. Douglas C.P. and Holt K.S. London: Institute for Research into Mental Retardation and Butterworth.

ILLINGWORTH R.S. (1975) Developmental testing and its value. Variations in individual fields of development. In *The Development of the Infant and Young Child: normal and abnormal*, 6th Ed, pp. 4, 193. Edinburgh: Churchill Livingstone.

IILLNGWORTH R.S. (1973) *Basic Developmental Screening 0–2 years*. Oxford: Blackwell Scientific Publications.

KNOBLOCH H. and PASAMANICK B., eds (1974) Validity of infant assessment. In *Gesell and Amatruda's Developmental Diagnosis*, 3rd Ed., p. 142. New York: Harper and Row.

NUFFIELD PROVINCIAL HOSPITALS TRUST (1968) *Screening in Medical Care: Reviewing the Evidence*. London: Oxford University Press.

SCOTTISH HOME AND HEALTH DEPARTMENT (1973) *Towards an Integrated Child Health Service*. Edinburgh: Her Majesty's Stationery Office.

SCRUTTON D. and GILBERTSON M. (1975) *Physiotherapy in Paediatric Practice*, p. 89. London: Butterworth.

SHERIDAN M.D. (1973) *Children's Developmental Progress: from birth to five years*. Windsor: National Foundation for Educational Research.

SHERIDAN M.D. (1975) The importance of spontaneous play in the fundamental learning of handicapped children. *Child care, health and development* 1, 3.

CHAPTER 5

Surveillance of Preschool Children in General Practice

Historical Background

With the introduction of the Stycar tests in 1958 and 1960 (Chapter 8) the stage was set for screening of development, hearing and vision for all preschool children. Gesell and Amatruda (1941) had already described the sequences of normal development, had delineated the norms and even more importantly had described carefully and comprehensively how to examine children in order to demonstrate normal development and the deviations that could signal disorder or retardation. Illingworth (1975) reviewed the controversy that has raged since, but concluded that 'developmental tests in infancy are of great value in that they can detect mental retardation and neurological conditions with a considerable degree of certainty'.

Soon Medical Officers of Health were instituting population screening in these three areas of development in infant welfare clinics, so that early diagnosis of disorder could be made in the under 5-year-old child population. It was agreed, amongst other things, that this enabled more effective treatment to be given.

Despite considerable evidence that this was the case, for over 16 years the position has remained unsatisfactory. The reasons are many. Inadequate training of personnel resulted in tests being poorly carried out. Too few staff led to the introduction of the At-Risk register (Lindon, 1961; Sheridan, 1962). It was thought possible to pick out at birth or in early infancy those most likely to develop disorders because of a history of familial disease, unsatisfactory home circumstances, adverse factors in the pre-, peri- or postnatal period or because of slow postnatal development. These children were offered routine screening. It was hoped that in the event of disorders presenting in children not included in routine screening, family and clinic doctors, parents or teachers would detect these, albeit usually at a later age.

In some parts of the country over-enthusiastic application of at-risk criteria placed more than one-half of newborns on at-risk registers and even then these might include fewer than two-thirds of infants subsequently found to have handicaps. In some areas health visitors were thought to provide the answer to man-power problems. However, health visitors are not trained as paediatricians and cannot be expected to identify many children with disorders (Richards and Roberts, 1967; Roberts and Khosla, 1972). Nevertheless, without their invaluable help and, in the absence of trained medical personnel, many more children would have remained with their disorders undetected. Statistical evaluation suggested that the at-risk concept itself might be basically unsound (Alberman and Gold-stein, 1970) and it was evident from later studies that many children with disorders do escape detection. In the Isle of Wight survey (Rutter *et al.*, 1970) it was demonstrated that 1 in 10 of all 9–11-year-olds had a significant disability. However, in only 1 of 7 such children was this already known to parent, teacher or doctor. Finally Davie, Butler and Goldstein (1972) showed that only at the lowest resource levels was it justified to allocate all resources to high-risk groups. 'At-Risk' registers are now gradually being phased out.

Current Development Screening Practices

The plethora of examination forms in current use causes confusion. A personal collection of record forms from all parts of the UK and Europe demonstrates many misconceptions about developmental norms. In nearly every case records are laid out in inventory form, inviting a tick or cross to attest to the child examined having passed or failed to pass some developmental milestone. The milestones chosen are sometimes inaccurately dated and no space is allowed to comment on the manner of passing them.

In many parts of this country and in the rest of Europe, the urge to introduce screening programmes has not been followed by any attempt to structure the method of examination and recording. For this reason, and the varying degrees of skill of those completing the forms, the quality of examinations is uneven, examinations are sometimes incomplete and the information recorded of doubtful value. Computers, often used to run immunization programmes, are sometimes adapted to control screening programmes and this causes problems relating to quality of input generally and failure to update information going to the computer.

Some workers have not come to grips with the problem of non-attendance. Barber *et al.* (1976) mention that at the Woodside Health Centre, Glasgow, only 60 per cent of 18-month children were seen for their routine surveillance examination. In this programme health visitors were responsible for carrying out most of the examinations. Infrequent contact with the doctors working in the programme could cause parents to feel that attendance was not of great importance. In another study (Zinkin and Cox, 1976), with a take up rate of 85–96 per cent at six developmental examinations between 6 weeks and 3 years, childen who did not attend clinics were significantly more likely to have developmental problems than those who did. In this study non-attenders were examined at home.

For all these reasons the statistics produced to prove or disprove the merits of developmental screening are likely to be unreliable and perhaps in part explain the widely differing reported rates of disorder. It is also apparent that there are wide regional variations in disorder. It may be that disorder is diagnosed only when facilities exist for its treatment. In areas with an effective speech therapy service, speech delay is diagnosed and treated. In other areas where no services exist speech disorder seems to be accepted as a fact of life despite its effects on schooling (Butler, Peckham and Sheridan, 1973).

Despite this unsatisfactory state of affairs, screening is carried out successfully in many parts of the country and many children with disorders are detected as a result. The provision of services to back up screening programmes is another matter. The distribution of orthoptists, speech therapists, psychologists, physiotherapists and paediatricians working in assessment centres is very uneven. In some areas all that exists of an assessment centre is one hard-worked developmental paediatrician examining children in their own homes.

The Role of the Family Doctor in Developmental Screening

Over a long period general practitioners have been experimenting with comprehensive paediatric primary care including screening. For many years in Bristol, N.F. Cook ran an exclusively paediatric general practice offering to all children on his list routine surveillance, psychological assessment and careers guidance as well as traditional illness care service up to age 16 years. The inevitable problems associated with a small list (such as the likelihood of a small pension on retirement) brought the concept in its original form to an end, although much of the work continues. Naish (1954) reported on an experiment in comprehensive child care in general practice resulting in a 50 per cent reduction in admissions to hospital, which he ascribed to greater parent confidence and increased effectiveness and improved quality of his own care. The words of Sheldon (Ministry of Health, 1967) 'eventually the child health services will no longer be a distinct and separate entity but will become part of a family health service provided by the family doctor in a family health centre' have proved prophetic, and since 1970 many papers have appeared from general practice, describing the organization and practice of comprehensive medical and developmental surveillance including screening (e.g. Hutchison, 1973; Pollak, 1973; Bain, 1974; Starte, 1974, 1975, 1976; Rowlands, 1975; Stark *et al.*, 1975). All describe their more or less successful attempts to offer a comprehensive paediatric medical and developmental surveillance service. However, some in general practice are particularly critical of the concept of routine, structured developmental assessment (Carne, 1976; Bolden, 1976) and argue that any general practitioner can do this work without special training or organization. Examination of their data reveals clearly the reasons for this attitude. The prevalence of reported physical disorder and the virtual absence of developmental disorder, with the implication that special assessment clinics generate anxiety, show all too clearly the great problems of education that lie ahead, if general practitioners are to be brought into this field on any large scale (Curtis Jenkins, 1976a). Other critics have pointed out the importance of providing an efficient 24-hour illness care service before providing assessment clinics, and deprecate clinics that do not provide the time to discuss sore bottoms as well as developmental delay.

For effective screening on a national level the following criteria should be fulfilled (Curtis Jenkins, 1975).

(1) Following Gesell's excellent precedent no examination should take longer than 15 minutes to carry out. This would allow one doctor working two sessions

weekly to screen all the children in a total practice population of 9000, six times in the first 5 years of life. This is perfectly feasible.

(2) The examination must be effective in detection and the tests selected fulfil the criteria suggested by Frankenberg (1974) for acceptability, reliability and validity.

(3) The disorders detected should, in the main, be capable of amelioration and the prognosis improved by treatment. Adequate provision of specialist support services is therefore essential.

(4) If the condition detected cannot be altered by treatment then some person (many believe that this should be the general practitioner, Curtis Jenkins, 1976b) must be responsible for the day-to-day care and co-ordination of services designed to lift some of the burden placed on parents of handicapped children by present-day fashionable attitudes about community care. All too often this means quite simply, care in the home by the parents with inadequate help.

(5) If screening is to be carried out by family doctors, health visitor attachment is essential; without this nothing is possible.

In the absence of any effective alternative Starte (1974) developed his own screening tool for the examination of 7-month and 2-year-old children in his Guildford practice and showed how careful and meticulous construction and use could facilitate surveillance. Building on his work, the Ashford developmental paediatric research group produced the developmental profile examination forms (illustrated in Figs. 5.1–5.6) for use at 3 weeks, 7 months and 1, 2, 3 and 4½ years. An accompanying protocol is strictly adhered to.

Personal Experience in One Practice

In one practice these profiles have been in use since 1970 and many thousands of examinations have been carried out as part of the surveillance service offered (Curtis Jenkins, 1976c). The programme covers the well-care needs of the under-5 population in one practice. The number of children is falling, in line with the nationwide fall in birth rate and currently there are about 1200 children under 5 years old in our care. Eighty per cent have been followed from birth. Twenty per cent have joined the programme since birth, on registering with the practice. A community child care specialist and the practitioner work two sessions each weekly. Eighty per cent of the time is spent carrying out routine surveillance examinations at the ages mentioned and 20 per cent seeing children more frequently because of problems already detected or at the request of parents, health visitors or the children's own doctors.

Children are discharged to our care from maternity hospital with a variety of conditions and are seen as required. In addition every newborn baby is visited in the home to carry out the initial modified Brazelton type examination (Brazelton, 1973) and to describe to the mother what is offered; this raises the home visiting rate by about 15 per cent per annum. This examination is considered to be the most important one of all in motivating the mother to use the services provided and to counter misinformation given to her about her baby's capabilities in seeing, hearing and responding (Curtis Jenkins, 1976c).

OFFICE USE

Dr's Code [ ]
(1–2)

DR. ....

On Cols 3–13

Punch: First
8 letters of
surname

Surname _____ First Name _____

14

Date of Birth [ ][ ][ ][ ][ ][ ]   Birth Rank [ ]   20

First 3 letters
of first name

21   22

Father's Age [ ][ ]   Mother's Age [ ][ ]   23   24

Father's Occupation _____   25 [ ]

26 [ ][ ][ ][ ][ ][ ] 31

Exam. within **21 days** of Birth | Date ....

Date of Birth [ ][ ][ ][ ][ ][ ]   E.D.D. [ ][ ][ ][ ][ ][ ]

History

	Normal	Abnormal	
Ante Natal			32 [ ]
Natal			33 [ ]
Post Natal			34 [ ]

Breast Fed | No | Yes | 35 [ ]
36

Birth WT. [ ][ ][ ][ ] Grms.   [ ][ ][ ][ ]

	<36	<42	42+		Asymm. Symm.	40 [ ] 41 [ ]

Maturity [ ] [ ] [ ]

Low Medium High
Moro Response [ ] [ ] [ ]   42 [ ]

	No	Yes	
Grasp	No	Yes	43 [ ]
Walking	No	Yes	44 [ ]
Placing	No	Yes	45 [ ]
Sound Resp.	No	Yes	46 [ ]
Light Resp.	No	Yes	47 [ ]

Ventral Susp. [ ] [ ] [ ]   48 [ ]

PHYSICAL EXAMINATION

Weight   Height   H.C.

(49–52) [ ][ ][ ] Grms. (53–5) [ ][ ] | Cms. (56–8) [ ][ ] | Cms.

	Norm.	State Abnormalities	
Skull			59 [ ]
Ears			60 [ ]
Eyes			61 [ ]
Palate			62 [ ]
C.V.S.			63 [ ]
R.S.			64 [ ]
Abdo.			65 [ ]
Spine			66 [ ]
Hernia			67 [ ]
Fem. Pulses			68 [ ]
Genitalia			69 [ ]
Hips			70 [ ]
Limbs			71 [ ]
Tone			72 [ ]
Reflexes			73 [ ]
Skin			74 [ ]
Biochem			75 [ ]

Appearance

Comments   Card Code

Action   79 [1]

If tests incomplete because of child's
unco-operation put tick in box   [ ]   80 [ ]

Fig. 5.1. Profile examination form, age 3 weeks.

PAEDIATRIC DEVELOPMENT RECORD

DR. ....

Surname _____ First Name _____

Date of Birth 14 ☐☐☐☐☐☐ Birth Rank 20 ☐

Father's Age 21 22 ☐☐ Mother's Age 23 24 ☐☐

Father's Occupation _____ 25 ☐

26 ☐☐☐☐☐ 31

Exam. at 7 months | Date ....

		No	Yes	26					

Mother's Comments

		No	Yes	
	Happy	No	Yes	32 ☐
	Sleeps	No	Yes	33 ☐
	Chews	No	Yes	34 ☐

Illness since last exam. No | Yes 35 ☐
(If yes specify nature of illness)

....

Breast Fed ☐ mos. 36 ☐
Solids started No | Yes 37 ☐

Nursery No | Yes 38 ☐
Minder No | Yes 39 ☐
Hours worked per week (mother) ☐ 40 41 ☐☐

	No stability	Sits supported	Sits un-supported	
Sitting	No stability	Sits supported	Sits un-supported	42 ☐
Standing supported	No weight Bearing	Full weight	Weight alternates foot to foot	43 ☐
Prone	No weight on hands, head up	Shoulders up weight on hands	Knee up to crawl	44 ☐
1″ Brick	No grasp	Mouthing	Transfer	45 ☐
Pellet	Whole hand scrabble	Whole hand pick up	Finger-thumb pick up	46 ☐
Rolling balls	$\frac{1}{2}$″	$\frac{1}{4}$″	$\frac{3}{16}$″	47 ☐
Cover test	Squint	Doubtful	No squint	48 ☐
Hearing 3 ft.	Doubtful	Satisfactory	Good	49 ☐
Speech	Noise only	Purposeful sound	2 Syllables or more	50 ☐
Imitates shaking rattle	No interest	Interest and manipulation	Imitation	51 ☐
Reaction to Examiner	None	Resists	Co-operates	52 ☐
Attention	Poor	Variable	Sustained	53 ☐

PHYSICAL EXAM:

Weight (54–6) ☐☐.☐ K.grms. Height (57–9) ☐☐☐ Cms. (60–2) ☐☐☐ H.C. ☐☐☐ Cms.

Abnormality No/Yes (Specify below) .... 63 ☐

Appearance

Comments Card Code

Action 79 ☐ 2

If tests incomplete because of child's unco-operation put tick in box ☐ 80 ☐

Fig. 5.2. Profile examination form, age 7 months.

PAEDIATRIC DEVELOPMENT RECORD

DR._____

Surname _____ First Name _____

Date of Birth ☐☐☐☐☐☐   Birth Rank ☐
14   20

Father's Age ☐☐   Mother's Age ☐☐
21   22   23   24

Father's Occupation _____ 25 ☐

26   ☐☐☐☐   31

Exam. at **12 months**	Date....................

Mother's Comments

	No	Yes	
Happy	No	Yes	32 ☐
Sleeps	No	Yes	33 ☐
Eats	No	Yes	34 ☐

Illness since last exam. | No | Yes | 35 ☐
(If yes specify nature of illness)

....

Change in family circumstances | No | Yes | 36 ☐

Nursery | No | Yes | 37 ☐
Minder | No | Yes | 38 ☐
Hours worked per   ☐   39 40
week (Mother)   ☐☐

Reported Speech | 1 | 2 | 3 | 4 | 41 ☐

Gait	Creeps Crawls Hitches	Pulls to stand	Cruises Walks one hand held	Walks alone	42 ☐
1″ Brick	Withdraws	Transfers	Casts not looking	Casts looking	43 ☐
Pellet	Withdraws or fails	Whole hand pick up	Finger Thumb Apposition	Releases	44 ☐
Rolling balls	$\frac{1}{2}$″	$\frac{1}{4}$″	$\frac{3}{16}$″	$\frac{1}{8}$″	45 ☐
Cover Test	Squint	Doubtful		No squint	46 ☐
Hearing	Doubtful	Satisfactory		Good	47 ☐
Speech heard	No words	2 words or less	3 words or less with meaning	More than 3 words with meaning	48 ☐
Imitation rattle	No interest	Interest and manipulation		Imitation	49 ☐
Reaction to Examiner	None	Resists		Co-operates	50 ☐
Attention	Poor	Variable		Sustained	51 ☐

PHYSICAL EXAM.

Weight   Height   H.C.

(52–4) ☐☐·☐ K.grms. (55–7) ☐☐☐ Cms. (58–60) ☐☐·☐ Cms.

Abnormality No/Yes (Specify below)

....

....

61 ☐

Appearance

Comments   Card Code

Action   79 | 3 |

If tests incomplete because of child's   ☐   80 ☐
unco-operation put tick in box

Fig. 5.3. Profile examination form, age 1 year.

PAEDIATRIC DEVELOPMENT RECORD

DR...

Surname _____ First Name _____

Date of Birth ☐☐☐☐☐☐ **·20** Birth Rank ☐
14

Father's Age ☐☐   Mother's Age ☐☐
21 22   23 24

Father's Occupation _____ 25 ☐

26 ☐☐☐☐☐☐ 31

Exam. at **24 months**	Date...

Mother's Comments

		No	Yes		
	Happy	No	Yes	32	☐
	Sleeps	No	Yes	33	☐
	Eats	No	Yes	34	☐
	Imaginative play	No	Yes	35	☐

Illness since last exam. (If yes specify nature of illness)	No	Yes	36	☐

....

Changes in family circumstances		No	Yes	37	☐
Play group	No	Yes		38	☐
Nursery	No	Yes		39	☐
Minder	No	Yes		40	☐
Hours worked per week (Mother)	☐			41–2	☐☐

		1	2	3		
Bowel	D				43	☐
	N				44	☐
Bladder	D				45	☐
	N				46	☐
Sentences	1	2	3	4	47	☐

Kick ball	No kick	Runs into ball	Poor kick	Good directed kick	48	☐
Throw ball	No throw	2 hands poor direct.	2 hands good direct.	1 hand	49	☐
1″ Brick column	2 or less	3 – 4	5 – 7	8+	50	☐
Screws on table	2 or less up	3 up	4 up	5 up	51	☐
Rolling balls	$\frac{1}{2}$″	$\frac{1}{4}$″	$\frac{3}{16}$″	$\frac{1}{8}$″	52	☐
Cover test	Squint		Doubtful	No squint	53	☐
6 Toy hearing	4 and under		5 – 6 with hesitation	6 Immediate	54	☐
Recognition	no yes	no yes	no yes	no yes	no yes	no yes	55 60
Comprehension	Spoon in cup	Ball to mummy	Car on brick	Doll	Brick under cup	Cup	· · · ·
Ladybird vocab.	2 or less	3 – 8	9 – 14	15+	61	☐
Sentences observed	None	Occasional connected words	3–4 words	5+words	62	☐
Form board	2 or less in	3 in after mistakes	3 in immediately straight	3 in immediately reversed	63	☐
Attention	None	Poor	Variable	Sustained	64	☐

PHYSICAL EXAM.

Weight (65 – 8) ☐☐☐ Cms.   Height (69 – 70) ☐☐ Cms.

Abnormality	No/Yes (Specify below)	71	☐

.... Dominant Foot   R L   72 ☐
.... ,, Hand   R L   73 ☐
.... ,, Eye   R L   74 ☐

Appearance
Comment
Action

Card Code 79 ☐ 4

If tests incomplete because of child's unco-operation put tick in box	☐ ☐	80	☐

Fig. 5.4. Profile examination form, age 2 years.

DR...

OFFICE USE

Dr's Code
(1–2) ☐☐

On Cols 3–13

Punch : First
8 letters of
surname

First 3 letters
of first name

Surname _____ First Name _____

Date of Birth **14** ☐☐☐☐☐   Birth Rank **20** ☐

Father's Age **21 22** ☐☐   Mother's Age **23 24** ☐☐

Father's Occupation _____ **25** ☐

26 ☐☐☐☐☐ 31

| Exam. at **36 months** | Date... | ☐☐☐☐☐ |

Mother's Comments

		No	Yes	
	Happy	No	Yes	32 ☐
	Sleeps	No	Yes	33 ☐
	Eats	No	Yes	34 ☐

Illness since last exam.   No   Yes   35 ☐
(If yes specify nature of illness)

....

Change in family circumstances   No   Yes   36 ☐

Play group	No	Yes		37 ☐
Nursery	No	Yes		38 ☐
Minder	No	Yes		39 ☐

Hours worked per   ☐   40 41
week (Mother)   ☐☐

			1	2	3	
Eating Mode	⎧	Knife				42 ☐
	⎨	Fork				43 ☐
	⎩	Spoon				44 ☐
Bowel	⎰	D				45 ☐
	⎱	N				46 ☐
Bladder	⎰	D				47 ☐
	⎱	N				48 ☐
		Dressing				49 ☐

Kick ball	Runs into Ball	Poor kick	Good direct kick	50 ☐
1" Brick ⊓⊔	Does not try	Tries but fails	Succeeds	51 ☐
Rolling balls	¼"	³⁄₁₆"	⅛"	52 ☐
Cover Test	Squint	Doubtful	No squint	53 ☐
7 Toy hearing	4 and under	5 – 6 with hesitation	7 Immediate	54 ☐
Ladybird Book	Speech	Less than 15 pictures	16 – 20 pictures	21 or more pictures	55 ☐
	Compre- hension	Less than 5 actions	6 – 10 actions	11 or more actions	56 ☐
Articulation	Not Under- stood	Under- stood with difficulty words in- complete	Under- stood minor errors only	Clear and under- stood	57 ☐
Story answers	0	1	2	3	4	5	6	7	58 ☐
Questions to Child	Name	Sex	Age	Address	Number correct	1	2	3	4	59 ☐

PHYSICAL EXAM.   Weight   Height

(60–2) ☐☐·☐ K.gms. (63–6) ☐☐☐·☐ Cms.

Abnormality No/Yes (Specify below)   70 ☐

.... Dominant foot   R   L   71 ☐

....   ,,   Hand   R   L   72 ☐

....   ,,   Eye   R   L   73 ☐

Appearance

Comment   Card Code

Action   79 ☐ 5

| If tests incomplete because of child's unco-operation put tick in box | ☐ | 80 ☐ |

Fig. 5.5. Profile examination form, age 3 years.

DR...

OFFICE USE

Dr's Code ☐☐
(1–2)

On Cols 3–13

Punch: First
8 letters of
surname

First 3 letters
of first name

Surname _____ First Name _____

Date of Birth (14) ☐☐☐☐☐☐ (20) Birth Rank ☐

Father's Age (21) (22) ☐☐ Mother's Age (23) (24) ☐☐

Father's Occupation _____ (25) ☐

26 ☐☐☐☐☐ 31

Exam at **54 months**	Date....................

Mother's Comments

Happy	No	Yes	32	☐
Sleeps	No	Yes	33	☐
Eats	No	Yes	34	☐

Illness since last exam. No | Yes 35 ☐
(If yes specify nature of illness)

....

Change in family circumstances No | Yes 36 ☐

Play group	No	Yes	37 ☐
Nursery	No	Yes	38 ☐
Minder	No	Yes	39 ☐

Hours worked per ☐ 40 41
week (Mother) ☐☐

		1	2	3		
Eating Mode	Knife				42	☐
	Fork				43	☐
	Spoon				44	☐
Bowel	D				45	☐
	N				46	☐
Bladder	D				47	☐
	N				48	☐
Dressing					49	☐

Heel-toe walk	Steps wider than 15 cms. or more than 1 step to side	Gap 5–10 cms. or 1 step to side	4 steps all less than 5 cms. gap		50 ☐
Matches in box	All in 3 or more corrections	All in less than 3 corrections	All in both hands		51 ☐
6 Brick pyramid	Fails	At least 3 bricks in relation	Succeeds after more than 1 at-tempt	Succeeds 1st attempt	52 ☐
Vision R	6/36	6/24	6/12	6/9	6/6	53 ☐
Vision L	6/36	6/24	6/12	6/9	6/6	54 ☐
Cover test	Squint	Doubtful	No squint		55 ☐
Hearing Toy	4 and under	5 – 6 or hesitation	7 Immediate		56 ☐
Articulation	Not under-stood	Under-stood with difficulty Words in-complete	Under-stood min- or errors only	Clear and under-stood	57 ☐
Story answers	0 1	2 3	4 5	6 7	58 ☐
Questions to child	Name Sex Age	Address Number correct	1 2 3 4		59 ☐
Draw a man	0 – 4	5 – 10	11 – 14	15+	60 ☐

PHYSICAL EXAM.

Weight Height

(61–3) ☐☐|☐ K.gms. (64–7) ☐☐☐|☐ Cms.

Abnormality No/Yes (Specify below) 70 ☐

.... Dominant foot R | L 71 ☐
.... „ hand R | L 72 ☐
.... „ Eye R | L 73 ☐

Appearance

Comment Card Code

Action 79 ☐ 6

If tests incomplete because of child's unco-operation put tick in box	☐	80 ☐

Fig. 5.6. Profile examination form, age 4½ years.

Every child is seen. Non-attendance for routine surveillance examination is one of the best at-risk indicators we have. Careful follow up of non-attenders, running at 8–10 per cent for first appointments, reveals unsuspected problems such as marital strife and illness in the mother.

The detection rate of disorder varies from year to year. In a representative year about 1100 children are seen for routine examinations using the profile system. In 1975–6, 158 disorders were detected. The detection rate was 10 per cent at 7 months, 6 per cent at 12 months, 19 per cent at 2 years, 30 per cent at 3 years and 31 per cent at $4\frac{1}{2}$ years (Appendix 5.1). The 3-year-old examination is a selective one depending on findings at the 2-year assessment, a history of convulsions, speech delay, middle ear infections and any other factors thought significant by the doctor, health visitor or parent. In 1975, 40 per cent of 3-year-olds were seen for these reasons.

From these figures it would appear that the 1-year-old examination was the least important; yet if it had not been done three children with cerebral palsy would have been missed, only one with a history in any way suspect. Decisions about what age groups to examine need to be carefully taken in the light of such findings and should not depend on arbitrary decisions taken by examination of gross data. Findings confirm other available evidence that every effort should be made to provide as full a service as possible to all children as often as is possible (Davie *et al.*, 1972) and certainly a great deal more frequently than is often stated as desirable (Curtis Jenkins, 1976a).

As many others have stated, it has been difficult to confirm that at-risk children show more disorders than children with no at-risk factors. Careful examination of *all* children must be the aim of any programme and the programme organized in such a way as to make this the invariable practice.

Finally, it is important to mention the beneficial effect that such a programme has on the quality of overall paediatric care in a practice which offers such a service. That 15 per cent of children seen were found to have disorders (7 per cent severe enough to warrant specialist opinion) is not the raison d'être of the service provided. It is much more important that over 900 children were found to be entirely normal and their parents told so. In addition, positive health educational advice is given as part of the service. The parents are quick to realize the close involvement with both the community child health services and the local hospital. This last is obvious to them when they meet paediatric resident staff sitting in the clinics to learn about normal children. The personal impact has been considerable. The main effect has been due to seeing children and their parents in a 'well' situation, freer from anxiety than the traditional illness consultation. Parents and children have taught in turn, a great deal about the loss of confidence and the provoking of anxiety that we as doctors tend to cause in patients by behaviour in sickness consultation. The patients have altered their demands in a subtle fashion as a result of their perception of our new role. A preliminary data analysis of the last 5 years of consultations suggests that the episode consultation rate is falling in the 0–5 year age group whilst remaining stationary at other ages. Certainly the outpatients referral rate shows a 30 per cent reduction compared to the national figures, although unlike Naish (1954) the inpatient referral rate is only marginally lower than the national average. The ability to resist the urge to treat has also become stronger. A recent analysis shows that my prescribing rate is half that of my partners (total number of prescriptions issued) and my costs are half that of the national average per patient on my practice list. The not infrequent question 'You are not going to give him an antibiotic are you doctor? which my partners now report from parents of their child patients, shows how wrong we can be when trying to analyse why parents bring their children to see the doctor. The traditional view is that parents will not be satisfied unless an antibiotic is prescribed for all infections, yet by altering the emphasis of cure towards care a fundamentally different attitude can be encouraged. The future of this new aspect of general practice is exciting. The considerable problem of changing the attitudes to care of both patients and their doctors must be faced. Adequate training programmes and motivation, efficient organization and lastly, but most importantly, the provision of services to treat the disorders discovered as the result of such programmes are all consumers of money, time and energy (Appendix 5.2). It would be regrettable if it was decided that this country could not afford these services.

References

ALBERMAN E.D. and GOLDSTEIN H. (1970) The at-risk register, a statistical evaluation. *British Journal of Preventive and Social Medicine*, **24**, 129.

BAIN D.J.B. (1974) The results of developmental screening in general practice. *Health Bulletin*, **32**, 189.

BARBER J.H., BOOTHMAN R. and STANFIELD J.P. (1976) A new visual chart for pre-school developmental screening. *Health Bulletin*, **34**, 80.

BOLDEN K.J. (1976) Developmental screening clinics are a luxury. *Proceedings of the Royal Society of Medicine*, **69**, 385.

BRAZELTON, T.B. (1973) *Neonatal Behavioural Assessment Scale. Clinics in Developmental Medicine. No. 50.* London: Heinemann.

BUTLER N.R., PECKHAM C. and SHERIDAN M. (1973) Speech defects in children: A national study. *British Medical Journal*, **1**, 253.

CARNE S. (1976) The case against developmental screening in general practice. *Update*, **12**, 535.

CURTIS JENKINS G.H. (1975) The preschool child. In *Screening in General Practice*, Edinburgh: Churchill Livingstone.

CURTIS JENKINS G.H. (1976a) Developmental and paediatric care of the pre-school child. *Journal of the Royal College of General Practitioners*, **26**, 795.

CURTIS JENKINS G.H. (1976b) The content of care. In *Child Care in General Practice*. Edinburgh: Churchill Livingstone.

CURTIS JENKINS G.H. (1976c) The case for developmental and medical surveillance of the pre-school child. *Update*, **11**, 777.

DAVIE R., BUTLER N. and GOLDSTEIN H. (1972) *From Birth to Seven.* pp. 90, 186. London: Longman.

FRANKENBERG W.K. (1974) Selection of diseases and tests in pediatric screening. *Pediatrics* **54**, 612.

GESELL A. and AMATRUDA C.S. (1941) *Developmental Diagnosis.* New York: Hoeber.

HUTCHINSON J.H. (1973) An experiment in the developmental screening of young children. *Health Bulletin*, **31**, 156.

ILLINGWORTH R.S. (1975) *Development of the Infant and Young Child: Normal and Abnormal*, 6th Ed. Edinburgh: Churchill Livingstone.

LINDON R.L. (1961) Risk Registers. *Bulletin of Cerebral Palsy*, **3**, 481.

MINISTRY OF HEALTH. STANDING MEDICAL ADVISORY COMMITTEE (1967). Chairman, Sheldon W. Child Welfare Centres, p. 23. London: Her Majesty's Stationery Office.

NAISH C. (1954) An experiment in family practice within the National Health Service. *Lancet*, **i**, 1342.

POLLAK M. (1973) *Today's Three Year Olds in London*. London: Heinemann.

RICHARDS I.D.G. and ROBERTS C.J. (1967) The at-risk infant. *Lancet*, **ii**, 711.

ROBERTS C.J. and KHOSLA, T. (1972) An evaluation of developmental examination as a method of detecting neurological, visual and auditory handicaps in infancy. *British Journal of Preventive and Social Medicine* **26**, 94.

ROWLANDS P. (1975) Developmental assessment in general practice. *Update*, **10**, 379.

RUTTER M., TIZARD J. and WHITMORE K. (1970) *Education, Health and Behaviour*. London: Longman.

SHERIDAN M.D. (1958) Simple clinical hearing tests for the very young or mentally retarded children. *British Medical Journal*, **2**, 999.

SHERIDAN M.D. (1960) Vision screening of very young and handicapped children. *British Medical Journal*, **2**, 453.

SHERIDAN M.D. (1962) Infants at risk of handicapping conditions. Monthly Bulletin. *Ministry of Health and Public Health Laboratory Services*, **21**, 238.

STARK G.D., BASSETT W.J., BAIN D.J.G. and STEWART F.I. (1975) Paediatrics in Livingstone New Town. Evolution of a child health service. *British Medical Journal*, **4**, 387.

STARTE G.D. (1974) The developmental assessment of the young child in general practice. *Practitioner*, **213**, 823.

STARTE G.D. (1975) The poor communicating two year old and his family. *Journal of the Royal College of General Practitioners*, **25**, 880.

STARTE G.D. (1976) The results from a developmental screening clinic in general practice. *Practitioner*, **216**, 311.

ZINKIN P.M. and COX C.A. (1976) Child health clinics and inverse care laws: evidence from a longitudinal study of 1878 pre-school children. *British Medical Journal*, **3**, 411.

Appendix 5.1

Costing of a Nationwide Development Surveillance Programme

In 1971 under Section 22 of the National Health Service Act 1946 (England and Wales) 246 000 sessions were held in local authority clinics at a cost of £13 000 000.

171 740 were staffed by medical officers employed by the local authorities concerned.

73 569 were staffed by general practitioners.

1 337 were staffed by hospital medical staff.

If a nationwide scheme was instituted along the lines described above, with 7 month; 1 year; 2 year; a selective 3 year and a 4½ year examination, 280 000 sessions would need to be provided (ten children being seen at each session) to cover the surveillance requirements of the child population of England and Wales. If one in six general practitioners worked one session weekly providing 160 000 sessions annually, and the community health services provided 170 000 sessions, then the needs of the child population would be more than adequately met. The total cost of such a service in 1977 would be £34 000 000. This figure is the cost of existing child health clinics with the addition of a notional £11.00 sessional payment to the general practitioners working in the service (the same payment that part-time community paediatricians receive per session).

This figure does not include cost provision for a computer-assisted programme, as in the author's opinion nothing replaces the up-to-date and accurate information and local knowledge of those working at the interface between patient and the service; nor does it include the cost of back-up services to provide treatment for children detected as a result of such a programme.

Appendix 5.2

Results of 12 Months Surveillance Examinations, April 1975 to March 1976

Total children seen   1064 (864 in clinics)
Total disorders detected or suspected (excluding neonatal) 158: 14.8 per cent
Total disorders referred for specialist assessment*   77: 7.2 per cent

First examination within 3 weeks (at home)
Modified Brazelton examination
  Infants seen   200
  Infants followed regularly to 7 months   40
    (on account of birth history, inadequate bonding, major handicapping condition)

Second examination at 7 months
  Total children seen   192: 97 boys, 95 girls
  Failed first appointment   13: 6.8 per cent
  Failed 2 or more   6: 3.1 per cent.

Disorders detected	Boys	Girls	Total No.	Per cent
Hypotonia	—	1	1	0.5
Hypertonia	2	1	3	1.6
Intention tremor	1	—	1	0.5
Motor delay	2	3	5	2.6
Strabismus	2*	2*	4	2.1
Failure to thrive	—	1*	1	0.5
Talipes equinovarus	1*	—	1	0.5
Balanitis (requiring circumcision)	1*	—	1	0.5
Obesity	—	2	2	1.0
Maternal deprivation	1	—	1	0.5
Total	10	10	20	10.4

Third examination at 12 months
  Total children seen   194: 94 boys, 100 girls
  Failed first appointment   23: 11.9 per cent
  Failed 2 or more   5: 2.6 per cent

Disorders detected	Boys	Girls	Total No.	Per cent
Motor delay	—	2	2	1.0
Cerebral palsy (initial diagnosis)	2*	1*	3	1.6
Strabismus	1*	1*	2	1.0
Myopia	1*	—	1	0.5
Behaviour disturbance	1	—	1	0.5
Battered baby (failed 3 appointments)	1*	—	1	0.5
Maternal deprivation (new patient)	1	—	1	0.5
Total	7	4	11	5.7

Fourth examination at 2 years

Total children seen	173: 82 boys, 91 girls
Failed first appointment	33: 19.1 per cent
Failed 2 or more	9: 5.2 per cent

Disorders detected	Boys	Girls	Total No.	Per cent
Intention tremor	1	—	1	0.6
Strabismus	2*	1*	3	1.7
Myopia	—	2*	2	1.2
Hearing loss	2*	5*	7	4.0
Behaviour disturbance	3	1	4	2.3
Global developmental delay	—	1*	1	0.6
Language and speech delay	7	7	14	8.1
Heart murmur (initial detection)	—	1*	1	0.6
Total	15	18	33	19.1

Fifth examination at 3 years

Selection based on results at 2 years and at request of parent, health visitor or other agency (e.g. child minder)

Total population of children	204
Total children seen	89 (44 per cent of total population): 52 boys, 37 girls
Failed first appointment	15: 16.9 per cent
Failed 2 or more	nil

Disorders detected	Boys	Girls	No.	Total Per cent seen	Per cent total population of 3 yr-olds
Hypotonia	—	1*	1	1.1	0.5
Strabismus	—	1*	1	1.1	0.5
Myopia	—	1*	1	1.1	0.5
Hearing loss	—	1*	1	1.1	0.5
Behaviour disturbance	1	2	3	3.3	1.5
Global retardation	1*	—	1	1.1	1.5
Language and speech delay	13*	5*	18	20.2	8.8
Undescended testicle	1*	—	1	1.1	0.5
Total	16	11	27	30.3	13.3

Sixth examination at 4½ years

Total children seen	216:	102 boys, 114 girls
Failed first appointment	37:	17.1 per cent
Failed 2 or more	4:	1.9 per cent

				Total
Disorders detected	Boys	Girls	No.	Per cent
Hemiplegia	—	1*	1	0.5
Intention tremor	1	—	1	0.5
Fine motor inco-ordination	3	2	5	2.3
Strabismus	1*	2*	3	1.4
Myopia	7*	2*	9	4.1
Colour blindness	1	—	1	0.5
Hearing loss	2*	1*	3	1.4
Behaviour disturbance	4	2	6	2.7
Retardation (new patient)	1*	—	1	0.5
Speech delay	5*	5*	10	4.6
Auditory sequencing disorder only	1	2	2	0.9
Crossed cerebral dominance, sequencing disorder, family history of illiteracy	7+	—	7	3.2
Crossed dominance, no other signs of possible reading/writing disability	10+	6	16	7.4
Ectopic testicle	1*	—	1	0.5
Obesity	—	1	1	0.5
Total	44	23	67	31.0

* Referred for specialist advice.

+Invited to return after 12 months at school for Aston Index Screening (a classroom test for screening and diagnosis of learning difficulties, age 5–14 years), Learning Development Aids, Park Works, Norwich Road, Wisbech, Cambridgeshire PE13 2AX. Also see NEWTON, M.E. (1975) Primary reading difficulty. In *Reading: What of the Future*, ed. Moyle, D. London: Ward Lock.

CHAPTER 6

Psychological Assessment

General Considerations

Psychological assessment is used primarily to evaluate a child's capacity to take his place and develop normally in a normal world. The purpose of psychological tests and developmental scales is to determine to what extent a child's development in various areas is normal for his age.

Psychological investigation is carried out in order to assess as far as is possible the child's present level of functioning. While it is obviously useful to have an estimate of a child's level of functioning, the idea of using some figure to fulfil an administrative need to classify children, particularly those whose development is deviant or those who are clearly handicapped in certain areas of development, can result in quite unsuitable provision, unrelated to their real needs, being planned for them. A much more systematic evaluation is needed in order to analyse and understand deviations in development and the child's special needs for help to overcome his handicaps, as far as is possible.

In recent years there has been an increasing emphasis on the developmental aspects of paediatrics. Infants are screened early for visual, gross and fine motor, auditory and language development. There is an increased awareness of the need for early assessment, particularly when problems are found which may impair total development. Even more importantly, infants and young children are increasingly referred to children's assessment units when deviances of development make them difficult to assess. As a result many more handicapped children are identified earlier, long before school entrance and the whole question of guidance to parents, treatment and future educational provision has developed a much greater immediacy.

In the light of recent advances in knowledge and understanding of the learning process in children, psychological investigation seeks to draw up a blue-print of the pattern of mental functioning within the child to present a guide to his strengths and his disabilities. The purpose of this kind of investigation is to be able to balance the factors of mental growth against physical condition in all areas of functioning. In this way it is possible to get some guidance as to how weaknesses can be supported or modified by strengths. It is only from this kind of information that suitable plans for helping the child's later development can be made.

During the early years even normal infants and young children vary widely in their rates of growth in different areas of development. The problem of the predictability of test results obtained through careful testing is discussed elsewhere (p. 44). However, it should be further stressed that the predictability of results obtained from infants and young children is very poor. The reason for this is because the growth of intelligence in young children is a dynamic succession of developing functions, the more complex of them depending on the maturing of the earlier and simpler ones, always provided that the child has had satisfactory conditions for growth, i.e. physical and emotional nurture as well as suitable opportunities and stimulations.

We do not know with certainty how the kinds of skills measurable in an infant relate to the skills needed later for formal learning in a normal school situation. Nor do we know how widely a young child can deviate in specific areas of development and still remain within the norm. Infants and young children do not develop evenly in all areas; they often 'stand still' in one area while exercising other skills. For these reasons it is important to record not only success or failure in any particular test item, but also the characteristics and the quality of the child's attempts. Even more important is regular follow-up from which the examiner can judge the child's rate of development.

Psychological assessment of infants and pre-school children differs in many ways from the approach to assessment of school age children. Tests measure different groups of functions at different age levels, each growing out of a previously matured behaviour pattern. If the tests are properly administered and good co-operation is obtained from the child, one can expect to get a reasonable indication of the child's level of functioning, but only for age of testing.

There are other factors to be considered in the assessment of young children. They have not yet made the big break with home (to the world of school) and many cannot easily go alone with a comparative stranger. Mother should be allowed to be present provided she understands that she must not actively help the child. Much can be learnt from observations of the mother–child relationship, the emotional support given by mother and her acceptance of the child.

Young children are much more at the mercy of their emotional moods and inner fantasies than older children. Links with inner fantasy can make them 'take against' a test. They are also more totally affected by their state of well-being at the time of testing; anxieties and fears can easily break through.

These difficulties are more exaggerated in testing handicapped preschool children. In addition these children are generally more quickly fatiguable and one should be prepared to discontinue the test and complete it later if necessary.

It is not easy to assess the full extent of the damage handicapped children may have suffered and how much of what remains to them might be used to develop new patterns of learning. In young children there has been little time to assess the effects of environment and physical and emotional nurture.

In choosing suitable tests and making a reliable report on the results, it is important to have a knowledge of relevant points in the child's medical history, sensory equipment (vision and hearing), experience through sensory channels, times spent in hospital, history of convulsions and whether the child is taking anticonvulsant drugs, which are often a distorting factor.

Assessment Procedures Suitable for
Infants and Children under 3 Years of Age

Gesell Developmental Scales (Gesell and Amatruda, 1947; Knobloch and Pasamanick, 1974)

Most of the so-called baby tests now in use owe a great debt to the work of Gesell. Many items included in other tests were drawn, with some modifications, from Gesell's scales. On the basis of many years of study and observation of normal infants, Gesell and his co-workers produced developmental scales which provided norms of development from 4 weeks to 6 years, presented in four areas of behaviour; namely, motor, adaptive, language and personal–social. These schedules have been described by Anastasi (1961) as 'a refinement and elaboration of the qualitative observations routinely made by paediatricians and other specialists concerned with infant development'.

Although the standardization and reliability of the scores have been questioned in comparison with the more usual psychological tests, there is no doubt that Gesell and his colleagues laid the foundations of a most valuable approach to the developmental assessment of infants and young children. Of great importance is the fact that no single score is computed for the entire behaviour schedule. More appropriately suitable developmental levels in months are indicated separately for each area of development by comparing the child's behaviour with that given as typical of the normal children studied in Gesell's sample. The value of this approach to the assessment of a child's level of development in separate areas is inestimable when seeking to make an assessment of a severely handicapped young child.

Gesell's norms of development were based entirely on his study of American children. After a period of study with Gesell, Illingworth became one of the chief exponents in this country of Gesell's method of approach. Although firmly holding to his recognition of Gesell's basic philosophy Illingworth has, out of his own experience of British children, made some modifications in Gesell's norms (Illingworth 1962; 1975).

Gesell type tests are found useful by many developmental paediatricians.

Denver Developmental Screening Test (Frankenburg and Dodds 1967, 1970)

Developmental screening scales, which are used mainly in the first 3 years, differ in character from more formally structured psychological tests (p. 115).

A general example of these is the Denver Test which gives scores in four different areas of development, viz. gross motor, fine motor-adaptive, language, personal–social individual behaviour. The scale was standardized on 1036 American children, ranging in age from 2 months to 6 years 4 months, chosen from a group thought to be representative of the general population of children living in Denver, Colorado. The test is based on 105 items out of an originally evaluated 240 potential test items, which require no elaborate equipment and are easy to administer and score.

The test aims to provide a clinically useful tool for the detection of infants and preschool children with possibly serious developmental delays. It claims to be suitable for use by persons who have had no training or supervised experience in psychological testing.

Despite the fact that efforts to predict intellectual functioning from measurement or observation of infant behaviour have proved disappointing and unreliable, this screening test is being used in a number of hospitals clinics with the specific purpose of detecting children with serious developmental delays. The psychological assessment of infants and young children is probably one of the most difficult areas of assessment, requiring special training, supervised practice and considerable experience and understanding of very young children. A psychological test or the simplest of screening tools is only as good as the sensitivity of its user to the characteristic behaviours of the young child. Since most requests for assessments arise from the paediatrician's doubts or uncertainty about the normality of a child's development, quite clearly the use of a screening tool such as the Denver is not likely to present an adequate picture of the pattern of the child's total development. It is also doubtful whether the authors' claim is justified that 'in a few hours' training almost any adult can administer this test competently'.

For paediatricians and other workers in this country, more useful screening devices are those prepared by Egan and colleagues (1969), Sheridan (1973) and Illingworth (1973).

More highly skilled psychological assessment may be requested in more complicated cases. The tests described below would normally be given and the results analysed and interpreted by a trained clinical psychologist. However, it is useful for the paediatrician referring the child to be familiar with the more frequently used of these tests and to understand the meaning of the information they offer. Most of these tests have been formally constructed and their scoring standardized. The better known and more generally used are described briefly here:

The Cattell Infant Intelligence Scale (Cattell, 1940)

This scale, which ranges from 2–30 months, was an attempt to extend downwards the Stanford–Binet Scale. The test is scored in terms of Mental Age and IQ and was designed to link up with the Stanford–Binet Scale at the 3-year level. It is an American test standardized on American children.

The Bayley Scale of Infant Development (Bayley, 1969)

This is another American infant scale which has been widely used as a research tool in the US. The age in months at which developmental performance is normally found is given for each test item. The scores for mental and motor development are presented separately in terms of the standard deviation from the mean. The test was originally devised for an age range of birth to 18 months and later extended to 30 months. This test, like Cattell's, was standardized on a population of American children. An exploratory study with an English sample carried out on the 0–15 months age tests (Francis-Williams and Yule, 1967) showed some differences between the English and American samples, which seemed to be related to differences in child-rearing practices in the two cultures.

The study emphasized the importance of standardization based on samples of children similar to those with whom the test is to be used.

As a useful addition to the Mental and Motor Scales, Bayley has added an Infant Behaviour Record. Of this she says 'The setting and situations established for the purpose of assessing an infant's mental and motor development also afford an excellent opportunity to assess his characteristic behaviour patterns'. This infant behaviour record consists of a number of descriptive rating scales for types of behaviour characteristic of children up to 30 months of age. The record is usually completed immediately after the Mental and Motor tests are finished and the mother and baby have left. These infant behaviour ratings are found by Bayley and her co-workers to give much more objective criteria than vague and ill-defined clinical impressions. She believes that, aside from their possible prognostic value, the ratings provide useful information about the current developmental status of the child and the adequacy of his adjustment to the environment.

The Griffiths Mental Development Scales (Griffiths, 1954, 1970)
The first Griffiths Scale is the only infant scale standardized wholly on English children. The items of this test are divided into five sub-scales; locomotion, personal–social, hearing and speech, eye and hand and performance. The results can be presented in the form of a profile and the total as a global score or a development quotient. The presentation of a profile showing levels of development in the five different areas tested is a useful conception, but with young and handicapped children, who show wide variability in their various areas of development, an overall general developmental quotient may be not only meaningless but also misleading.

Griffiths suggested that an uneven pattern of development on the sub-scales of her test may be of diagnostic value. Unfortunately, there are no standardized data on the significance of differences in the sub-scale scores, but there is some evidence (Munro, 1968) to suggest that the 5 sub-scales, in spite of the face validity of the divisions, are only sampling three main areas of ability, viz. locomotor, manipulative and verbal. It is possible that the overall infant test may act as a pointer to defects of sight or hearing or in restricted areas of functioning such as verbal development. These findings would point the way to the need for tests of specific sensory modalities discussed below.

This developmental scale for babies (0–2 years) is not well standardized and, particularly in the testing of babies in the first year of life, there are a number of items which could be open to misinterpretation, e.g. crawling reactions at 6 months and stepping reactions and dancing movements at 7 months could be manifestations of minor neurological abnormality and due to a prolongation of primitive responses; similarly rolling from side to side, normal at 5 months, is seen at 2–3 months in infants with minor neurological impairment.

For this author, an overall criticism of the test lies in the unquestioning way in which scoring is made from the mother's history, e.g. the acceptance of the mother's report of 1, 2 and 3 clear 'words' at 9, 10 and 12 months, or 'enjoys a bath' at 3 months, which, incidentally, seems to have little to do with developmental status. This contrasts with the more rigorous scoring of the Bayley

Infant Scale where the only recognized scores are based on what the examiner has seen and heard.

In contrast to the Bayley, the Griffiths test takes little note of the quality of the infant's response, his alertness and his interest in the surroundings, all of which contribute to the general impression gained by the examiner and give possible clues to the child's mental potential.

Later, Griffiths extended her scale to children of 8 years, and she published a further manual (1970) for use with this extension.

On her death manuals and test materials were left in the care of a trust (The Association for Research in Infant and Child Development). The purchase of this material is limited to those who have taken the course of training in using the first infant scale.

Assessment Procedures Suitable for
Older Preschool and Early School-age Children

The McCarthy Scales of Children's Abilities (McCarthy, 1972)
This fairly recent American test promises to be a very useful scale for children ranging in age from 2½–8½ years. It is based on a carefully representative and standardized sample. The test covers a wide range of abilities:

(1) Verbal scales; which draw on pictorial memory, word knowledge, verbal memory, verbal fluency and opposite analogies.

(2) Tests involving perceptual performance; block building, puzzle solving, tapping sequences, right–left orientation, draw a design, draw a child, conceptual grouping.

(3) Quantitative; involving number questions, numerical memory, counting and sorting.

(4) Tests of memory; pictorial memory, tapping sequence, verbal memory, numerical memory.

(5) Tasks involving motor skills and co-ordination.

The scores on most tests are combined to provide a General Cognitive Scale which claims to provide a measure of the child's overall cognitive functioning. Scores on motor co-ordination, leg and arm co-ordination and imitative action are not included in the General Cognitive Scale because they involve gross motor rather than cognitive ability. This test has not been used very widely yet in the UK, but it is described here because it appears to have promise.

The Minnesota Preschool Scale (Goodenough *et al.*, 1940)
This other useful American test gives a reasonably well-standardized scale for the measurement of mental ability of children between the ages of 18 months and 6 years of age. The test has been found useful as a research tool because it yields measures of verbal and non-verbal categories of ability at a very early age.

The Stanford–Binet Scale, L–M Revision (Terman and Merrill, 1961)
This has been the most generally used scale for many years. Although the test is heavily weighted with verbal items, there are in the preschool ages (2–6

years) a fairly representative number of items which tap non-verbal abilities, such as the simple three-hole form board, identifying parts of the body, building towers and bridges with blocks, threading beads, delayed responses, copying circle and square, comparison of length of sticks and paper folding.

However, the test is essentially verbal and it is inappropriate if the child has a marked verbal handicap. It is important, as with all formal intelligence tests, that it should be administered and scored according to the rubric. Because no formal allowance can be made in the scoring of the Stanford–Binet Scale for refusals or omissions, it is obviously a test of limited value for children whose levels of functioning vary widely from area to area of development.

The Merrill–Palmer Scale of Mental Tests (Stutsman, 1931)

In the standardization of this test allowances are made for refusals and omissions. It is chosen as the test most likely to clarify the situation regarding possible mental ability of children who are not yet speaking or have language delays.

The Merrill–Palmer Scale is of interest to the preschool child. It is heavily weighted with performance items and the language tests are relatively few. The latter consist mainly of memory span for words and for meaningful word groups, and simple questions such as 'What does a doggie say?' 'What is this?' (pencil), 'What is it for?' and also a number of verbal action–agent associations, e.g. 'What runs?' 'What cries?' 'What burns?'

Many of the non-verbal tests assess sensori-motor co-ordination, e.g. throwing a ball, pulling a string, crossing the feet, standing on one foot, closing fist and moving thumb, cutting with scissors and buttoning, solving practical problems involving visuo-spatial abilities (such as reconstruction of cut-out picture puzzles), copying drawings of circle, cross and star and formboards, such as the Sequin Form Board and the Mare and Foal formboards.

The fact that most of the performance tests are timed and the speed with which the child carries out the task raises the level of his score, makes this a poor test for children with motor handicaps. Many cerebral palsied children have difficulties in visuo-spatial perception and this test is heavily weighted with tasks that depend for their success on good perceptual ability. Exploratory studies with English children suggest also that this scale tends to overestimate ability.

Nevertheless, used with a recognition of its limitations, the Merrill–Palmer Scale frequently proves to be a valuable tool in the psychological assessment of young children with known specific language difficulties.

The Wechsler Intelligence Scale for Children (Wechsler, 1949)

While this test gives much useful additional information regarding a child's functioning, it is not as suitable an all-round tool of assessment of children below 7 years of age as is the Stanford–Binet.

The Wechsler Preschool and Primary Scale of Intelligence (Wechsler, 1963)

This more recently published test is useful for psychological assessment of overall, general level of intellectual function. It is a downward extension of the Wechsler Intelligence Scale for Children (WISC) and is standardized for children ranging in age from 4–6½ years. Like the WISC, this test consists of five sub-tests which combine to present a result in terms of a Verbal IQ and five presented as a Performance IQ. The total score (Full Scale IQ) is a weighted combination of the scores from the whole scale.

An empirical evaluation of the Wechsler Preschool and Primary Scale of Intelligence (WPPSI) with a British sample has been made by Yule *et al.*, (1969). The test battery was tried out with 150 5-year-olds living in the Isle of Wight in order to test the applicability of the scale to British children and to try out certain substitutes for some obvious 'americanisms' contained in it. On the evidence of this study the WPPSI was found to be a comparatively well-standardized test. In interpreting results with British children, it is suggested that the expected mean on the Full Scale IQ is about 105.

Supplementary Tests for Preschool Children with Specific Disabilities

Testing of children with visuo-motor and perceptual problems
Qualitative examination of the pattern of successes and failures in the child's responses to the general intelligence scale used for an overall assessment very frequently gives indication of specific difficulties in the child's level of functioning. If the Stanford–Binet is used it may show that the child's difficulties lie in visuo-motor and perceptual tasks such as the formboard, bead threading, copying forms, block building of a bridge or discrimination of forms. Similarly, if the test chosen is the Merrill–Palmer Scale, the child's special difficulties may again be shown in his attempts to complete formboards, to match shapes or copy forms. In the case of the WPPSI, difficulty with blocks designs, mazes or copying geometric shapes will alert the examiner to the possibility that the child may have a specific disability in these areas of learning.

Supplementary tests may throw light on these children's difficulties.

Frostig Developmental Test of Visual Perception (Frostig *et al.*, 1961; Frostig, 1964). This test has been experimented with fairly extensively in recent years. It is based on a normative study of the perceptual abilities of children between the ages of 3 and 9 years. It examines five separate areas of visual perception, viz. eye-motor co-ordination, figure–ground perception, perception of form constancy, perception of position in space, and perception of spatial relations.

Tests of eye–motor co-ordination require the child to follow, by drawing, paths of increasing complexity and gradually decreasing width. Figure–ground perception requires the child to find one of two or more intersecting figures; to do this he must be able to focus on the relevant aspects of the visual field and not allow himself to be distracted by the irrelevant background. Form constancy requires the child to find, e.g. all the squares on a page, regardless of colour, size, background or different tilts and angles. The child's perception of position in space is tested by requiring him, e.g. to pick out from a number of forms the one that is reversed or rotated. The test of spatial relations requires the child to reproduce a dot pattern by linking the dots; the patterns increase in difficulty and complication.

The Frostig test is only suitable for children who have adequate manual control. It is entirely a pencil and paper test and has limited interest for young children. The results, which should be interpreted with caution, are presented as a 'perceptual quotient'.

It is difficult to find formal tests which throw light on the problems of a young child who appears to have specific spatial disabilities and often a great deal more can be learnt through experienced and patient observation of these children (Holt and Reynell, 1967).

Testing of children with language problems

A qualitative examination of a general intelligence scale may suggest that the child is falling behind in language development. Careful observation of preschool children emphasizes the importance of the development of language, the manipulation of symbols and the use of language as a tool of thought. Where the child seems to show delayed language development a separate supplementary investigation can be of very great value in planning help for him.

There are various supplementary tests designed to assess areas of language development more specifically.

English Picture Vocabulary Test (Brimer and Dunn, 1966). This test, which is designed to assess a young child's capacity for understanding vocabulary, is probably the most frequently used in the UK. It was re-standardized on English children by Brimer in co-operation with Dunn, whose Peabody Picture Vocabulary Test was originally standardized on American children. The test ranges from 2½–18 years.

Reynell Developmental Language Scale (Reynell, 1969). This English test is a useful supplementary instrument for the investigation of language ability in young children. It ranges in age from 6 months to 6 years and consists of three scales:

(1) Verbal Comprehension A which uses objects and toys, requires no speech but does require some hand function.

(2) Verbal Comprehension B is an adaptation of Scale A for use with severely handicapped children who have neither speech nor hand function and most of the responses can be made by eye-pointing.

(3) The Expressive Language Scale is divided into three sections which may be scored separately or as a whole. They are: language structure, vocabulary and content.

By not requiring speech for the Verbal Comprehension Scales, comprehension can be assessed completely separately from expressive language. This is a useful distinction for assessing the language development of a young child, particularly in cases where the child has severe speech and language disorder.

The test has been constructed with the problems of assessment of severely physically handicapped children very much in mind.

Illinois Test of Psycholinguistic Abilities (Kirk *et al.*, 1968). Where language as a means of communication is at all possible for a handicapped child the ITPA offers great promise as a diagnostic procedure. It recognizes the two channels of communication (auditory and visual inputs and vocal and motor outputs) and it makes a clear distinction in central organization between that developed at a meaning or symbolic level and that developed at an automatic or sequential level. By means of carefully chosen test items it separates the child's ability to understand and appreciate auditory and visual symbols ('decoding' tests); the ability to relate symbols in a meaningful way at auditory and visuo-motor levels ('association' tests) and the ability to put ideas into words or gestures ('encoding' tests). This is not an easy test to use or interpret. It calls for the skill and understanding of an experienced psychologist but used competently it can offer useful pointers to the assets and deficits of children with language handicaps. There are still aspects of the test which call for improvement, for example auditory decoding tends to be heavily weighted for vocabulary rather than comprehension of sentence complexity.

Many children show severe language delay and while it is helpful, where possible, to relate this condition to the child's general overall intelligence and specific language difficulties, plans for treatment must be made in co-operation with the medical specialist who is specifically concerned with this aspect of the child's development (Chapter 9).

Testing of blind or partially sighted young children

Psychological assessment of young blind or partially sighted children is beset by difficulties. Our testing techniques are very inadequate and the differences in the upbringing of visually handicapped and normally sighted young children make any comparative assessment almost impossible. A period of observation is essential. Writing of blindness in preschool children, Norris *et al.*, (1957) say 'Qualitative, descriptive observations of the child were often more significant than his response to test items'.

Williams Test for Children with Defective Vision (1957). Perhaps the most useful formal test to date for children with defective vision is the Williams. This test is composed almost entirely of items selected from material already standardized on larger groups of seeing children. Nearly all the items are verbal but 'in order to furnish variety in the nature of tasks to be required from the younger subjects, it did seem essential to include a small number of items of the performance type in the lower part of the scale'. These are not scored but they certainly add interest and stimulation when assessing younger children.

Reynell and Zinkin (1975). This recent paper describes the thesis on which a new developmental scale for children with visual handicaps is being constructed. The techniques are designed for babies and young children who may have additional handicaps. For those who work with young visually defective children or who need to attempt to make developmental assessments of them, this paper is rewarding reading and promises the later publication of a useful assessment procedure.

Testing deaf children

One of the most useful tests for deaf or partially hearing children is the Snijders–Oomen Non-Verbal Intelligence Scale from 3–16 years of age (1959). This is a Dutch test which has been completely revised, enlarged and standardized on 1400 hearing and 1054 deaf subjects between the ages of 3 and 16. The whole test can be administered without the use of spoken or written language either on the part of the tester or the testee. Two sets of instructions are given and are placed in parallel in the manual but the two ways of presenting the test are virtually equivalent so that hearing subjects are not favoured in comparison with the deaf.

The Scale consists of eight sub-tests in four groups:

(1) tests of form (mosaic and drawing);
(2) arrangement and completion of pictures;
(3) tests of abstraction in sorting and analogies, and
(4) tests of memory (picture memory and cube tapping).

Each of these eight sub-tests contains problems over the whole age range. The test is not timed, so that children have a reasonable chance of completing it and the standard scores and mental ages provide for the sum of standard scores to be converted into intelligence quotients.

The second edition of this test will be further revised in the near future.

Testing of cerebral palsied children

Recent studies of cerebral palsy all emphasize the wide variation and extensiveness of the handicap suffered by cerebral palsied children. Since cerebral palsy arises from widespread cerebral dysfunction it is rare to find a cerebral palsied child with a motor handicap only. Indeed the combination of handicaps and their varying severity makes the cerebral palsied child a unique person with his own individual problems in coping with the demands of his world.

Physical handicaps impose severe limitations on achievement in testing many cerebral palsied children. These are mainly due to difficulties in eye–hand coordination and hand function and those imposed by limits in physical posture and sitting balance. In addition the cerebral palsied child may suffer from defects of vision and hearing, speech disorders, behaviour problems, perceptual and visuo-motor disturbances, mental retardation and epilepsy.

Speech difficulties range in severity from a complete inability to speak to a mild dysarthria. For purposes of assessment for educational advice it is important to determine whether the speech defect is due to mental retardation which causes delay in the development of speech, hearing difficulties, specific cortical damage which may cause aphasia or auditory agnosia, motor dysfunction of the tongue, lips and palate or to emotional causes, particularly breaks in a consistent mothering relationship in early childhood.

Other sensory and perceptual handicaps which are likely to affect school learning and which should be taken into account when making decisions regarding school placement include defects in kinaesthetic, proprioceptive and tactile sense areas, astereognosis and a wide variety of perceptual disabilities, among the most studied being spatial disorders of a visuo-motor type (Abercrombie, 1964; Wedell, 1973). It is important also to remember that perceptual and spatial disabilities are not necessarily in keeping with overall intellectual level.

In terms of general intelligence it is clear that an unduly high percentage of cerebral palsied children are mentally subnormal. Others suffer from epilepsy and problems of assessing these children are increased by the fact that many will have periods of medication and quite often at the time of testing are on anticonvulsant drugs.

From the above it will be clear that children with cerebral palsy differ so much in the range and severity of their handicaps, in the kind of care and management they have experienced and in their own personal attitude to their handicaps, that those who make decisions regarding their future educational treatment must be aware of the many factors that are likely to affect the educability of the child. For this reason it is important to approach the assessment with as much information as possible regarding the range and degree of involvement of each individual child. In assessing the child's level of intellectual functioning it is well to have some awareness also of the limitations in life experience that the child may have suffered, partly because of the limitations of movement caused by his motor disability, partly through intermittent periods of hospitalization and partly due to limits on normal social learning through association and play with unhandicapped children (Loring, 1968).

When the aim in testing a young cerebral palsied child is to assess those of his assets and disabilities that will be a guide for current management as well as for future provision, the real value of testing is not to produce an IQ figure but to chart the child's abilities in order to get some idea of his level of intellectual functioning. For this reason it is often helpful to supplement the standardized test chosen with tests that give the child an opportunity to demonstrate his abilities through other media. However, when the purpose in making an assessment is to advise on suitable educational provision, the core of our diagnostic procedure (and around which we construct our appraisal of what is possible and most suitable educational provision for a particular child) is a formal intellectual assessment, in so far as that can be arrived at despite the handicaps to communication from which the child may suffer.

The Wechsler tests are of limited usefulness as overall tests of general intelligence for cerebral palsied children since the Performance Scale has so many timed tests in which a child with a motor handicap and poor motor co-ordination inevitably scores badly. The Block Designs and Object Assembly sub-tests present serious difficulties to children with spatial and perceptual problems such as are experienced by many hemiplegics. The Stanford–Binet Intelligence Scale is accepted as the most satisfactory overall test for assessing the intelligence level of cerebral palsied children whose speech can be understood or who can make clear, even though in a most limited way, what their response is to questions and tasks.

Since there are a number of test items in the Stanford–Binet Scale to which the severely handicapped child cannot respond, there has been much controversy regarding the justification for making modifications in the test procedure.

In this country the view expressed by the Spastics Society's Sub-Committee on Intellectual Assessment (1958) would seem to be rightly the most generally accepted one. 'If intelligence test scores are to continue to mean anything the tests must be given and scored strictly in accordance with the rubric. Should the examiner feel that he would get some additional and helpful data by doing something other than strict administration this should be done apart from the normal test situation . . . and such 'results' should be recorded in a separate comment'.

Columbia Mental Maturity Scale (Burgemeister *et al.*, 1959). When a child is so heavily handicapped that he clearly cannot do himself justice in the Stanford–Binet, tests to which the child can respond by eye-pointing or yes–no cues can be used. It should be remembered that this is a very limited type of testing and the results on a single test interview should not be relied on to decide the long-term educational provision for any child.

An example of this type of test is the Columbia Mental Maturity Scale which can provide a valuable supplementary test for children ranging in mental age from 3 years 5 months to 13 years 11 months. This is a test of reasoning ability in which the child is presented with a series of cards on each of which are pictures of objects or variously coloured shapes and forms, all but one of which are tied together by a principle of grouping. The task is to select the one picture on each card that 'does not belong' with the others. The task becomes progressively more difficult requiring a higher level of abstraction for the solution of the problem.

There are 100 cards in all and many examiners find that the test tends to become tiring and tedious, particularly as many cerebral palsied children have a short attention span and are quickly fatiguable.

The Haeussermann approach. For those who are concerned to assess the educational potential of young cerebral palsied children, Developmental Potential of Pre-School Children (Haeussermann, 1958) makes rewarding reading. A systematized manual utilizing the Haeussermann approach to evaluation of the preschool child was published more recently (Jedrysek *et al.*, 1972). This is a most valuable manual for paediatricians, psychologists and teachers who seek to get an estimate of the level of functioning relative to educational potential of young handicapped children, particularly when formal assessment is not immediately available.

Testing children with uncomplicated mental retardation
Much of what has been said on the assessment of infants and young children will be seen to have relevance and application to problems of the psychological assessment of mentally retarded children without other defects.

When performance is equally depressed in all areas it is probable that the child is presenting a fairly reliable picture of his current level of functioning. Where, however, the pattern of successes and failures in a test is grossly uneven it is wise to investigate further into the child's functioning. In such cases the value of team discussions and specialist investigations (p. 16) cannot be over-estimated.

The psychologist who finds it difficult to get a formal test result often finds he can learn much and supplement his more informal findings by using such instruments as the Vineland Social Maturity Scale (Doll, 1953) or the Social Progress Assessment Charts (Gunzberg, 1966). These provide basic information on the child's skills and competence in specific areas of functioning. It must always be remembered that these various supplementary tests are not designed to replace the findings of a general intelligence scale. However, they can add information and insights which prove extremely valuable.

Since we should never determine a plan for the placement of a young child on the basis of test findings from one interview, the best judgements can be made from rates of improvement in various areas of development as seen from tests repeated at regularly defined intervals.

Early Identification of Children at Risk of Later Learning Difficulties

Recent years have seen a growing interest in the learning problems of young school children (Chapter 16). Increasingly interest is being shown in anomalies of functioning of children who have a known poor perinatal history and in the possibility of investigating the more subtle indications of potential future learning difficulty at a preschool age. In a research study, undertaken to examine the possibility of identifying children in the normal range of intelligence who were likely to have specific learning disorders arising from neurodevelopmental dysfunction, a battery of tests was developed including tests of verbal ability, visuo-spatial perception and concept formation (Francis-Williams, 1974). Children who had had minor neurological dysfunction in the newborn period scored significantly less well on a number of items than did control children. The findings suggested that difficulties of language development, including failure to use language symbols as well as lack of clarity in speech itself, separated the groups more significantly than did difficulties of visuo-spatial perception, general motor clumsiness or lack of precision in the execution of finer manipulations. Associated difficulties for children who had exhibited minor neurological dysfunction were seen in delayed sense of body-image, more than normal distractibility and limited attention span.

Follow-up examination at $8\frac{1}{2}$–9 years showed that a significant number were still falling behind, particularly in reading (Francis-Williams, 1976). This kind of study has also been carried out in a follow-up of low birth-weight infants (Francis-Williams and Davies, 1974).

These studies demonstrated very clearly how important it is to recognize that children who are educationally at risk may need the opportunity of a slow pace and quiet, small school group during the early school years.

Children identified as having considerable difficulty with visuo-spatial tasks benefit greatly from extra help in nursery class before school entry.

In all psychological testing of handicapped children, even though the tester has carried out what he would judge to be a satisfactory test and reached a reliable result, it is most important that he should try to understand and assess what significance the child's performance has in terms of his handcapping condition. What may appear to be slight differences in a psychological assessment result can present very real problems to the child. We do not always make enough allowance for the inroads on total functioning that even a clearly defined and limited handicap can cause.

References

ABERCROMBIE M.L.J. (1964) *Perceptual and Visuo-Motor Disorders in Cerebral Palsy. Clinics in Developmental Medicine No. 11*. London: Heinemann.

ANASTASI A. (1961) *Psychological Testing*. London: Macmillan.

*BAYLEY N. (1969) *Infant Scales of Development: mental, motor and behaviour profile*, Revised Ed. New York: Psychological Corporation.

*BRIMER M.A. and DUNN L.M. (1966) *English Picture Vocabulary Test*, 2nd Ed. London: National Foundation for Educational Research.

*BURGEMEISTER N., BLUM L.H. and LORGE I. (1959) *Columbia Mental Maturity Scale*, Revised Ed. New York: Harcourt Brace and World Book Co.

*CATTELL P. (1940) *The Measurement of Intelligence of Infants and Young Children*. New York: Psychological Corporation.

*DOLL E.A. (1953) *Measurement of Social Competence*. Minneapolis: Educational Test Bureau.

EGAN D., ILLINGWORTH R.S. and MAC KEITH R.C. (1969) *Developmental Screening 0–5 Years. Clinics in Developmental Medicine No. 30*. London: Heinemann.

FRANCIS-WILLIAMS J. (1974) *Children with Specific Learning Difficulties*, 2nd Ed. Oxford: Pergamon Press.

FRANCIS-WILLIAMS J. (1976) Early identification of children likely to have specific learning difficulties. *Developmental Medicine and Child Neurology*, **18**, 71.

FRANCIS-WILLIAMS J. and DAVIES P.A. (1974) Very low birthweight and later intelligence. *Developmental Medicine and Child Neurology* **16**, 709.

FRANCIS-WILLIAMS, J. and YULE, W. (1967) The Bayley infant scales of mental and motor development. *Developmental Medicine and Child Neurology* **9**, 391.

*FRANKENBURG, W.K. and DODDS, J.B. (1967) The Denver Developmental Screening Test. *Journal of Pediatrics*, **71**, 181.

FRANKENBURG, W.K., DODDS, J.B. and FANDAL, A. (1970) *The Revised Denver Developmental Screening Manual*. Denver: University of Colorado Press.

*FROSTIG, M. (1964) *The Marianne Frostig Developmental Test of Visual Perception*, 3rd Ed. Palo Alto: Consulting Psychologists Press.

FROSTIG, M., LEFEVER, D.W. and WHITTLESEY, J.R.B. (1961) Developmental test of visual perception for evaluating normal and neurologically handicapped children. *Perceptual and Motor Skills*, **12**, 383.

*GESELL, A., and AMATRUDA, C.S. (1947) *Developmental Diagnosis*, 2nd Ed. New York: Hoeber.

*GOODENOUGH, F.L., MAURER, K.M. and VAN WAGENER, M.J. (1940) *Minnesota Pre-School Scale Manual*. Minnesota: Educational Test Bureau.

†GRIFFITHS, R. (1954) *The Abilities of Babies*. London: University of London Press.

†GRIFFITHS R. (1970) *The Abilities of Young Children*. London: Child Development Research Centre.

GUNZBERG H. (1966) *The Progress Assessment Charts*, 6th Ed. London: National Association for Mental Health.

HAEUSSERMANN E. (1958) *Developmental Potential of Preschool Children*. New York: Grune and Stratton.

HOLT K.S. and REYNELL, J.K. (1967) *Assessment of Cerebral Palsy*, Vol. II. London: Lloyd-Luke.

ILLINGWORTH R.S. (1962) *An Introduction to Developmental Assessment in the First Year. Little Club Clinics No. 3.* London: Heinemann.

ILLINGWORTH R.S. (1973) *Basic Developmental Screening 0–2 Years.* Oxford: Blackwell Scientific Publications.

ILLINGWORTH R.S. (1975) *The Development of the Infant and Young Child: normal and abnormal,* 6th ed. Edinburgh: Churchill Livingstone.

JEDRYSEK E., KLAPPER Z., POPE L. and WORTIS J. (1972) *Psychoeducational Evaluation of the Pre-School Child.* New York: Grune and Stratton.

*KIRK S.A., McCARTHY J.J. and KIRK W.D. (1968) *Illinois Test of Psycholinguistic Abilities,* Revised Ed. Chicago: University of Illinois Press.

KNOBLOCH H. and PASAMANICK B. (1974) *Gesell and Amatruda's Developmental Diagnosis,* 3rd Ed. New York: Harper and Row.

LORING J., ed. (1968) *Assessment of the Cerebral Palsied Child for Education.* London: Spastics Society and Heinemann.

*McCARTHY D. (1972) *Scales of Children's Abilities.* New York: Psychological Corporation.

MUNRO J.A. (1968) Early abilities and their later development. *Advancement of Science,* 24, 464

NORRIS M., SPAULDING P.J. and BRODIE F.H. (1957) *Blindness in Children.* Chicago: University of Chicago Press.

*REYNELL J.K. (1969) *Reynell Developmental Language Scales.* London: National Foundation for Educational Research.

REYNELL J.K. and ZINKIN P. (1975) New procedures for the developmental assessment of young children with severe visual handicaps. *Child care, health and development,* 1, 61.

SHERIDAN M.D. (1973) *Children's Developmental Progress from Birth to 5 Years.* London: National Foundation for Educational Research.

*SNIJDERS J.TH. and SNIJDERS-OOMEN N. (1959) *Non-Verbal Intelligence Test.* Groningen: J. B. Wolters.

SPASTICS SOCIETY: MEDICAL ADVISORY COMMITTEE (1958) *Notes on the Assessment of Educational Needs of Children with Cerebral Palsy.* London: National Spastics Society.

*STUTSMAN R. (1931) *Mental Measurement of Pre-School Children: Merrill–Palmer Scale.* Yonkers: World Book Co.

*TERMAN L.M. and MERRILL M.A. (1961) *Stanford-Binet Intelligence Scale. Form L–M,* 3rd Revision. London: Harrap.

*WECHSLER D. (1949) *Intelligence Scale for Children.* New York: Psychological Corporation.

*WECHSLER D. (1963) *Pre-School and Primary Scale of Intelligence.* New York: Psychological Corporation.

WEDELL K. (1973) *Learning and Perceptuo-Motor Disabilities in Children.* London: John Wiley.

*WILLIAMS M. (1957) *Williams' Test for Children with Defective Vision.* Birmingham: Education Department, University of Birmingham.

YULE W., BERGER M., BUTLER S., NEWHAM V. and TIZARD J. (1969) The WPPSI: an empirical evaluation with a British sample. *British Journal of Educational Psychology,* 39, 1.

* Test materials distributed by National Foundation for Educational Research, Test Division, 2 Jennings Buildings, Thames Avenue, Windsor, Berkshire.

† Test materials distributed by Child Development Research Centre, 47 Hollycroft Avenue, London.

Further Reading

BOWLEY A.H. and GARDNER L. (1972) *The Handicapped Child. Educational and psychological guidance for the organically handicapped,* 3rd Ed. Edinburgh: Churchill-Livingstone.

MITTLER P., ed. (1970) *The Psychological Assessment of Mental and Physical Handicaps.* London: Methuen.

CHAPTER 7

Physical and Neurological Examination

Ideally, and particularly in the case of a child presenting with a possible handicapping condition, history taking and examination should be a fairly leisurely procedure, as relaxing as possible for the parents and fun for the child. At least on the first occasion, up to an hour or more should be allowed. Comfortable chairs, cups of tea and friendly staff all help to allay parental anxieties and to overcome the resentful, aggressive attitudes which may have been generated by the child's referral. Toys and drinks should be available for the child and his siblings while waiting. Measurements of weight and height should be deferred until after the examination on the first visit, if an infant is asleep on arrival and when the mother judges that the procedure will upset the child.

Gaining the child's confidence and co-operation is a vital part of the examination. Establishing friendly contact with the mother, making the examination a 'game' for the child and leaving until the end any potentially unpleasant procedures (such as examination of the mouth, throat, ears and fundi) usually ensures success. Unless unwell, tired or hungry, most infants up to 12–15 months are easy to examine, although from around 9 months many infants object to being placed supine and for parts of the examination (e.g. of the legs and hips) are more co-operative when half reclining on their mother's knees. From the second year onwards, getting down to floor level (on a warm carpet) is likely to be less threatening to the child than using an examination couch. Some children are shy, negativistic or disturbed to a degree which makes undressing and examination difficult. In these cases repeated out-patient attendances or examination after a short period of day attendance in a nursery setting may be necessary. For an experienced examiner, who is usually successful in gaining a child's co-operation, marked difficulty in carrying out the examination may be a useful sign of abnormality in the child.

History

Details of family history, pregnancy, delivery, the neonatal period, subsequent development and health are obtained as for any paediatric examination. For the child presenting with possible neurodevelopmental abnormality certain aspects of history taking require special attention.

When eliciting family history, the mother should be asked specifically if she has or has had any worries about the health or development of each of the siblings, which schools they are attending (if appropriate) and how they are progressing there. Significant differences in early handling and management, development and personality between the patient and siblings should be sought. Deviations from normal in the parents' own early development and any particular schooling problems should be discussed. A history of sinistrality or ambidexterity in parents and siblings should be recorded and also details of neurodevelopmental disorders in the wider family.

Involuntary infertility and the outcome of all pregnancies, normal and abnormal, should be noted as there is a known association between poor reproductive history and congenital neurodevelopmental handicap (Drillien *et al.*, 1964; Drillien, 1968). Details of the pregnancy, delivery and neonatal period should be confirmed and expanded from the obstetric and neonatal records. Specific questions should be asked about problems of management in the first few weeks at home (pp. 49, 340).

The method of obtaining a detailed developmental history is discussed elsewhere (p. 46). Independent confirmation of the mother's history may be possible where routine developmental screening has been carried out or from health visitor or hospital notes.

Details of significant past illnesses should be confirmed from case records if available. A history of seizures should be enquired for specifically. Since, to most parents, the term 'convulsion' means a major motor fit, phrases such as 'blank spells' and 'funny turns' should also be used.

The mother should be asked for her opinion of what (if anything) she feels is wrong with the child and what her main concerns are.

General Physical Examination

While the history is being taken from the mother much can be learned by simultaneous observation of the child. He may show abnormally clinging behaviour or, at the other end of the scale, demonstrate frank hyperactivity, reducing the consulting room to chaos. The toys he chooses to play with and the maturity of play should be noted. Although most children who have acquired speech tend to be silent during this initial stage, some will produce spontaneous speech at this point and later withdraw into silence when approached directly. Although the examination setting is not likely to demonstrate subtle abnormalities in the child–parent relationship, some idea of the basic healthiness or otherwise of this relationship can usually be obtained by observation.

The child's overall state of well-being should be noted. Chronic rash and ulceration in the nappy area, an excessive degree of grubbiness of the child or his clothes and lack of hair growth over the back of the head (indicating that the child spends long periods on his back) may be pointers to a mother who is not coping and to a poor non-stimulating home background. Bruising and other evidence of non-accidental injury should always be looked for (p. 400).

A general systematic examination should be carried out with emphasis as indicated by the history. The ears should always be examined.

The head
Head circumference is measured and charted. Differences in measurement due

to differing techniques can be minimized if the maximal circumference is taken. This is measured around the occiput and the area of maximum prominence of the forehead. Previous head circumference measurements should be obtained from developmental screening cards or hospital notes when possible, in order to assess the rate of growth. Head size must be considered in relation to the child's weight and height.

The size of the fontanelles and the degree of tension is noted. The anterior fontanelle is usually palpable until the end of the first year but may remain open until 18 months. The posterior fontanelle closes in the first few months of life. Large head size may be a familial feature and it is often useful to ask for photographs of other affected family members. Hydrocephalus is the commonest pathological cause of an enlarged and/or enlarging head. Associated features are the typical bulging shape of the forehead, enlargement and increased tension in the fontanelles, separation of the sutures, prominence of veins over the forehead, limitation of upward gaze and evidence of increased intracranial pressure on fundoscopy. Less common causes of a large head are subdural effusions, tumours, achondroplasia and megalencephaly.

Small head size (microcephaly) may also be familial but is more often associated with congenitally poor brain growth, as occurs in many of the mental deficiency syndromes (Chapter 13) and with cerebral atrophy following brain damage. In some cases of microcephaly the maximal head circumference is less affected than the size of the cranial vault.

Unusual head shape should be noted. Postural plagiocephaly (parallelogram skull) is common in infancy and is usually related to the preferred side of lying. A long, narrow head (dolicocephaly) is a usual finding in the pre-term infant. Flattening of the occiput (brachycephaly) commonly accompanies the microcephaly found with congenitally abnormal brains (as in mongolism) and is seen in its most severe form with premature closure of the coronal sutures. Other forms of craniostenosis produce abnormal head shapes, depending on the suture or sutures involved.

Minor physical stigmata
Throughout the examination note should be taken of any external features which might point to specific diagnoses, such as the increase in conjunctival vessels of ataxia telangiectasia, the dry skin and hair and coarse features of hypothyroidism, depigmented areas of skin and adenoma sebaceum of tuberose sclerosis and the multiple café-au-lait spots of neurofibromatosis. Numerous other examples could be given and a text such as *Recognisable Patterns of Human Malformations* (Smith, 1970) is recommended.

Certain combinations of minor or minor and major congenital physical anomalies, arising during embryogenesis, are well recognized as being indicators of specific disorders, the commonest example being Down's syndrome with its plethora of minor stigmata and frequent major anomalies. Many minor anomalies occur, usually singly and with low frequency, in otherwise normal individuals. Rarely a genetic cause can be presumed, the same anomaly being found in one or other parent, but usually no causal factor is known.

It is also recognized that the presence of several minor physical anomalies may be a non-specific indicator of neurodevelopmental disorder. Waldrop and her co-workers (1971) demonstrated a significant relationship between high anomaly scores and deviations of behaviour in a group of normal 2½-year-olds. The boys with high scores were more likely to show the behaviour patterns found in hyperkinetic children, i.e. they were aggressive, overactive and intractable. Girls with high scores also tended to be intractable but they showed more inhibition, moved around less, were more fearful and clung more to adults. Further studies confirmed and expanded these initial findings. On follow up at age 7½ the anomaly scores tended to remain stable and those with high scores still showed the same behavioural disturbances. In addition the high scoring children tended to be clumsy, to have lower IQ levels and to be below average in verbal ability. It was also shown that elementary school children, identified by their teachers as being hyperactive, had significantly more minor anomalies than controls and the more hyperactive the child the higher the anomaly score.

Using the same anomalies and scoring system, Rosenberg and Weller (1973) found no significant correlation in first year school children between anomaly scores and personality factors or performance IQ but verbal IQ was significantly lower in children with high scores and a very strong correlation was found between high scorers and the teacher's recommendation that the child should repeat the first year.

Dental enamel defect of the primary dentition should also be considered as a minor physical anomaly. The position of the defect on the teeth allows the causative pre- or perinatal disturbance to be timed (Via and Churchill, 1959). Cohen and Diner (1970) showed a significant relationship between dental enamel defect and neurological impairment. In a later study Cohen *et al.* (1975) looked for dental anomalies and other minor physical stigmata in children referred with motor, language, behaviour or intellectual deficits. Of those found to be neurologically impaired (over 80 per cent) about 60 per cent had three or more stigmata as opposed to only 30 per cent of the neurologically intact children.

Some minor physical anomalies are detailed in Table 7.1; those used by Waldrop are asterisked.

Examination of the Cranial Nerves

The eyes

These are inspected at rest. Roving or nystagmoid movements signify defective vision. The 'setting sun' sign, with the eyes displaced downwards leaving the sclera visible above the iris, is seen in raised intracranial pressure. A minor degree of sunsetting may occur transiently as a normal finding in the first few weeks of life. Any ptosis of the eyelids is noted. Equality of pupil size and response to light is checked, as is pupillary response to accommodation.

Light from a pen torch can also be used to assess ability to fixate centrally with both eyes (p. 428). To assess eye movement the light is then moved horizontally and vertically while holding the child's head still. The smoothness and extent of following is assessed and whether the eyes move conjugately (p. 421). Young

TABLE 7.1. Some minor physical stigmata (*indicates used by Waldrop, 1971).

Hair
   *Fine 'electric' hair
   always 'standing up' and untidy
   *Extra whorls on crown
   one whorl is the normal finding
   Low hairline
   back or front

Ears
   *Low set
   i.e. when the anterior part of the helix joins the skull below a horizontal line drawn
   backwards from the outer angle of the eye (Fig. 7.1)
   Slanting
   i.e. when the ear slopes upwards and backwards more than 10° to 15° from the vertical
   (Fig. 7.1)
   Simple
   lack of normal convolutions
   *Lack of lobule
   the lobule normally extends below a horizontal line drawn through its point of contact
   to the skull (Fig. 7.2)
   Prominent
   'bat' ears
   *Dissimilar (asymmetrical)
   distinct difference in shape or size between the two ears
   Pre-auricular skin tags (accessory auricles), pits or sinuses

Eyes and eyebrows
   *Epicanthic folds
   vertical skin folds covering the inner canthi, usually bilateral, very common in infancy,
   often disappearing later
   *Hypertelorism
   abnormally wide spacing of the eyes as measured either by inner canthal and outer
   orbital dimensions (Laestadius *et al.*, 1969) or inter-pupillary distance (Pryor, 1969)
   Slanting palpebral fissures
   laterally and upwards (mongoloid) or laterally and downwards (anti-mongoloid)
   Brushfield spots
   white speckles near the periphery of the iris, found in 20 per cent of general population
   Small and/or deep set eyes
   may be familial
   Coloboma
   defect or notch in the upper or lower eyelid (usually at junction of inner and middle thirds)
   and/or in the iris
   Bushy eyebrows
   tendency to meet in the midline
   Long straight eyelashes

Nose
   Broad root
   Beaked nose
   Anteverted nares

Mouth and Lips
   Macro/micro stomia
   Long upper lip
   increased distance between nose and upper lip margin

Triangular or 'fish' shaped
down turning at corners, usually associated with thin lips

Teeth
Enamel dysplasia
mild degrees show chalky spots of hypoplasia; in severe forms the enamel is aplastic. Abnormalities are most obvious on the incisor teeth, canines and first molars. They may be present as pits, grooves or bands of dysplasia.
Abnormal shape or spacing

Tongue
*Furrowing
one or more grooves other than the centre groove; age related and more frequent among older than younger children.
Macroglossia

Palate
*High arched
tented or smoothly arched
Low flat
Bifid uvula

Jaws
Malocclusion
associated with hypoplasia of maxilla/mandible or protrusion of the mandible with distortion of the usual pattern of bite

Skin
Skin dimples
over bony prominences, e.g. around the elbow and shoulder
Multiple pigmented or vascular naevi

Hands
*Abnormal palmar creases
Simian, single complete transverse crease; Sydney, complete transverse crease with a partial ulnar transverse crease distally (Figs. 7.3a, b and c.)
*Incurving 5th finger
Single flexion crease 5th finger
Broad palms and short stubby fingers
Partial syndactyly (webbing)
most commonly of third and fourth fingers
Polydactyly
varying from a small nub of tissue (usually on ulnar side) to complete replication
Constriction bands of fingers
Hypoplasia of nails

Feet
*Wide separation of 1st and 2nd toes
gap more than half the width of the 2nd toe
Prominent plantar crease
between 1st and 2nd toes
First toe longer than 2nd
*3rd toe equal to or longer than 2nd
age dependent, commoner in younger children
*Partial syndactyly
usually between 2nd and 3rd toes, minor degrees very common
Hypoplasia of nails

TABLE 7.1. Some minor physical stigmata (*indicates used by Waldrop, 1971).—*continued*

Neck
  Short neck
  Webbing

Spine
  Midline anomaly
    lipoma, vascular naevus, hairy tuft, pit, sinus or deviation of natal cleft

External Genitalia
  Minor forms of hypospadias
  Hypoplasia of scrotum and/or penis
  Small soft testes
  Undescended testes

Chest
  Pectus excavatum
  Shield shaped chest
  Pigeon chest

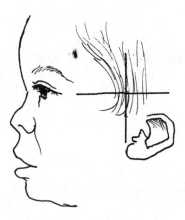

FIG. 7.1. Low set slanting ears.

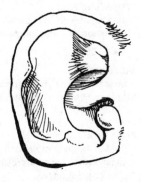

FIG. 7.2. Lack of ear lobule.

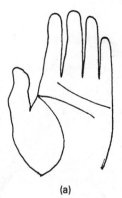 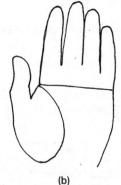 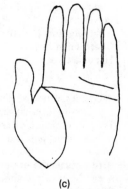

(a)   (b)   (c)

FIG. 7.3. Palmar creases: (a) normal; (b) Simian; (c) Sydney.

infants of 1–2 months or so will more readily fixate on and follow the examiner's face or a dangling ring or ball (p. 151). Limitation of lateral eye movements is most commonly seen in 6th nerve paralysis. Limitation of upward gaze occurs with raised intracranial pressure in infants and may also be seen in dyskinetic cerebral palsy.

During these manoeuvres strabismus and nystagmus may be noted. Types of strabismus and methods of testing are discussed in Chapter 21. Searching nystagmus, either coarse and roving or slow, pendular to and fro movements on attempted fixation, occur in severe visual defects. Regular rhythmic nystagmus with slow and fast components (which occurs with cerebellar or labyrinthine disease) is looked for as the child follows vertically, horizontally and obliquely. This type of nystagmus is described according to the direction of the fast component.

Visual acuity and methods of testing at different ages are discussed elsewhere (pp. 151, 428). When severe visual defect or blindness is suspected in young or mentally retarded infants, the presence of opticokinetic nystagmus on rotation indicates that vision is present. Holding the infant facing him in vertical suspension and tilted slightly forward, the examiner rotates quickly two or three times. During rotation the infant's eyes will open and nystagmus can be observed, the quick phase in the opposite direction to rotation. Nystagmus continues after rotation stops but in the reverse direction. Opticokinetic nystagmus is seen in the normal infant from 2 weeks post-term. Blink response to threat may also be useful in suspected blindness. The examiner moves his hand, with the fingers extended, rapidly towards the child's eyes. The extended posture of the fingers cuts down any air draught which might stimulate the corneal reflex and produce a blink.

Testing of visual fields is discussed on p. 154.

Examination of the fundi is best left until the end of the examination except in co-operative older children. Dilatation of the pupils with mydriatic drops (e.g. cyclopentolate 0.5 per cent) is often necessary, particularly in young infants. Some infants and young children co-operate better when seated on their mother's knee, others when lying supine with their mother's face visible above them, when they are less likely to look directly at the ophthalmoscope light. With increased intracranial pressure the margins of the optic disc may be blurred or the whole disc may be raised with frank papilloedema. The veins are distended and tortuous and haemorrhages may occur, radiating out from the disc. Retinal haemorrhages also occur in subdural haematoma. In optic atrophy the disc is whiter than normal, the margin very distinct and the vessels are narrowed and decreased in number. The causes of optic atrophy are discussed on p. 426. Areas of chorioretinitis may be found in congenital toxoplasmosis and cytomegalic virus infection. Excessive retinal pigment can occur as a normal variant but is also seen in the rubella syndrome and in the chorioretinal degenerations (p. 424). Retrolental fibroplasia is discussed on p. 426. The macula should be examined to exclude the cherry red spot of Tay-Sachs disease. Ophthalmological opinion should be sought when abnormalities of the fundus are found.

The face

Symmetry of the face at rest and on movement, both voluntary and involuntary (e.g. laughing or crying) is noted. In lower motor neurone 7th nerve paralysis both the upper and lower parts of the face are affected. On the affected side the palpebral fissure may be widened, the nasolabial fold is less marked and the corner of the mouth droops. The child will show decreased movement when requested to wrinkle the forehead, close the eyes, show his teeth, blow out his cheeks or purse his lips as in whistling. Movement of the affected side will also be absent or diminished on laughing or crying. In upper motor neurone lesions, because of the bilateral innervation of the upper part of the face, brow wrinkling and eye closure are not affected and involuntary movements of the lower part of the face will be retained.

The liveliness of the child's facial expression is noted. A characteristically mask-like expression is seen in myopathies, such as dystrophia myotonica, myasthenia and some forms of muscular dystrophy (Chapter 19).

Children under 5 are seldom able to co-operate well enough for accurate sensory testing of the 5th nerve supply to the face but, if indicated, the ophthalmic division of the trigeminal nerve can be tested by using the corneal reflex. The eye will blink when the lateral side of the cornea or conjunctiva is touched lightly with a small twist of cotton wool; the child is encouraged to look in the opposite direction to prevent a visual blink. In young or highly unco-operative patients, a small puff of air directed towards the eye will stimulate the reflex.

The jaw jerk tests the motor and sensory elements of the 5th nerve. With the child's mouth slightly open, the examiner places one forefinger over the centre point of the chin and taps the finger gently with a tendon hammer. The masseter muscles contract and the jaw elevates. Excessive briskness of response is found in supranuclear lesions. Depression or absence of the response may be a normal finding.

Hearing and vestibular function

Testing of hearing at various ages is fully discussed in Chapters 8 and 21. Formal hearing testing should always be carried out when hearing loss is suspected from the history, when multiple handicaps may be present (e.g. in cerebral palsy), if the mother expresses any doubt about the child's hearing and in any child with delayed or disordered language. Further pointers to possible hearing loss may be obtained from the history or during examination. These are: a decrease or lack of social–vocal response in the first few months of life, although it should be remembered that even a deaf child may vocalize fairly normally up to 6 months of age; monotonous vocalization replacing the normal inflectional pattern of sounds; a screeching cry making it difficult to distinguish, from the sound alone, whether the child is pleased or distressed, and appropriate response to speech only when the child can use visual clues. In the last case the mother may, unconsciously, be increasing her use of these clues.

Testing of vestibular function is not carried out routinely. If indicated the child should be referred to an Ear, Nose and Throat department. The only test which can be used easily in the consulting room is the elicitation of opticokinetic nystagmus on rotation (already described as a test of vision in young infants, p. 133) and this is only suitable in the first year or so when the child is still light enough to be rotated safely.

The mouth and throat

Pointers to possible abnormal pharyngeal, laryngeal and palatal function should always be sought from a history of the child's early feeding behaviour. Prolonged tube feeding may have been required at birth or the mother may give a history of poor sucking, frequent choking, nasal escape of fluids and a weak cry. Excessive or prolonged drooling may be noted at examination or may have occurred in the past.

The soft palate is examined at rest for symmetry of the palatal arches. In unilateral paresis of the nerves to the palate (mainly the vagus nerve) the arch of the affected side will droop at rest. If the child can co-operate in saying 'aah' or if the child is crying during the examination, movement of the soft palate and uvula can be seen and any asymmetry noted. In a unilateral paresis the palate is drawn towards the normal side. In bilateral paresis movement of both sides is reduced or absent. Movement of the palate may be apparently reduced by enlarged adenoids and in palatal pharyngeal disproportion, where either the soft palate is congenitally short or the nasopharyngeal aperture disproportionately large.

The palatal reflex is tested by stimulation of the uvula or soft palate with a spatula. The soft palate elevates and the uvula retracts. The gag reflex is elicited by touching the back of the tongue or the pharyngeal walls when there is normally a brisk response of contraction and elevation of the pharyngeal muscles, with some distress to the child. The afferent impulses of both reflexes are carried in the glossopharyngeal nerve and the motor response in the vagus nerve.

The degree of nasality of the child's speech should be noted. Bilateral vagal paresis, palatal pharyngeal disproportion and submucous cleft of the palate will produce hypernasality similar to that heard with cleft palate speech. Hyponasality is most commonly associated with enlargement of the adenoids or rhinitis. Disorder of the neuromuscular control necessary for speech sound production is discussed in Chapter 24.

The tongue is examined at rest within the mouth for evidence of unilateral or bilateral atrophy, signifying a lower motor neurone lesion. Fasciculations (p. 390), occurring in motor neurone disease, are most easily seen in the tongue muscles. They are small, rapid, asynchronous rippling movements. Larger involuntary movements may occur in dyskinetic cerebral palsy. Voluntary movements of the tongue can only be tested in older co-operating children. The child is asked to protrude the tongue as far as possible, to attempt to touch his chin and nose and to move the protruded tongue laterally to the angles of the mouth. Any asymmetry or weakness is noted. In unilateral paresis the tongue deviates towards the affected side on protrusion. If the child is reluctant to move his tongue on request, he may be willing to carry out the movements in pursuit of a sweet held in the appropriate direction.

Examination in Supine, Prone, Vertical and Ventral Suspension

Supine

Supine posture should be inspected in the infant and young child. The amount, symmetry and smoothness of spontaneous movement is noted. Normal supine postures expected at different ages are discussed in Chapter 4. With marked generalized hypotonicity, as in the floppy infant syndrome, the infant may assume a 'pithed frog' posture (p. 30).

The asymmetric tonic neck reflex (ATNR) (pp. 29, 181, 275) should be looked for, both on active head turning by the child and passive head turning by the examiner. Normally the reflex is seen most fully and frequently between the ages of 2 and 4 months and fades completely by 5–6 months. The arm postures are usually more obvious than those in the legs. In normal infants the reflex is never obligatory or fixed, i.e. it does not occur every time the head is rotated and, when it does occur, the infant easily breaks the pattern by turning his head in the opposite direction. Some asymmetry of response may be a normal finding in infants who persistently lie with their heads to one side and it is then usually associated with some degree of postural plagiocephaly. However, marked asymmetry is abnormal.

A brisk, obligatory or fixed ATNR and retention beyond the age of 5–6 months are indicative of delayed or disordered maturation of centres above the brain stem. Exaggeration and retention of the ATNR is seen classically in spastic and dyskinetic forms of cerebral palsy and the longer the reflex is retained the more severe the condition. Exaggeration and retention of the reflex often occurs as a transient phenomenon in the dystonic syndrome (p. 343). The ATNR may reappear in later acquired severe damage or degenerative diseases of the brain.

In the presence of an ATNR, particularly when it is abnormal, care should be taken to keep the head central while assessing tone and reflexes in the limbs, hand function and the Moro reflex.

The tonic labyrinthine reflex (TLR) (pp. 182, 275) is anotherre flex which may impose an abnormal posture in supine. The significance of this reflex in the normal child is uncertain, but it is often found in spastic and dyskinetic cerebral palsy. In supine it causes a generalized increase in extensor tone, so that the child lies with the neck and spine extended, shoulders retracted and the legs in extension and adduction. In severe cases the posture may be fixed.

Pull-to-sit and head control. The pull-to-sit manoeuvre is appropriate until the child can get up to sitting voluntarily. Gripping the hands gently, and with minimal assistance, the child is pulled up to the sitting position from supine, noting head lag and the amount of active neck, shoulder and arm flexion, the extent to which the child anticipates the action and the ease with which the sitting posture is achieved. The normal progression of development has been described (p. 54) and any delay should be noted.

Conditions causing hypotonicity and all forms of cerebral palsy are likely to cause delay. In addition, infants with the dystonic syndrome and in the dystonic stage of cerebral palsy show a tendency to come up to the standing rather than the sitting position with this manoeuvre, because of the increase in extensor tone of the trunk and legs.

Once in the sitting position, head control is noted in infants. This should be complete by 5 months and the infant should be able to maintain his head erect without 'bobbing' movements, on gentle displacement of the trunk in any direction.

The Moro reflex (pp. 36, 276) should be tested in infants. It is elicitable in normal infants until 3–4 months of age. It may be decreased or absent in severe cerebral damage and with marked hypotonicity. Excessive briskness of response and retention beyond the normal age is found in the dystonic syndrome and in spastic and dyskinetic cerebral palsy. Asymmetry occurs in hemiplegia and in lower motor neurone conditions such as Erb's palsy.

Prone
Posture in prone should be examined in infants and in older children with delayed development. The normal progression of milestones in the prone position has been described (p. 54). Delay in achieving these milestones is noted.

In the early months, apparently advanced development in prone posture with excessively good head raising for age, particularly if combined with delayed head control on pull-to-sit, is abnormal and a sign of the increased extensor tone found in infants with the dystonic syndrome and in the early stages of some forms of cerebral palsy. The abnormalities of tone and posture seen in the prone position in the later stages of spastic and dyskinetic cerebral palsy depend on the interaction of the tonic labyrinthine reflex and the symmetrical tonic neck reflex (STNR) (pp. 181, 276) and often it is difficult to differentiate their effects. In prone the TLR tends to increase flexor tone generally or at least reduce extensor tone. The STNR produces extension of the legs and flexion of the arms when the head is flexed and vice versa when the head is extended.

Vertical
Vertical suspension is a useful position for examination before the child has achieved independent walking. The examiner holds the child around the upper chest, suspended in mid-air. In the early weeks of life the infant shows semi-flexion and adduction of the limbs. This flexed posture gradually becomes less marked over the succeeding months and voluntary movements, particularly cycling and kicking movements of the legs, are seen.

The increased extensor tone of the dystonic stage of cerebral palsy and the dystonic syndrome is well shown in vertical suspension, particularly in the legs which are strongly extended at the hips and knees with plantar flexion at the ankles and, in some cases, spontaneously up-going first toes. Adductor tone is increased at the hips and the legs may scissor. The arms may be held internally rotated at the shoulders and extended at the elbows or they may be flexed up to the chest. The hands are held closed in either position.

Some infants, when suspended vertically, will hold their legs flexed to 90° at the hips with the knees in extension (p. 70). This seems to be a normal variant in a few cases but is seen more often in some infants showing a mild non-specific delay in motor development associated with hypotonicity. Such infants are usually noticeably slow in weight-bearing.

Downward parachute. While the child is held in vertical suspension the downward parachute response of the legs is tested by lowering him fairly quickly towards the floor, feet first. The legs abduct and extend and the feet point down in plantar flexion. The response is normally present by 5–6 months of age. It is delayed or absent in cerebral palsy and other conditions causing delay in motor development of the legs.

Placing reactions of the legs. These can conveniently be tested next (p. 35), noting any asymmetry in response. The significance of an absent response is discussed on p. 281. Increased extensor tone produces a rapid stereotyped response and both feet are placed at the same time.

Weight-bearing. The ability to bear weight varies throughout infancy. The positive supporting reaction of the newborn usually wanes between 2 and 4 months, to be followed by the development of voluntary weight-bearing. With increased extensor tone the positive supporting reaction is exaggerated and retained beyond the normal age. An exaggerated response, when the infant seems to spring into extension as soon as his feet come into contact with a firm surface, is known as an extensor thrust. It will be noted that this term is used differently in Chapter 3 (p. 35).

Primitive or primary walking (p. 36), like the other primitive reflexes exaggerated by increase in extensor tone, may be more easily elicited or prolonged beyond the normal age of 6 weeks in the dystonic syndrome and in the spastic and dyskinetic forms of cerebral palsy.

Ventral suspension

Posture in ventral suspension, with the infant held prone in mid-air, should be noted. In the normal infant there is a gradual progression from the generally flexed posture of the newborn, with only occasional head lifting to the horizontal plane. Through the influence of the labyrinthine righting reflex (p. 275), which is present from 2 months of age, there is increasing ability to extend the neck, to hold the head in line with the trunk and later (by 3 months) above the body plane. Ability to extend the spine and lower limbs also increases.

The Landau reflex can be demonstrated after 3 months of age. In ventral suspension the head, spine and legs automatically take up an extended posture. With passive neck flexion extensor tone is lost and the spine and legs flex. When passive neck flexion is removed, the extended position is resumed.

Poor posture in ventral suspension and absence of the Landau reflex are seen in conditions causing hypotonicity, and also in cerebral palsy when the flexed position is maintained due to the overactive tonic labyrinthine reflex.

Examination of the Limbs

Inspection

The limbs should be inspected for evidence of muscle wasting. The neuro-muscular disorders affecting young children (Chapter 19) are more likely to produce proximal rather than distal muscle wasting. Fasciculation, indicative of irritative lesions of the anterior horn cells, such as spinal muscular atrophy, may be seen in the small muscles of the hand, particularly the first dorsal interosseus.

Apart from the wasting seen in association with the obvious condition of myelomeningocele (Chapter 18), lower motor neurone wasting may occur in the lower limbs in spina bifida occulta where there is associated myelodysplasia. Here the wasting affects the distal muscles and is often confined to one limb or affects one limb more than the other. Depending on the part of the cord involved there may be loss of muscle bulk, reduction in leg length and disparity in foot size.

Muscle wasting, associated with shortening of the limb, may also be seen in hemiplegia. Usually the delay in growth does not become obvious until a year or more after the onset. In cases of mild hemiplegia the minor difference in size may be noticeable only by comparing the digits and nails.

Leg lengths may be compared visually if there is no tilting of the pelvis, i.e. if the anterior superior iliac crests are in the same horizontal line, and if any postural deformities at the knee and ankle can be corrected and the legs satisfactorily aligned. In cases of doubt the legs should be measured from the anterior superior iliac crest to the medial malleolus of the ankle.

Relative dwarfing of the pelvis and lower limbs is seen in cerebral diplegia, again usually becoming noticeable during the second year of life.

Any abnormality of posture in the limbs is noted and described. In doing so the influence of the child's position in space and the primitive reflexes, described above, should be remembered.

Tone

Tone is assessed while the child is fully relaxed by moving the limbs through the full range of passive movement at each joint and also during general handling of the child.

A useful assessment of shoulder girdle tone, particularly in the first year or two of life, is obtained by holding the child in vertical suspension. From the newborn period onwards this should be a secure way of holding a young child, the examiner's hands being 'hooked' in the child's axillae by the normal adductor tone in the shoulders. With reduced muscle tone the child's arms tend to abduct and the examiner has the feeling that the child is slipping through his grasp. Alternatively adductor tone may be increased and less than the normal amount of grip may be needed.

Hypotonicity at the elbow is judged by lowered resistance to passive movements and whether the elbow can be overextended. In marked hypotonicity, as the elbow overextends, the examiner may feel that the limit of extension is imposed not, as is usual, by the muscle tone and soft tissues but by the bony and cartilaginous elements. Movements around the elbow provide the easiest way of judging the type of increased tone in the upper limbs. In the 'clasp-knife' type of hypertonicity, found in the spastic forms of cerebral palsy, resistance is maximal at the beginning of passive movement, is maintained smoothly and then suddenly gives way. In the 'lead-pipe' hypertonicity of extra-pyramidal lesions, resistance is maintained smoothly throughout the movement. 'Cog-wheel' rigidity, in which tone alternatively increases and decreases throughout the movement, is a less common manifestation of extra-pyramidal lesions in childhood.

To test tone in the pronators of the forearm, the examiner steadies the child's arm below the elbow with one hand, grips the base of the child's thumb with the other and fully supinates the forearm. As the grip on the thumb is smartly released the forearm will pronate back to a position of rest. The speed and extent of this return is increased when the tone of the wrist pronators is raised and such an abnormal response is referred to as a 'pronator catch'.

A useful method of testing tone at the wrist is for the examiner to grasp the middle of the child's forearm and shake the hand so that it flaps back and forward several times. Most children from 18 months onwards find this manoeuvre amusing and do not, therefore, resist and voluntarily increase their muscle tone as they may do in more formal testing. An idea of the normal amount of 'flappability' is obtained from experience.

The degree of passive extension of the wrist and fingers should also be noted. Extension will be more difficult or limited where flexor tone is increased and hyperextension is possible in hypotonicity.

There is a wide normal range of degree of hip abduction but it usually lies somewhere between 50° and 70° from the vertical, when tested with the hips flexed to a right angle and the knees flexed. In hypotonicity the hips may be fully abductable to 90°. With increased tone (as in the spastic forms of cerebral palsy), apart from the increased resistance felt to passive movement, an adductor 'catch' may be elicitable on rapid bilateral abduction.

Asymmetry of hip abduction occurs in hemiplegia, in asymmetrical involvement in the other spastic forms of cerebral palsy and in hip dislocation.

When examining for dislocation of the hip, inequality of leg lengths (as detailed above) and asymmetry of thigh creases should also be looked for. In infants the tests of Ortolani and Barlow are applied. To carry out Ortolani's test (Fig. 7.4) the infant is laid supine and the hips flexed to a right angle. With the flexed knees grasped, one in each hand, and held together the hips are taken separately through the full range of adbuction. During this manoeuvre the femoral head on the dislocated side can be felt slipping back into the acetabulum and this may be heard as a 'clunk'. In Barlow's test (Fig. 7.5) the legs are held in the same starting position and then semi-abducted. Each hip is tested separately. Pressure applied with the fingers over the greater trochanter of the femur will cause a dislocated femoral head to return to the acetabulum and pressure from the thumb on the

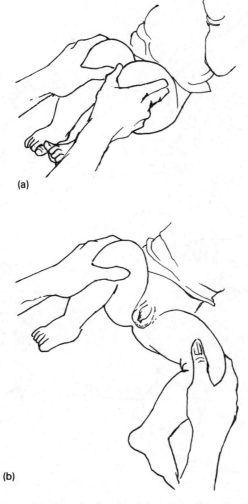

(a)

(b)

FIG. 7.4 a and b. Examination for dislocation of hip. Ortolani's test.

medial side of the femur, in the opposite direction, will dislocate an unstable hip. These tests will not be positive when a dislocation has become fixed.

An attempt should be made to bring the feet up to the head in infants and young children. Normal infants of 6–9 months often achieve this posture spontaneously, putting the toes into the mouth, but some degree of knee flexion is always present. When the posture is imposed in hypotonic children the knee over-extends and it may be possible to place the feet behind the ears.

The ankle can normally be dorsiflexed to 20°–30° beyond a right angle, except in the first month or so of life when the angle achieved is usually greater. In hypotonicity it may be possible to dorsiflex the foot as far as the anterior surface of the tibia.

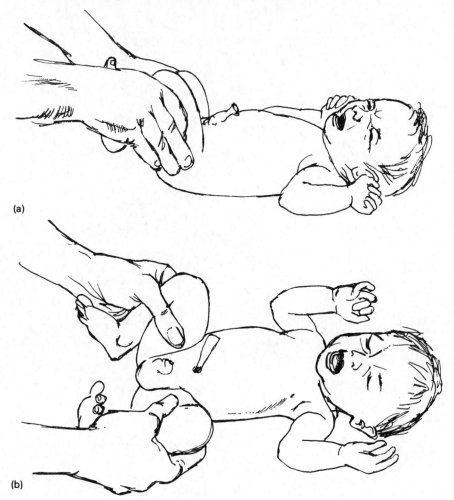

(a)

(b)

FIG. 7.5 a and b. Barlow's test for dislocation of hip.

Power

Attempts to carry out formal testing of power using the MRC grading (p. 187) are likely to be very time consuming or unsuccessful except in co-operative older children near 5 years. In younger children full voluntary power will be shown when the child is crying and struggling and, if this situation arises during the examination, a rough estimate of power can be obtained.

Tendon reflexes

Testing of the biceps, triceps and supinator reflexes and the knee jerk are carried out as in the neurological examination of the adult. To elicit the ankle jerk in infants and young children it is often easier for the examiner to tap his own fingers where they are held over the plantar surface of the child's toes to maintain dorsiflexion (Fig. 7.6). This gives a more obvious point of contact for the tendon hammer than the rather small tendo-achilles.

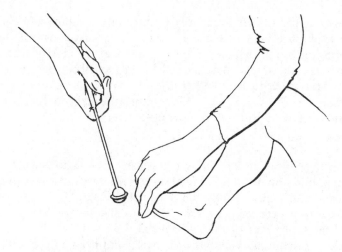

Fig. 7.6. Eliciting the ankle jerk in a young child.

Any clonus is noted and whether it is sustained or nonsustained (1 or 2 beats only). Clonus is most likely to be elicitable as the ankle jerks are tested. In the spastic form of cerebral palsy a crossed adductor response is often obtained with the knee jerk, i.e. with elicitation of one knee jerk the opposite thigh adducts reflexly.

Plantar responses
These are obtained by firm pressure beginning at the heel, moving along the lateral border of the sole and then over the metatarsal heads. An extensor plantar response is found in most normal children up to the age of 18 months to 2 years but thereafter it can be taken as evidence of a pyramidal lesion as in the adult. As mentioned earlier (p. 137) a spontaneous extensor plantar response is sometimes found in the dystonic syndrome and in cerebral palsy.

Sensation
Even with a bright co-operative 5-year-old, testing of sensation is likely to be unrewarding as the child is liable to lose interest in the proceedings. Except for specific instances, e.g. defining the upper level of anaesthesia in paraplegia, testing of pain sensation by pinprick is seldom justifiable.

Gross Motor Abilities

An integral part of every neurological examination in young children is to determine whether or not the child has reached the appropriate developmental level for his age. The normal stages of development in gross motor abilities are discussed fully in Chapter 4 and will not be repeated here.

Rolling

The infant's ability to roll voluntarily from prone to supine and back again, normally established between 6 and 8 months of age, develops from the earlier neck righting reflex (pp. 184, 276). The smoothness, ease and frequency of rolling should be noted and whether the child rolls equally to either side. The persistence of other reflexes, such as the ATNR and TLR, makes rolling difficult or impossible in some cases of cerebral palsy. Where there is inequality of function between the two sides the child will roll towards the weaker side.

Sitting

The acquisition of full sitting ability takes many months to achieve, from the earliest stage of propping up to the final stage when the child is able to adopt the sitting position at will and maintain it completely steadily for as long as he wants. Apart from determining which stage the child has reached, certain other aspects of the sitting posture should be noted.

Retention of the primary curve of the back, with delay in acquisition of the normal lumbar lordosis from the 5th month onwards, is found in conditions which cause generalized hypotonia. Such a child may also flop forwards and place his head between his feet. Retention of the primary curve is also found in those types of cerebral palsy where there is an increase in extensor tone in the trunk, which interferes with the amount of hip flexion required for sitting. Later on in the spastic forms of cerebral palsy limitation of knee extension, due to increased knee flexor tone, will cause further difficulty and the child sits unsteadily, balanced on the sacrum rather than on the ischial tuberosities.

Steadiness in sitting, including the ability to pivot, requires efficient functioning of the equilibrium reactions of the trunk and limbs (p. 186) and parachute responses of the arms (p. 185). The sideways parachute response is usually acquired by 6–7 months, the forward parachute by 7–8 months and the backward parachute by 10–11 months. The response should be observed for speed and completeness, as it may be present but too slow to be effective or extension of the arm may be present without full opening of the hand. Asymmetry of response is a fairly subtle test for minor degrees of suspected hemiplegia or for confirming the more involved side in asymmetrical cerebral plasy.

Sitting between the heels, with the knees flexed and the hips internally rotated ('W' sitting, p. 303) is the sitting position adopted for choice by many children with problems of motor control and balance. The position provides a wider and more secure base, but in spastic cerebral palsy it is considered to intensify the already increased adductor and internal rotator tone at the hip joints and to increase the danger of dislocation.

Methods of progression other than walking

The method by which the child chooses to progress across the floor and the ease and speed with which he does so is noted. Continuous rolling or 'sealing' with the abdomen on the floor, can be seen as fairly transient stages in normal children but may be the only methods available for a prolonged period for the child with cerebral palsy. Sealing is particularly typical of cerebral diplegia when the main propelling force is supplied by the arms, the extended adducted legs being dragged along behind.

Hand–knee crawling is particularly difficult for children with spastic forms of cerebral palsy. When both sides of the body are involved it is difficult for the child to move the legs independently. In these cases 'bunny hopping' (which is also used by some normal children) is often adopted as it allows both legs to be moved together. Bottom-shuffling or hitching is also a normal variant of progression but it is the preferred method for many hemiplegic children who hitch on the side of their unaffected limbs.

Stance

The child's stance is observed either in free standing or, in the case of children who are not yet walking, in supported standing with the minimum of assistance. This is a convenient point at which to look for any abnormalities of the spine, such as scoliosis or excessive lordosis. The width of the child's base, his degree of steadiness and the presence of any postural deformities are noted.

In all forms of cerebral palsy with increased adductor tone at the hips, the base is narrow. In ataxic cerebral palsy and other conditions causing hypotonicity the stance is wide based. Ataxic children may show bobbing or wobbling of the trunk or legs and may curl their toes strongly as if to get a better grip on the floor. The arms may be held up for balance as in the normal younger child who has recently started to walk alone.

Other deviations from normal stance should be noted, e.g. abnormal degrees of flexion or internal or external rotation at the hips, genu valgum or varus and flexion or hyperextension postures at the knees, valgus or varus at the ankle and any tendency to stand on the toes.

Some degree of genu valgum (knock knee) is normal after the age of 3 disappearing over the next 2–3 years. It is commoner in over-weight and hypotonic children. When the degree of genu valgum, as measured by the distance between the medial malleoli with the knees together and extended, is between 5 and 10 cm regular observation and measurement is necessary to confirm that the condition is resolving. If the measurement increases or the distance is greater than 10 cm, further investigation is necessary (Sharrard, 1976). Genu varum (bow leg), of less than 5 cm between the medial femoral condyles with the ankles together, is common in late infancy and the early toddler stage. More severe degrees require investigation (Sharrard, 1976). Flat foot is another common postural deformity which occurs when a child begins to weight bear, the heel being tilted into eversion. The posture may be more pronounced or retained longer when there is associated hypotonicity.

In children of 3 years and over, who have achieved steady walking, the ability to balance on one foot without support is assessed and timed. The length of time that normal children, from 3–5 years, can balance on one foot is given in Table 4.4. Between these ages balancing movements of the arms are usually needed. The child will often show a preference for and perform better on one side than the other. This is usually but not always the dominant side. Marked asymmetry is abnormal. Delay in this ability in a child with no obvious neurological defect (including mental retardation) is most usually found as part of the general motor clumsiness of 'minimal cerebral dysfunction'.

Gait

Gait is observed in walking, running and if possible on stairs. As with stance, the width of the base, the degree of co-ordination and any postural deformities should be noted. The presence or absence of the normal associated movements in the arms and any abnormal movement of the limbs should also be noted. The abnormalities mentioned under stance are likely to be more pronounced when the child walks, e.g. the child who stands on a narrow base due to increased adductor tone at the hips may show further narrowing of the base on walking; the child with increased calf tone is more likely to go up on his toes while walking and more so while running. Unless he has learned to lift his feet high enough, such a child is likely to catch the toes of his shoes, particulary when running. Any degree of unsteadiness will become more obvious especially on changing direction.

Asymmetry of involvement, as in hemiplegia, may produce a limping gait to the affected side. Weakness of the hip abductors produces a waddling gait.

The child's shoes should be examined for evidence of excessive wear on the inner and outer borders of the heel or the uppers and for scuffing of the toes.

More skilled aspects of gait can be tested, when this is appropriate, in children of 3 years and over. By 3 years most children can walk on tiptoe when requested. The child is also asked to hop on one foot. At this stage he will do so by hopping forwards as the ability to hop on the spot does not usually develop until after 5 years. Normal children begin to hop during their fourth year, can manage 5–8 hops by 4 years and 9–12 hops by 5 years. The child may perform better on his preferred leg but, again, marked asymmetry is abnormal. As with ability to stand on one leg, the level of achievement is often decreased in children with 'minimal cerebral dysfunction'.

Involuntary Movements

Athetoid and choreoid

These movements occur classically in dyskinetic cerebral palsy and are seen in combination in its commonest form. Athetoid movements are slow, writhing movements involving the distal parts of the limbs and are most easily recognized in hand and wrist with successive combinations of abduction, adduction, hyperextension and flexion of the fingers and flexion, hyperextension, pronation and supination at the wrist. Choreoid (choreiform) movements are jerky, more rapid and are seen proximally in the limbs and also in the face. The movements are not present in the earlier stages of dyskinetic cerebral palsy, usually first appearing during the 2nd and 3rd years. They occur when voluntary movement is attempted and with emotion. Athetoid movements of the hand and wrist may also occur in spastic forms of cerebral palsy, particularly hemiplegia.

Choreiform movements may be seen in children of 3–5 who are classified as suffering from the 'minimal cerebral dysfunction' syndrome. The movements are seen most easily in the arms and hands when the child is asked to extend his arms out in front of him (with the fingers abducted and extended) and to maintain the posture for 20 seconds or so. The assumption of a 'dinner-fork' posture is also typical with flexion of the wrist and hyperextension at the meta-carpo-phalangeal joints.

Another less common type of involuntary movement occurring in established dyskinetic cerebral palsy is tension, in which tone in both the agonist and antagonist muscles suddenly increases on voluntary movement.

Tremor

Tremor occurs classically in the ataxic forms of cerebral palsy and other condi-tions causing cerebellar and proprioceptive dysfunction. It occurs on voluntary movement and may be seen in the trunk when the child is attempting to main-tain balance. Tremor may also be seen, less commonly, in the dyskinetic and spastic forms of cerebral palsy.

Dystonia

This is an involuntary increase in extensor tone, particularly of the trunk and lower limbs and is a common finding in the dystonic syndrome and the early stages of all forms of cerebral palsy other than hemiplegia and pure ataxia. When the basic tone, with the child relaxed and in supine, may be within normal limits or hypotonic, dystonic posturing occurs on handling of the child, particu-larly in the following situations: a sudden change in position, the head allowed to fall back into extension, assumption of the vertical position and when the feet touch a firm surface. It may occur as a response to loud or sudden noise and attempted voluntary movement may also be a trigger.

The underlying mechanism of dystonia is not fully understood but from the stimulae which produce it and the movements observed in the child, it is possible that a number of primitive reflexes are involved including the positive supporting reaction and the tonic labyrinthine reflex.

The ease and frequency with which dystonic posturing can be elicited decreases with time and in inverse proportion to the severity of the condition but, even in the cerebral palsied child who has obtained some sitting and even some stand-ing balance, sudden stiffening in response to threatened loss of balance or to loud noise may still be seen.

Associated movements

Many of these movements, such as swinging of the arms with walking and screwing up of the face during muscular effort, are normal throughout life but associated movements are particularly common in the normal young child, e.g. when the child is concentrating on a skilled hand task exaggeration of facial expression, such as frowning, and movements of the tongue, such as protrusion, are common. Mirror movements is the name given to a variety of associated movements, where voluntary movements of one side of the body (particularly of the hand) are copied simultaneously on the other side. They are also normal in young children.

Absence of associated movements may occur in all forms of motor disorders. Asymmetry is particularly noticeable in hemiplegia. Abnormally exaggerated associated and mirror movements and retention beyond the normal ages are seen commonly in children with 'minimal cerebral dysfunction'.

Handedness and Footedness

At 4–5 months, when an infant first begins to use the hands for reaching, the approach is often two-handed or he will use the nearest hand to the object and the other hand will be brought up. A tendency to use one hand more than the other for complicated skills such as self-feeding with a spoon may emerge at the beginning of the 2nd year but fully established handedness is not usually present until the end of the 2nd year (p. 76).

Apart from obtaining the mother's opinion on the child's handedness, the child should be observed while playing. In testing infants, attractive objects should be presented centrally while the child is held securely with both hands free. The hand used for reaching is noted on a number of occasions. From the age of 12 months or so, any preference for one hand can be noted at the same time as testing hand co-ordination with cubes (see below). Older children, who have begun to use crayon or pencil, can be tested by placing the pencil centrally on a sheet of paper and noting whether the child consistently uses one or other hand or alternates.

From the age of 2 years foot preference can be tested by observing the child kicking a ball several times. As with the hand, dominance is not usually established before 2 years and any marked preference before this age is likely to be abnormal. Such a preference might be noted if the child consistently leads off with one leg in crawling, pulling to standing or in assisted or unassisted walking.

Hand Function

The child's degree of co-ordination in hand function is observed while he is playing with toys or, more formally, in tests appropriate for his age. In the young infant from 4–5 months hand function is observed while he is reaching, grasping and transferring objects such as rattles. From 8–9 months a small object (1 cm diameter) can be used to observe the developing pincer grip, remembering that after he has secured the object the infant will automatically take it to his mouth unless prevented. From 12–15 months children are usually keen to play with brightly coloured 1-inch cubes, putting them in and taking them out of a mug and beginning to build towers. Presenting a small sweet held in mid-air at his chest height is also a useful way of encouraging the child to demonstrate hand function at this age.

By 3–4 years most children will co-operate in some form of finger-tip-touching test. The younger child can usually be persuaded to place his index finger on a sweet or a specific part of a toy (e.g. a doll's eye or nose) held in varying positions in front of him. By 4–5 years more formal finger–nose tests can be used. With his index finger the child touches the tip of the examiner's index finger and then the tip of his own nose (the examiner demonstrating touching his own nose at the same time). The manoeuvre is repeated 3 time and both hands are tested. Once dominance is established the dominant hand is usually slightly but noticeably more skilful on these tests. However, any marked difference between the two sides is abnormal.

The normal sequence of development of hand function has been described (p. 56) and a lag in development should be noted. Abnormal features should also be looked for. Particularly in children with the spastic types of cerebral palsy the hand may not open fully on reaching, movements of the thumb being most restricted. In the dyskinetic forms of cerebral palsy and in some children with a predominantly spastic type of cerebral palsy the fingers over-extend and splay out on reaching, and athetoid movements become obvious. Intention tremor is most obvious in ataxic forms of cerebral palsy but can occur in other types as well.

Even if none of these specific abnormalities are present, the child's hand function may appear clumsy with lack of smoothness in combining various parts of a movement (dyssynergia), or poor control of muscular power and the speed of movement (dysmetria) with overshooting. Clumsiness which is not explainable by abnormalities of tone, muscle power, cerebellar or proprioceptive function or the presence of involuntary movements, is referred to as dyspraxia or apraxia (p. 286) and is due to higher, central defects in planning and control.

References

COHEN H.J. and DINER H. (1970) The significance of developmental dental enamel defects in neurological diagnosis. *Pediatrics*, **46**, 737.

COHEN H.J., DINER H. and DAVIS J.G. (1975) Stigmata, dental defects and dermatoglyphics as aids in neurological diagnosis. *Developmental Medicine and Child Neurology*, **17**, 365.

DRILLIEN C.M. (1968) Studies in mental handicap: some obstetric factors of possible aetiological significance. *Archives of Disease in Childhood*, **43**, 283.

DRILLIEN C.M., INGRAM T.T.S. and RUSSELL E.M. (1964) Further studies of the causes of diplegia in children. *Developmental Medicine and Child Neurology*, **6**, 241.

LAESTADIUS N.D., AASE J.M. and SMITH D.W. (1969) Normal inner canthal and outer orbital dimensions. *Journal of Pediatrics*, **74**, 465.

PRYOR H.B. (1969) Objective measurement of interpupillary distance. *Pediatrics*, **44**, 973.

ROSENBERG J.B. and WELLER G.M. (1973) Minor physical anomalies and academic performance in young school-children. *Developmental Medicine and Child Neurology*, **15**, 131.

SHARRARD W.J.W. (1976) Knock knees and bow legs. *British Medical Journal*, **1**, 826.

SMITH D.W. (1970) *Recognisable Patterns of Human Malformation*. Philadelphia: W.B. Saunders.

VIA W.F. and CHURCHILL J.A. (1959) Relationship of enamel hypoplasia to abnormal events of gestation and birth. *Journal of the American Dental Association*, **59**, 702.

WALDROP M.F. and HALVERSTON C.F. (1971) Minor physical anomalies and hyperactive behaviour in young children. In *The Exceptional Infant*, vol. 2. ed. Hellmuth J. New York: Brunner and Mazel.

Further Reading

PAINE R.S. and OPPÉ T.E. (1966) *Neurological Examination of Children. Clinics in Developmental Medicine Nos. 20/21.* London: Heinemann.

CHAPTER 8

Development and Assessment of Vision and Hearing

In connection with research into developmental progress from birth to 7 years in 1960 it was necessary to devise tests of vision, hearing and language applicable to normal infants and young children and those with mental and multiple handicaps. The tests needed to possess high validity, provide as much information as possible concerning everyday capabilities and with handicapped children point the way to therapeutic management. The STYCAR series of tests (Sheridan Tests for Young Children and Retardates) were designed with these aims in view.

All tests for children whether designed to assess motor capacity, vision, hearing, language development or social progress must conform to certain rules. They must be within the child's comprehension, providing challenge without strain; engaging, but not so interesting as to distract attention from the test itself; not so long-drawn out as to be boring and finally, capable of application and recording so that results can be interpreted and repeated by independent examiners.

Every normal infant enters life with equipment enabling him simultaneously to develop in body, mind and personality as a unique individual, while adapting to the cultural usages of his social environment. He is subject to an array of sensory stimulations which stream into his central nervous system, through receptors which cope with sensations from outside his body (sight and sound), near to it (touch, temperature, taste, smell) and within it (proprioceptive, visceral). Although this chapter is concerned with vision and hearing it needs to be remembered that development of everyday visual and auditory competence cannot be considered in modal isolation, since both depend upon a moment-to-moment selective integration of complex sensory intake.

Vision

Everyday visual competence involves the integration of two separate processes, seeing and looking (Sheridan, 1976a).

Seeing is the reception by the eye of mobile and static patterns of light, shade and hue and the transmission of this intaken information to the central nervous system, i.e. it is mainly a physiological process and depends upon adequately functioning optical equipment. Seeing not only relates to colours, contours and shapes which are followed or fixated within an individual field, but also to binocular fusion and three-dimensional perception.

Looking is paying attention to what is seen with the object of interpreting its meaning, i.e. it is mainly a psychological function. Looking (like listening) involves the simultaneous appreciation of a number of complex mental activities occurring in time and space. These include recognition (i.e. matching) of presently incoming visual patterns against memories already centrally registered, coupled with awareness of novel elements; interpretation of familiar and novel elements in the situational context and finally the promotion of appropriate co-ordinated motor response (expression), e.g. reaching for an observed object, manipulating it, combining it with similar objects, copying its shape in drawing, miming its action or speaking its name. Naming of objects implies facility in use of spoken language, thus involving additional cognitive factors. Objective electro-physiological procedures employing electronic instruments test seeing rather than looking, so that subjective clinical tests must always be included in the assessment of visual competence.

BIRTH TO 6 MONTHS

In the course of normal development a child's attentional world (i.e. the three-dimensional space which he learns to hold in continual visual and auditory awareness) increases in size as a gradually expanding sphere from within a radius of about half a metre at 2–3 weeks to full adult range by 2–3 years (Catford and Oliver, 1973). The clinical assessment of visual competence after 6 months becomes comparatively reliable. Before 6 months, however, even experienced examiners can misinterpret behavioural responses. Normal stages may be summarized as follows:

The neonate has not seen before birth but rapidly adapts. Pupils react to light, lids close against intense light. Eyes and head turn towards diffuse light. Limited powers of accommodation produce relatively fixed focal length of 8–12 inches until 4–6 weeks. Eyes and head follow a dangling ball briefly at focal distance. Eyes often 'corner' reflexly in direction of a sound-source; examiners should therefore test vision using silent objects. Intermittent glancing at mother's nearby face is present from birth, progressing to consistent watching during feeding from about 2 weeks.

At 1–3 months the infant regards a nearby care-giver's face with intense pre-occupation, scans surroundings when held upright with no face in view and follows attentively a slowly moving dangling ball at 6–10 inches from his own face. Defensive blink is usually present from about 4–6 weeks and convergence of eyes for finger play from 10–12 weeks.

At 4–6 months the infant demonstrates smooth following eye movements for a dangling ball in all directions. He is visually alert for near and far, watches movements of his own hands together and singly from about 4 months and, a week or two later, movements of his feet. From about $4\frac{1}{2}$ months he reaches accurately for a toy, grasps firmly and regards closely and regards a small pellet on table-top, a few weeks later approaching with extended hand and spread fingers.

6 MONTHS–$2\frac{1}{2}$ YEARS

The STYCAR graded balls tests, which are applicable from 6 months, are used to test three visual functions (assuming eye movements in all directions are normal); these are ability to follow movement of very small objects (rolling balls), ability to fixate (mounted balls) and peripheral vision (mounted balls). In order to obtain satisfactory results it is necessary to apply STYCAR tests strictly according to the instructions (Sheridan, 1969; 1976a).

Rolling balls test

This test takes advantage of the infant's ability to follow visually from start to finish objects moving within his uninterrupted gaze. This ability can be demonstrated from about 6 months, which is 6–8 weeks before he looks for an object leaving his field of vision, however briefly. Outward directional cues are avoided by rolling from the side. Observers watching this test for the first time usually comment that the child is receiving directional cues from the examiner's arm movements, but in fact he does not look for a ball unless it leaves the examiner's hand. In catching and holding attention coloured or patterned balls have no advantage over plain white; black balls on a white surface are less easily distinguished than white balls against dark, because of dazzle effect.

Initially, six white plastic balls were used with diameters of $2\frac{1}{2}$, 2, $1\frac{1}{2}$, 1, $\frac{3}{4}$ and $\frac{1}{2}$ inches respectively, but finding that many infants of 9–12 months were able to fixate and follow even smaller balls, four more were added with diameters of $\frac{3}{8}$, $\frac{1}{4}$, $\frac{3}{16}$ and $\frac{1}{8}$ inches.

An incidental finding was that deaf infants, notoriously visually alert, seemed to cultivate their peripheral vision more effectively than normal hearing infants, so that the slightest movement well to one side, which would be ignored by normal infants, immediately caused turning to look.

Binocular testing is always carried out first in order to determine the child's everyday visual competence. Later, if considered desirable (e.g. when squint is present or unequal vision is suspected) monocular testing must be patiently attempted.

Procedure. The mother (M) is requested to sit on a low chair with the child (C) seated on the floor at her feet, or if she prefers may sit on the floor close beside him. To facilitate rolling and eliminate sounds a strip of dark coloured carpet or baize (at least 1 foot wide and about 13 ft long) can be fastened to the floor at the measured distance.

The examiner (E) stations himself at a measured distance of 10 ft from C, well to one side. With inattentive or retarded children a 'training run' at 5 ft may be required. C's attention is drawn to E's face and hand movements by calling his name (if he can hear) or by tossing the largest ball a foot or so in the air and catching it. When his attention is fully engaged the first ball is rolled slowly along the floor horizontally across his line of vision for a distance of 8–12 ft. E carefully observes C's orienting response. His usual reaction is to watch the ball intently until it comes to rest and then, if mobile, to make rapidly and delightedly towards it. If he has enough understanding of speech he should be instructed: '(Name) get it and give it to Mummy.' When he returns to her M should be instructed to hold him firmly until the next (smaller) ball has been presented and ceased to roll. If C does not watch the first throw he may be given a second chance.

It is essential to vary speed, distance of roll and side from which the ball is cast, otherwise intelligent children quickly learn to anticipate end-position. The record should show the sizes of balls to which C gave full attention.

These manoeuvres, although they appear to be very simple, require considerable practice before they become smooth in execution and reliable in result. Hence the test should not be delegated to inexperienced or unsupervised ancillary staff. If the clinician considers it appropriate in any individual case he may reduce testing by using fewer balls. Most suitable sizes for this abbreviated form of application are 2, 1, $\frac{1}{2}$, $\frac{1}{4}$, $\frac{1}{8}$ inches. This concession also applies to the mounted balls test.

Mounted balls test

Everyday visual competence for static as distinct from moving objects not only involves visual acuity but accurate fixation and intelligent appreciation of foreground–background relationships. Developmental aspects of stereoscopic vision are imperfectly understood but practical experience indicates that it is well advanced by 4–5 months when a child begins to reach for toys, although it is probably functionally restricted to a spatial world within a few feet of his eyes.

It appeared obvious that the simplest way to test infants' ocular fixation and visual acuity for small, still objects was to use the same series of balls mounted on rigid sticks. In order to prevent the usual shifting of gaze from test object to human face (which occurs at $4\frac{1}{2}$–6 ft when an examiner slowly withdraws while presenting a still fixed object), or to more interesting nearby stimuli, the examiner should set out to attract attention to the test object itself as before and then disappear from view behind a screen provided with a narrow viewing slit through which the child's reactions can be observed, while the visual 'bait' continues to be displayed. Behind the examiner's chair is a large black curtain against which the white balls stand out clearly, whilst their black sticks become invisible.

Procedure. The testing is carried out at 10 ft. With a distractible child it is sometimes necessary to attract his attention from shorter distance. E must allow C to be fully aware of his hidden but active participation in the procedure or C may quickly lose interest in the game. Consequently E draws C's attention to himself and screen by calling C's name and momentarily showing his face with the first mounted ball close beside it, before disappearing behind the screen, leaving C regarding the ball. The ball is held completely still at a few inches beyond the edge of the screen for 2–3 seconds, then rapidly removed and presented again for 2–3 seconds in a position at the opposite edge of the screen. In response C usually swiftly moves his eyes to fixate the ball in its new position. The ball is similarly presented above and below the edge of the screen. Through the narrow viewing slit C's successive eye fixations are clearly seen so that the slightest abnormality of movement or tendency to squint is obvious.

The balls should be presented in order of decreasing size and in random starting positions, otherwise children over 9 months may learn to anticipate where the ball will regularly appear. The ball must be completely hidden behind the screen while in motion and E's hands should not be in sight at any time.

Test of peripheral vision
Since this test must be applied from behind the child, the examiner needs an assistant (A).

Procedure. A suitable pair of mounted balls are those of diameter ½ inch and ⅜ inch. With C seated on M's lap facing him, E lightly attracts his visual attention to the front while A, holding the sticks about 10–12 inches on either side of the child's head at eye level, silently brings forward one of the balls, gently agitating it as he does so. Usually, when the moving object enters C's peripheral visual field he turns immediately to look at it. The procedure is repeated from the opposite side and at any other angle E chooses. This simple procedure has proved of considerable value in testing severely handicapped children for suspected field defects.

Standards
Owing to the 'free-field' nature of the testing procedures and the unpredictable variability of young children's individual responses, it has been impossible to submit findings to conventional statistical analysis, but from extensive clinical experience, the following conclusions about normal infants have been reached.

6–8 months. Infants may be expected to watch rolling balls down to ¼ inch diameter at 10 ft. Under 8 months they do not usually follow the two smallest balls and it is difficult to secure their attention for mounted balls of under ½ inch diameter at 10 ft. It is noticeable, however, that infants of 6 months can often fixate at 5 ft a mounted ball which is less than half the diameter of one which is ignored (i.e. out of their visual world) at 10 ft indicating that the difficulty is not one of visual acuity but results from immaturity of visual attention-span in space and time. Response to the peripheral-field test is brisk and unmistakable from 6 months onwards.

8–12 months. Infants watch eagerly, almost automatically, the full range of rolling balls and can usually be persuaded to fixate the full range of mounted balls.

12–24 months. Infants become more difficult to test owing to their high distractibility and mobility and also perhaps because they are now passing from the stage of finding sufficient satisfaction at a purely perceptual level (intake), to a capacity for early conceptual appreciation (interpretation) of observed phenomena, so that they need to have a recognizable reason, a primitive 'definition-by-use' built into their experiences. The next stage, which quickly follows, is a need for some resulting 'aim-in-view', i.e. opportunity for appropriate motor response (expression) such as retrieving of the rolled balls, or pointing at the mounted balls. Older handicapped children pass through the same stages, and are often easier to test than normal children of similar mental age because they are more ambulant and have better understanding of spoken or mimed instructions. When encouraged they enter enthusiastically into the game. Rolling balls are endlessly interesting to all groups, but they provide less information than correctly presented mounted balls.

After 2 years. Testing becomes easier again after 2 years because children are more able to comprehend and willing to obey interesting simple instructions.

Near vision
This can readily be tested from the age of 9 or 10 months when the child visually fixates a very small object close by, and usually pokes at it with a forefinger. Suitable test objects include crumbs or tiny sweets which will not harm him if he swallows them. If his mother covers up one eye at a time with her hand, uniocular testing is usually accepted by a young child.

2–5 YEARS

Miniature toys vision test
This test was evolved for use with severely handicapped children, particularly those with low intelligence and those with such limited previous opportunities to learn from experience that they were unable to match two-dimensional letters or coloured pictures, but could recognize, match and sometimes name, solid balls, coloured wooden cubes, toy motor cars and aeroplanes and a variety of doll's house-sized domestic objects. The test is also applicable to normal children from about 21 months until the age when letter-cards can be applied.

Procedure. At conversational distance E asks C to name and/or match the toys shown. Even the youngest children usually know and match the car, doll, chair and spoon. By 2 years most can cope with all 7 toys. Having confirmed C's understanding, E withdraws to 10 ft and presents one of the toys, asking 'what's this'? The toy should be presented at C's eye level and stand out clearly against its background, e.g. against a strip of black velvet. Each item must be removed before the next is presented. If C cannot speak intelligibly he is given a duplicate set and requested, by signs if necessary, to indicate the matching toy. In this case E's coloured toys should be differently coloured from C's (e.g. E blue car and C red) or C will probably match by colour rather than form. This fortunately does not apply to the toy cutlery which provides very fine visual discrimination, e.g. between prongs of fork and bowl of spoon.

Near vision can be tested by requesting the child to pick up very small sweets, crumbs, scraps of cotton wool, pieces of thread etc. Vision for far and near with each eye separately must be recorded in descriptive terms.

Standards
Optical experts consulted considered that ability to distinguish between the larger fork and spoon at 10 ft approximates to about 6/9 vision and between the smaller fork and spoon to at least 6/6. A child who cannot distinguish all seven toys (with larger cutlery) at 10 ft with each eye separately requires immediate ophthalmological examination. It is desirable to follow-up within 3–6 months those who cannot distinguish between smaller fork and spoon at 10 ft. All handicapped children should be re-examined at regular intervals (Harcourt, 1975).

Letter matching test for children under 5 years
Letter matching procedure, with the same seven reversible letters described

below, can be used with all normally intelligent children of 4 years. Approximately 80 per cent of 3-year-olds can match five letters (A and U omitted) as can 50 per cent of 2½-year-olds. With preliminary matching practice the percentage of testable 2- and 3-year-olds can be considerably increased.

At this age test letters are presented singly on cards, 5 inches square, at a distance of 10 ft. Two extra 'lines' (6/4.5 and 6/3) are provided for this purpose.

If the child cannot match the smallest letters (Snellen equivalent of 6/6) with each eye separately, it is wise to retest again within 3–6 months. If he cannot match the letters equivalent to 6/9 with each eye he should be referred forthwith for expert opinion.

TESTS FOR SCHOOL ENTRANTS

Snellen letter tests
The history of vision-testing charts since Snellen's original publication in 1862 has been well discussed by Bennet (1965). Snellen's original calculations remain valid and many authorities still discuss visual competence solely in terms of Snellen fractions.

Investigations in which several hundred 5- to 7-year-olds were tested originated in the need for a reliable chart to test school entrants of 5 years. Picture tests then available proved unsatisfactory, especially for retarded children who found difficulty in comprehending crowded lines of highly stylized black and white pictograms.

The Illiterate E test and Landolt's broken rings test, applied under controlled conditions in school clinics, gave better results, particularly the broken rings test. In school screening conditions, however, the E test frequently fails to retain children's interest beyond the 6/12 line. It is very monotonous to apply and is often difficult for the examiner to interpret responses which are indicated with hand or model. There are other serious drawbacks to E and Landolt tests (and to the later Sjögren Hand Test) which are unnecessary to discuss here.

Choice is very limited since only the four cardinal positions can be employed with young children. Confusion of right and left positions and even of up and down are common under the age of 7 years. This directional difficulty is particulary marked in neurologically handicapped children. Although the illiterate E conforms to Snellen measurements the bar-pattern presented is constant, so does not give further information regarding the child's ability to discriminate differences in configuration.

STYCAR letter test
Having discovered from experience that most 5-year-old children first learn to sound, write and name letters based on vertical and horizontal lines, circles and part-circles, crosses, squares and part-squares and triangles, I incorporated the nine most favoured letters (T, L, H, O, C, X, V, U, A) in the design of the charts. Experienced examiners are able to test vision in over 95 per cent of normal 5-year-old school entrants. The untestable group includes mentally retarded children and a few who are unusually anxious or resistive. Very occasion-

ally a child with definite visuo-spatial difficulties is encountered. All non-responders are therefore in need of prompt expert investigation.

The charts provide a rapid and interesting screening test for normal children up to 7 years. They are not suitable for children over 7 years, who require less easily memorized material. The chart should be hung flat against a plain wall, in good light, at children's eye level. Reading distance (20 ft or 10 ft in a mirror) must be accurately measured. The eye not under test must always be effectively occluded.

Procedure at 20 ft. E will require an assistant (A), preferably a familiar, to stay near the child (C), who sits at a small table or stands with his feet touching a marked line. His left eye is then effectively covered (a wooden spoon held in his left hand makes an excellent occluder) leaving his right hand free. It is inadvisable to tell C to cover his eye with a hand as he invariably peeps through his fingers, or kneads his eyeball and is later unable to use it effectively for some minutes. Demonstrating a large plus sign in the air with his index finger E then points to top letter with one simple instruction, 'Draw this.' When C has done so E says 'Good . . . now this . . .'. At least one letter on each line should be presented and the two bottom lines in their entirety. If C falters before the bottom line E should go back to discover the lowest line he can see completely. Each eye is tested separately. If C is wearing corrective lenses his vision should be recorded without spectacles and then with them.

It is noteworthy that children who know their letters invariably spontaneously name them. Hence the following simple rule-of-thumb can be applied:

Advanced performance: names letters at 20 feet
Average performance: copies letters in the air or on paper at 20 feet
Immature performance: matches letters at 20 feet (or 10 feet in a mirror)

Some immature children of 5–7 years find it difficult to maintain rapport with an examiner at 20 feet. For these children, the modified procedure of testing in a mirror at 10 feet, or by using smaller letters, should be employed.

Testing in a mirror at 10 feet entails discarding the two irreversible letters C and L on the charts and using the block of seven single-letter cards, to be drawn or matched on a corresponding seven-letter key-card or with solid letters.

Sitting side-by-side with C facing the mirror, E holds up the single-letter cards in turn immediately above or beside C's head (i.e. out of C's direct line of vision), so that in order to read them C is obliged to look into the mirror, thus doubling the distance.

Standards

Normal vision of school entrants at 5 years is R. 6/6, L. 6/6, i.e. the child should be able to read the bottom line on STYCAR charts at 20 ft (6 m) with each eye separately. All children reading only R. 6/9, L. 6/9 should be considered sub-optimal or border-line, as should any refusing at first trial, and should be recalled in 3–6 months time. If the child is only reading 6/9 and has (or has ever had) squint or a family history of myopia, it is wise to refer him for full ophthalmological examination without further delay, together with all those who read only 6/12 or worse in one or both eyes. The reason for referral should always be clearly recorded in the case notes (Harcourt, 1971).

Near test

Many ophthalmologists consider it unnecessary to test the near vision of children routinely. However, this was done to obtain some information concerning relative child–adult competence, to discover whether certain children with poor distant vision were similarly handicapped close by and to evolve some standard way of recording recovery of near vision in young children with an amblyopic eye under treatment (Stuart and Burian, 1962). I had already observed that when his amblyopic eye is responding to treatment, a child usually manifests recovery of near vision before distance vision, in other words he retraces the normal developmental stepping-stones of visual learning. A card of graduated letters was therefore specially prepared which has proved useful with very young children, and with non-speaking or illiterate older children. It was found that normal 4-year-old children and many $2\frac{1}{2}$–3-year-olds were able to match down to the smallest letters with each eye separately, although the use of print as small as this in children's books would be inadvisable.

The record should state the test-name and line of smallest letters read, as my standardization differs slightly from that of Law (1951; 1952).

Colour vision test

A useful colour vision test for young children, using the same letter matching procedure, was designed by Gardiner (1973).

TESTS FOR PARTIALLY SIGHTED CHILDREN

Partially seeing children constitute a severely handicapped group whose visual difficulties are complex, difficult to analyse and seldom fully appreciated (Harcourt, 1975). The Panda Test has recently been designed for assessment of such young children, employing nine white letters or figures on black ground (Sheridan, 1976a).

In addition to determining visual acuity for near and distance, other aspects of the visual competence of partially seeing children should be investigated such as eye movements, ability to fixate, stereopsis, peripheral fields, appreciation of colour, shape, size and perspective, co-ordination in locomotion and manipulation of eyes, body and limbs. At school age, difficulties in reading, writing and drawing must also be investigated. Preferred level of illumination needs to be determined. The indefinable qualities of 'drive' and visual comprehension are all-important. Direct observation of a child's performance in clinical and social situations is always more revealing than any hearsay report. A large proportion of visually handicapped children suffer from additional, often obscure, neurodevelopmental disabilities. Their emotional problems are also highly individual and complicated (Lansdown, 1969, 1975; Zinkin, 1975).

The difficulties of assessing the complicated problems of visually handicapped infants and young children on the fringe of a busy out-patient clinic are insurmountable. Reliable results can only be obtained when comprehensive testing procedures are carried out by paediatrically experienced professionals in friendly surroundings (Reynell and Zinkin, 1975). The interests of individual handicapped children can only be served if close co-operation between ophthalmologists, paediatricians, psychologists, educationalists and therapists in planning treatment and training is not only discussed but put into everyday practice.

Hearing

Previous investigations regarding the development of everyday auditory competence in babies and young children (Sheridan 1976b) taught the need to differentiate between the mainly physiological aspects of sensory functioning (hearing) and the mainly psychological aspects (listening). To this end the following terminology is employed.

Hearing is reception of sound by the ear and its transmission to the primary auditory area of the cerebral cortex. It therefore depends upon effectively functioning peripheral and intracranial structures.

Listening is paying attention to what is heard in order to interpret its meaning. It develops in close association with cognitive and affective maturation and depends upon favourable opportunities to learn from experience.

In connection with auditory competence it is also desirable to distinguish between language and speech.

Language is the use of one or more coding systems for the purpose of interpersonal communication.

Speech is the use of systemized, articulated vocalizations for audible expression of words.

The nature and acquisition of the four principal forms of language-code has been described in detail (Sheridan, 1976c). By reason of its auditory implications this discussion is mainly concerned with spoken, verbal language.

PHONETIC AND PSYCHOLOGICAL PRINCIPLES

Without entering into details regarding acoustic properties of sound and physiology of speech, a brief account of underlying phonetic and psychological principles will help examiners to understand the potentialities and limitations of tests. Natural sounds, including noise, musical tones and phonemes are highly complex, possessing components over many octaves. Fundamental notes, deprived of their overtones, can be instrumentally produced as 'pure-tones' for testing hearing. All sounds, pure-tone or complex, possess qualities of pitch, intensity, duration and, in everyday life, occur sequentially and in space.

Pitch of a sound depends upon its frequency, i.e. the number of waves or cycles per second (cps or Hertz, usually abbreviated to Hz) which it initiates in the air. The 'speech range' stretches over some seven octaves from approximately 64 Hz, which is about 2 octaves below the fundamental note of middle C on the piano to 8192 Hz which is 5 octaves above middle C, i.e. 1 octave above the piano keyboard. Normal human ears can appreciate musical and other sounds below and above speech range.

For convenience the speech range is arbitrarily divided into three sections: the low frequencies below about 500 Hz, the high frequencies above about 3000 Hz and the middle frequencies between these. Frequencies below 1200 Hz provide most of the carrying power and emotional quality of speech, while those above 1200 are mainly responsible for intelligibility.

Excepting the long /ee/ (as in 'feet') and its shorter form /i/ (as in 'ship'), which have important components in the upper frequency bands, the characteristic components of all the vowel sounds are in the lower and middle frequencies, the sound /oo/ being the lowest of all in pitch. The chief components of consonant sounds are in the middle and high frequencies. The principal components of the nasal sounds /m/n/ng/ border on the lower frequencies. Those of the /r/w/l/y/ group of continuants are somewhat higher in the middle frequencies. The plosives /b/d/g/ and their voiceless equivalents /p/t/k/ are still higher in scale, bordering on the upper frequencies, while the sibilants /z/sh/s/ and the fricatives /f/v/th/ are the highest of all. The average vowel pitch of women is about 250 Hz and of men approximately one octave lower. High-pitched consonant components in both male and female voices are much the same.

Intensity of sound is measured in decibels (dB). The decibel level at which a vocal sound is delivered, therefore, determines its energy, loudness and carrying power. Vowels possess higher decibel intensity than consonants. The vowel /aw/ possesses the strongest power and vowel /ee/ the least. Sibilant and fricative consonants possess the lowest decibel intensity and, therefore, have weak carrying capacity. The weakest speech sound is the voiceless /th/. The difference in intensity level between /aw/ the strongest and /th/ the weakest of the phonetic units (phonemes) is approximately 30 decibels.

Thus, every ordinary spoken phrase requires the listening ear to appreciate sequences of complex sounds which swing rapidly over differences of 7 octaves in pitch and 30 decibels in intensity. For practical purposes one may assume that a conversational voice at 3 ft carries to the listening ear sound intensities varying between peaks at 55 to 60 dB and troughs at 25 to 30 dB. The most difficult sounds to hear are /s/p/f/th/ being highest in pitch and weakest in intensity.

Duration of speech sounds has important bearings on intelligibility. The short plosives /p/t/k/ are often more difficult to appreciate than the continuants /ch/sh/s/ which possess components in even higher frequency bands. The split-second timing of vocal cadence, pauses and stress contributes significantly to auditory comprehension. How stereophonic hearing assists intelligibility is still imperfectly understood.

HEARING TESTING OF YOUNG CHILDREN

Tests in use at present fall into two broad categories:

Screening devices used in large-scale surveys to sort out quickly and effectively individual children requiring further investigation.

Diagnostic procedures to define more precisely the nature and severity of individual hearing and listening disabilities.

Considerable research has been carried out on both types of test. Notable British authorities include Ewing (1957), Taylor (1966), Whetnall and Fry (1964), Murphy (1964), Rutter and Martin (1972), Beagley (1973), Martin and Martin (1973) and Fisch (1974).

General considerations

To make sure that a child possesses adequate hearing over the full range of sound waves essential for speech recognition it is necessary to test his response to spoken utterances. His reaction to other meaningful sounds possessing similar characteristics in pitch, intensity, duration and stereophonic properties provide useful supporting evidence regarding his auditory acuity and his ability to interpret the world of sound in which he lives. However, until he has given unmistakable evidence that he hears, that he can imitate, and that he can correctly articulate and sequence separate phonemes to form words and sentences, it is not possible to be certain that he possesses normal auditory discrimination. From about $4\frac{1}{2}$ months onwards a child's own spontaneous vocalizations provide valuable clues to his capacity for appreciating the cadences and phonemic elements of spoken language. His utterances should, therefore, be carefully noted and the mother's report of his speech and hearing habits must always be obtained. Even when reliable pure-tone testing becomes possible, clinical speech tests are essential (Sheridan, 1948; Fisch, 1974).

It needs to be kept constantly in mind that hearing for pure-tones and hearing for speech, although closely related, are not identical. Sophisticated electro-physiological procedures now available (Beagley, 1973) provide valuable information regarding the severity of hearing loss, the sound cycles involved and the location of blockage in the complex auditory relay system between cochlea and cortex, but they cannot show how any individual child interprets what he does hear. Some children with poor auditory discrimination and gross speech defects produce normal audiograms. Other children with appreciable loss for pure-tones function as adequately hearing individuals. Therefore, while it is desirable to apply and compare results of both tests it is essential to determine hearing for speech in the acoustic conditions and situations of everyday life.

Since the primary aim of testing is to obtain information regarding the child's everyday hearing, materials employed and conditions of application should be graded according to the child's developmental level, general understanding and experience.

Capacity for sustained auditory attention of infants and young children for distances beyond 4 or 5 ft tends to be inconsistent, although it is possible to demonstrate prompt response to exceptionally alerting auditory stimuli at considerably greater distance. For this reason only near tests are given to children under 15 months, the distance varying from $1\frac{1}{2}$ ft at 6 months to 3 ft at 9 months, and up to $4\frac{1}{2}$ ft after 12 months. Recording of testing distance is essential.

A child normally learns to speak first from constantly listening to spoken words, addressed directly to him in meaningful situations (i.e. mother-teaching at mother-distance), then by imitating utterances he has already come to recognize when they recur in similar context, and finally by spontaneously using them in appropriate new situations. Hence the child's own vocal communications provide good evidence of his ability to hear, comprehend and employ spoken language.

The STYCAR procedures
These tests are intended to provide information regarding the presence and extent of everyday hearing. The sounds and words used were carefully selected both for their acoustic properties and for their psychological significance in relation to expected mental capacity, emotional maturity and social experience. Originally designed for handicapped children, they have proved equally useful for normal children. They can be carried out in any quiet room and the material required is familiar and easily replaceable. They are simple enough to be readily grasped by young children, but when correctly applied provide clear-cut evidence regarding auditory capabilities. For valid interpretation the tests must be carried out by appropriately experienced professionals, closely observing the child's individual responses. They are essentially clinical in nature and not amenable to conventional statistical analysis.

The mental age-levels given are approximate and, although the procedure provides useful information concerning developmental status, the series is not designed as an intelligence scale. The terms pass and fail do not apply. Children manifesting deviation from the pattern of hearing and speech behaviour considered to be appropriate for their chronological ages require immediate referral for full diagnostic investigation.

The following general rules for application of testing procedures are necessary to give valid results. The mother (M) or other familiar adult should be present. Although it is permissible to vary the spoken carrier phrases and (sometimes) the order of application, the prescribed materials and methods used must not be varied.

Vocalizations or speech personally observed by the examiner (E) during the interview should be recorded. An account should be sought from mother about the child's everyday hearing and speech behaviour and this clearly recorded as hearsay evidence.

After age 2 years application of tests appropriate to the child's chronological age should be attempted first, having checked recognition of test items at conversational distance (3 ft). If the child shows the slightest confusion in recognition the test should be discarded in favour of an easier one in the same series.

It is also essential to test the child's visual competence since this is important for early localization of sound and later for lip-reading.

The record should state test used, distance, and results obtained.

BIRTH TO 6 MONTHS

During the past decade the auditory responses of young infants including neonates have been extensively studied. Instrumental testing procedures employed demand sophisticated equipment and trained personnel, but careful observation in everyday situations fortunately provides very useful information. An infant's span of selective visual and auditory awareness is fragmentary in time, and limited in space to the confines of care-giving activities. Hence until the infant is able to sit up and move head and limbs freely, soft, varied, meaningful sounds close by are more likely to evoke consistent responses than loud, featureless noises farther away. From 12–14 weeks unmistakable, discriminatory localizing responses to nearby meaningful sounds, particularly a human voice, can be evoked.

The more formalized testing procedures given below are broadly classified according to age groups, allowing for considerable overlapping.

6–12 MONTHS

Infants of this age are comparatively easy to test, particularly those between 9 and 12 months. The infant has already learned to associate certain sounds with human beings and meaningful events but he cannot yet take the source of these sounds for granted. Consequently he is impelled to support his uncertain powers of auditory recognition and localization with visual reinforcement. Hence his immediate response to an alerting sound is to turn with a look of enquiry towards the person or object originating it. This localizing reaction probably plays a necessary part in normal stereoscopic and stereophonic learning in space and time.

Procedure. E should stand 1–3 ft to the side of C but outside his range of peripheral vision. To ensure consistent results the first sound stimulus should be given at ear level. Until about 8 months sounds below horizontal plane are not easy to localize and above it even harder (Murphy, 1964). Sounds in midline behind or above the head are difficult to locate at any age.

Infants of 6–7 months are friendly and curious but later the near approach of strangers is unwelcome. Hence E should not make boisterous frontal overtures but while keeping in sight at respectful distance, engage in introductory conversation with M. The gestural, visual, auditory and vocal reactions of C to E's voice and to M's will be instructive.

Sound-makers employed are high-pitched 'Nuffield' rattle (Kemp, 1977), spoon in cup, tissue paper, handbell and selected speech sounds delivered very quietly. The rattle must be positioned, held and moved correctly (Sheridan, 1976b). The other objects are applied at distances of 1½ ft (at 6 months) to 3 ft (8 months and upwards), paper rustled very softly, handbell tinkled very gently and spoon merely stroked round the inside brim of cup. Sounds are applied for 2–3 seconds. Each sound should be separated from the next one by a silent interval of at least 2 seconds. Speech test sounds are the low-tone vowel 'oo' repeated in sing-song cadence, two to four times (e.g. 'Oo-oo John, oo-oo') and high-tone consonants 's-s, t-t, ps-ps-ps, pth-pth-pth', repeated rapidly four to six times.

Ambient noise in ordinary rooms is very variable so that monitoring with a portable sound level meter is desirable.

With normal infants of 6 months and upwards first application of the stimulus usually provokes instant turning, often with a delighted smile, and when the sound is repeated on the other side of his head the infant will promptly localize it in the new position. Younger infants are slower to react and may show discrepancy of 1 or 2 weeks in acquisition of ability to localize between right and left ears.

If the infant gives clear-cut response to any four of the five test sounds, including rattle and high-tone consonants, it may be assumed that he possesses adequate hearing for speech, but it must be remembered that these tests are not fine enough to exclude partial deafness (particularly high-tone loss) with absolute certainty. All doubtful responders and infants known to be 'at risk' require careful follow-up.

Normal development of vocalization and speech is dealt with elsewhere (Chapter 9). It is only necessary to mention here that appreciable delay in appearance of tuneful babbled strings of repetitive syllables such as 'daa-dad, baba, mama', normally beginning about 7–8 months, is a significant pointer to possible hearing and speech difficulties and should be closely followed up.

12–14 MONTHS

Children of this age are often very difficult to test. Hence when response to a first test is unrewarding all children considered to be at risk should be referred for expert opinion without further delay. At this stage a child is actively exploratory and resentful of restriction, especially in strange surroundings. He probably has sufficient auditory experience to localize and interpret the foregoing sound-makers without needing to repeat visual verification. Having conceded one brief glance, he may show no further interest. If the child is not yet able to co-operate in simple 'give and take' toy tests (described below) response to his mother's or the examiner's quiet voice across the room and the tonal quality of his own spontaneous utterances will provide useful information of hearing for speech.

14 MONTHS TO 2 YEARS

First toy test
Material includes the four familiar objects (not miniatures) listed below.

Procedure. Addressed by name at conversational distance C should be requested courteously but firmly to hand to E in this order the cup, ball, toy motor car and dolly. At this age definite commands are more likely to produce results than gentle suggestions. Similar quiet instructions to hand the objects to M may then be made at 7–10 ft. Following this an unexpected sounding of rattle or high-tone consonants will usually provoke a well-defined response.

Five toy test may be attempted after about 20 months. Objects employed are the same cup and ball with a miniature motor car and baby doll and a small coloured wooden brick. These objects provide information about the child's hearing and speech.

Procedure. With C facing at conversational distance, E presents the objects slowly in the following order, saying 'Here is a cup' (the responsive child will delightedly echo 'tup'). 'Here is a ball and a motor car', then presenting the doll E says 'What's this?' and waits for C to say 'dolly' or 'baby'. If C does not speak E says 'A dolly, and here is a brick' (the word brick is acoustically essential and must not be altered to block.) Then holding out his hand flat (not suggestively cupped) E instructs in order 'Give me the ball please . . . the brick . . . the car . . . the dolly'. Replacing the toys, E slowly retreats to 7–10 ft as before, continuing instructions to hand toys to M.

Children of this age can usually recognize and name parts of the body and items of clothing. The following 'doll vocabulary' provides a useful test involving discrimination of most common vowels and consonants. Suggested order of delivery is: shoe, hair, nose, foot, eye, arm, mouth, leg, ear, teeth and, if desired, the more difficult high-tone words chin, cheek, knee, wrist, may be added.

CHILDREN OF 2–3 YEARS

At this age tests of hearing and speech become increasingly reliable. Play audiometry may be possible (Sheridan, 1976b). In addition to the five toy test and doll vocabulary the following clinical test is applicable.

First cube test is applicable from about 2½ years onwards and occasionally earlier.

Procedure. E places the cup and six wooden 1 inch bricks before C saying 'Now we're going to play another game. See these bricks? When I say in . . . in . . . in I want you to put a brick in the cup. It will get quieter and quieter, like this (demonstrating) . . . You try.' E gradually drops out the vowel and sounds only the consonant; 'in . . . in . . . n . . . n . . . n. Good.' 'Now I'm going over there and when I say lift, lift, I want you to lift a brick out of the cup and put it on the table. It will get quieter and quieter like this (demonstrating). Try.' Having made sure that C understands the procedure, E moves 10 ft from C's right ear. 'Ready? Lift, lift, ift, -f, -th- (the voiceless /th/ as in thin). Good.' E then repeats the test for left ear. C must not be allowed to lip-read. Sounds are delivered at irregular intervals in order to prevent automatic performance. Clinically it is usually exceedingly simple to monitor C's manipulations. Children greatly enjoy this game and it is a very sensitive test. Effective occlusion of ear not under test is advisable whenever possible (see below).

Whether or not the child appears to hear normally if he shows any deviations from the expected development of spoken language he should be referred immediately for expert examination. He may be generally retarded, or high-tone deaf, or suffering from one of the developmental language disorders. Denied normal ability to speak, he may express his frustration in tears and tantrums, or take refuge in silence and social withdrawal. Such children, unhelped, are seriously at risk of wrongful diagnosis.

CHILDREN OF 3–4 YEARS

Seven toy test is applicable from about 3 years onwards, holding interest to 6 or 7 years, and up to 16 years with mentally handicapped children.

The 7 objects employed were selected, after extensive research in hospitals, training schools and nurseries, for everyday familiarity and acoustic properties of names.

Procedure. Sitting opposite C at a table E slowly places the toys in front of C from C's right to left in the following order: car, plane, fork, spoon, knife, doll, ship. He requests C to name each in turn. If C remains silent E speaks the name clearly, requesting C to repeat it, checking auditory and speech performance again at the end of the row. If C still shows uncertainty it is best to discard this test in favour of the easier 5 or 6 toy test. If response is satisfactory, E, using a quiet conversational voice, says 'Where is (or show me) . . . the spoon, doll, fork, car, knife, plane, ship, the spoon, the car, the ship'. For acoustic reasons related to the vowel scale it is essential that the words should be spoken in this order. Still facing C but retreating to 10 ft E covers his mouth to prevent lip-reading and repeats the list.

To provide a more refined test of hearing each of C's ears is occluded separately by an assistant (A) who steadies C's head with one hand while firmly pressing the tragus of the ear not under test inwards with the other hand. Then from the appropriate side but out of C's visual range, E, having first warned C what to expect, repeats the words in a whisper at 10 ft.

Second cube test provides a more sensitive although slightly more difficult test of hearing for isolated high-tone consonants.

Procedure. Presenting eight wooden bricks E instructs as follows, 'Whenever I say a little sound, /oo/sh/t/ anything—I want you to take out a brick and put it on the table like this (demonstrating) -/ooo/-/ee/ . . . Now you do it. . . . /sh/t/s/p/f/th/—Good. . . . Now I'm going over there. . . .' Each ear is tested separately at 10 ft from the ipsilateral side, the other ear being occluded. Increased sensitivity depends upon the inclusion of the two plosives t and p with the unvoiced continuants /sh/s/f/th/ thus necessitating auditory discrimination for brief duration as well as pitch. In order to keep the consonant sounds at their highest pitch, E should imagine each as being preceded by the short vowel 'i' as in 'ship', e.g. (i)sh, (i)p, (i)th. It is essential to avoid 'ter' or 'per'.

Picture vocabulary tests can usefully be applied from 3 years onwards. Selective pictures for high-tone discrimination with standardized word lists and sentences, employing all the common vowels and consonants for recognition and repetition, are provided in both the STYCAR Hearing and Language (Sheridan, 1976c) Tests. Puretone testing using play-audiometry can be reliably applied from this age by experienced people.

5–7 YEARS

Children in their first 2 years in school readily co-operate in instrumental pure-tone and other audiometric tests as well as in clinical speech tests using pictures, selected word lists and sentences. Correlation between clinical and pure-tone tests is high but both should be routinely applied (Sheridan, 1976b).

The need for detailed history-taking and, whenever possible, for personal observation of a child's auditory responses and social competence at home, at school and at play requires no emphasis.

References

BEAGLEY H.A. (1973) Electro-physiological tests of hearing. *Journal of Disorders of Communication*, **8**, 115.

BENNET A.G. (1965) Ophthalmic test types. *British Journal of Physiological Optics* **22**, 238.

CATFORD G.V. and OLIVER A. (1973) Development of visual acuity. *Archives of Disease in Childhood*, **48**, 47.

EWING A.W.G., ed. (1957) *Educational Guidance and the Deaf Child*. Manchester: University Press.

FISCH L. (1974) Conditions for audiometry. *Proceedings of the Royal Society of Medicine*, **67**, 697.

GARDINER P.A. (1973) A colour vision test for young children and the handicapped. *Developmental Medicine and Child Neurology*, **15**, 437.

HARCOURT B. (1971) Functional and organic visual defects: the differentiation in school children. *Proceedings of the Royal Society of Medicine*, **64**, 619.

HARCOURT B. (1975) Clinical ophthalmic assessment in visually handicapped children. *Child care, health and development*, **1**, 315.

KEMP D. (1977) The Nuffield Rattle. *British Journal of Audiology*, (in the press).

LANSDOWN R. (1969) What the research doesn't know. *Special Education* **58**, 20.

LANSDOWN R. (1975) Partial sight, partial achievement? *Special Education, Forward Trends* **2**, 11.

LAW F.W. (1951) Standardization of reading types. *British Journal of Ophthalmology*, **35**, 765.

LAW F.W. (1952) Reading types. *British Journal of Ophthalmology*, **36**, 689.

MARTIN J.A.M. and MARTIN D. (1973) Auditory perception. *British Medical Journal*, **1**, 459

MURPHY K. (1964) Development of normal vocalisation and speech. In *The Child Who Does Not Talk. Clinics in Developmental Medicine No. 13*, eds. Renfrew C. and Murphy K. London: Heinemann.

REYNELL J. and ZINKIN P. (1975) New procedures for the developmental assessment of young children with severe visual handicaps. *Child care, health and development*, **1**, 61.

RUTTER M. and MARTIN J.A.M., eds. (1972) *The Child with Delayed Speech. Clinics in Developmental Medicine No. 43*. London: Heinemann.

SHERIDAN M.D. (1948) *The Child's Hearing for Speech*. London: Methuen.

SHERIDAN M.D. (1969) Vision screening procedures for very young or handicapped children. In *Aspects of Developmental and Paediatric Ophthalmology. Clinics in Developmental Medicine No. 32*. London: Heinemann.

*SHERIDAN M.D. (1976a) *Manual for the STYCAR Vision Tests*, 3rd Ed. London: National Foundation for Educational Research.

*SHERIDAN M.D. (1976b) *Manual for the STYCAR Hearing Tests*, 3rd Ed. London: National Foundation for Educational Research.

*SHERIDAN M.D. (1976c) *Manual for STYCAR Language Tests*. London: National Foundation for Educational Research.

STUART J.A. and BURIAN H.M. (1962) A study of separation difficulty: its relationship to visual acuity in normal and amblyopic eyes. *American Journal of Ophthalmology*, **53**, 471.

TAYLOR I.E. (1966) Hearing in relation to language disorders in children. *British Journal of Disorders of Communication*, **1**, 1, 11.

WHETNALL E. and FRY D.B. (1964) *The Deaf Child*. London: Heinemann.

ZINKIN P. (1975) The paediatrician's role in comprehensive assessment of the visually handicapped child. *Child care, health and development*, **1**, 335.

*The STYCAR Vision, Hearing and Language Tests (copyright) are published by The National Foundation for Educational Research, address NFER Publishing Co. Ltd., 2 Jennings Buildings, Thames Avenue, Windsor SL4 1QS. Berks.

A series of relevant colour slides/audio-tapes are available from the Medical Recording Service Foundation (MRSF), Kitts Croft, Writtle, Chelmsford CM1 3EH, Essex.

CHAPTER 9

Speech and Language Development and Assessment

'Language is a cognitive skill with affective components which performs a communicative function in a social context' (Rutter and Bax, 1972).

Normal Language Development

Knowledge of the range and sequence of language development in normal children is an essential prerequisite for understanding speech problems. This applies to comprehension of language (competence) as well as speech (performance).

Ingram (1969) offered a very useful approach to the study of language by suggesting that three aspects be borne in mind: phonological, syntactical and semantic. Phonology is the sound system of language which distinguishes between the different sounds and the intonation, rhythm and stress with which they are produced. Syntax represents the meaningful relationships of words to each other in an individual utterance. Semantics covers the meaningfulness of the child's language, whether described in words, gesture or play. In normal development these three aspects progress in a combined logical sequence, but in the child in whom one aspect is particularly distorted it is helpful in diagnosis to separate them in this way; e.g. in the common mild developmental speech disorders the syntax and semantics of the child's language are normal while phonology is slow in developing.

The first year

The newborn baby responds positively to a wide variety of sensory stimuli and shows a particular preference for the sight of his mother's face and the sound of her voice. Evidence for this is seen in quieting to her voice and in head and eye turning. Babies have distinct types of vocalization denoting pain, hunger or pleasure and mothers can recognize the individual characteristics of their own baby's cry. A clinical assessment is rarely requested or required at this age except when siblings or parents suffer from congenital deafness, but the mother's recollection of this period may be of considerable importance in assessing later development.

In the first few months of life infants show a great deal of interest in voices, even when they cannot see who is speaking. Even in the early weeks they can discriminate between very similar sounds such as /b/ and /g/ or /i/ and /a/. (Todd and Palmer, 1968). The amount of vocalization produced in response is affected by what the infant hears. This is a time when parents' interplay with their infant is most important. Language stimulation may be affected by puerperal depression, and in addition some adults feel that verbal contact with babies is beneath their dignity.

By 8–12 weeks spontaneous vocalizations are beginning to take over from the initial repertoire of cries, yawns, sneezes, gurgles, belches and coughs. The earliest sounds are described as 'cooing' as they consist mainly of vowels with occasional guttural sounds, e.g. 'arghroo-oo'. At around 4 months the infant begins to make sounds at the front of the mouth, e.g. 'ebe ebeb ebebeb' and 'aba abab'. Possibly these sounds are related to the development of a hard alveolar ridge and the imminent eruption of the incisor teeth. Certainly after 6 months the infant loves to produce long runs of this repetitive babble. As it contains the inevitable 'mum mum mum mum' or 'dad dad dada dad' there is frequently a markedly positive response from the respective parent and erroneous reporting of the child's first words. The first meaningful words other than mama and dada are usually said around 12 months of age but their appearance in normal children can vary from 8–18 months (Morley, 1965). Language comprehension normally precedes language production. An example of this is the child's understanding of and response to the request to wave bye-bye several months before he can say the words.

The second year

A child's passive and active vocabulary expands rapidly during the second year of life. Studies have shown (Smith, 1926; McCarthy, 1954) that by the age of 2 years a child will have 200 words or more on average in his active vocabulary. This progression does not take place in a regular fashion and it is not uncommon for parents to say that the child has stopped progressing or even gone back at times during the second year. This is particularly likely if the child goes through a stage of intensive jargoning, which so many do in the middle of this year (p. 78). While it may be interesting in an individual case for the parents to write down all the words that they hear the child pronounce and compare their lists at intervals, this arithmetical approach is not generally helpful, since it is not at all unusual to find normal 2-year-olds who have only 10–20 words in their active vocabulary. It is likely that the range of what normal children understand is less variable than the range of words which they produce.

During the second year many children start to enjoy completing the lines of songs and nursery rhymes. They are, however, unlikely to respond to requests to repeat words after an adult in the 'say after me' approach.

Use of words also develops a great deal during this period. Nouns are the first words acquired and they become less restricted in their meaning as the year progresses. An example of this is first naming the household pet (e.g. 'pussy cat'), then extending the use of 'cat' to other members of the feline race and finally naming a picture of a cat. Towards the end of the second year verbs, adjectives and adverbs are used increasingly. Pronouns usually appear just before 2 years and prepositions just after.

Initially when words are combined in phrases this is in the form of telegrammatic speech. Various 'pivot' words are used in conjunction with 'open' words (Braine, 1963). The pivot words are used repeatedly in different situations and are attached to a wide variety of objects in the open class. An example of this would be the expression 'Daddy gone' where 'Daddy' is the open word and 'gone' is the pivot word. The pivot can be used in other expressions such as 'Teddy gone' or 'potty gone'.

The marked increase in the depth of understanding of language is shown by the child's response to commands and instructions. He understands the difference between getting up and sitting down and when asked he will look for something to bring to an adult. He enjoys stories and takes a very active part in following the pictures in a story book, particularly if it is well known to him. He shows understanding of the uses of common household objects by mimicking their use in play. By the end of the second year play in a household setting can be quite complex, putting dolls in and out of bed, pretending to bath and feed them, using toy telephones and tea-sets.

2–5 years
The rapid advance of speech during this period is evidence of very complex development in the child's language. He progresses from the toddler stage when speech tends to accompany action to that of the 4-year-old whose command of language enables him to describe abstract ideas and use speech as a formidable weapon in preschool psychological warfare. By the time he goes to school the child has several thousand words in his active vocabulary and the length of his sentences rises from approximately two words at 2 years to around five words at 5 years. This does not mean that every sentence of a 5-year-old has five words in it as many utterances are much longer and many are shorter. The child begins to use conjunctions and the definite and indefinite articles (the, a) at about $2\frac{1}{2}$ years and these words are in common use by 3 years.

It is useful to note when a child uses the questions 'what?' (around 2 years), 'where?' and 'who?' (3 years) and 'why?' (by the age of 4 years). These questions become a game which can go on all day and elicit a great deal of spoken language from adults with accompanying attention (and sometimes frustration).

In the toddler age group it is not unusual to hear children echo the last few words of a sentence spoken to them. In most cases it is a transient phase which is often wrongly interpreted by parents as a sign of 'brightness'. In the child with persistent echolalia this is evidence of poor understanding of language and is frequently noted in the hydrocephalic child with a 'cocktail party personality'.

Children between 3 and 4 years (especially when excited and trying to describe an event which has just taken place) frequently develop marked dysrhythmia, either blocking of words or frank stuttering. The impression given by the child is that he has so much to say, so little time to say it and is still ill-equipped in his verbal repertoire. This common occurrence, which is usually described as 'cluttering', is a normal phase of development and does not indicate that the child will develop a stutter.

The articulation of words steadily improves to adult norms. The majority of children are readily understood from the time they start to speak, in spite of the typical consonant substitutions, but about one-third go through a phase when they are largely unintelligible even to their families. The production of vowel sounds relates more to the regional accents but consonant sounds and their gradual clarification appear to vary little from area to area and can be followed by repeated assessments on the Edinburgh Articulation Test (p. 173).

The development of syntactical rules progresses over this time and is shown by the way children treat irregular verbs as regular; e.g. 'I digged the garden' and their appreciation of nonsense sentences such as those in the ever popular Doctor Seuss books; e.g. 'Sam I am', 'Great Day for Up'.

After 5 years

Normally a child has mastered all the basics of spoken language by the time he goes to school but after this there is a continuing progression in the complexity of its use, particularly in relation to abstract thought. IQ tests make use of this gradual progression in the verbal aspects of their scores.

Some important influences

As a general rule girls show a faster pattern of speech maturation than boys but the difference is so small compared with the normal range that no special account need be taken of it. Certainly this is not a reason for disregarding a boy's slow language development.

Institutional care can have a profound effect in retarding language development (Tizard, 1969) and this retardation persists throughout childhood. The most likely explanation is the small amount of adult–child interaction in many institutions. The same effect may be seen in children brought up at home as there is no doubt that later born children from large families are slower in language development than children from small families.

Studies have repeatedly shown that twins are slower in their use of spoken language than singletons (p. 79) and this difference persists throughout childhood (Day, 1932).

In households where more than one language is used the child may be slow to learn to speak either or both languages. An added complication may be that one language is spoken with an unusual and difficult accent or even in a pidgin form. Children of such families may be further subjected to social deprivation and isolation. That this may well be a more important factor than the language problem is indicated by studies which show that early development of speech is little delayed when parents of different nationalities speak to the child each in his/her own language.

Social class differences are important. Early language milestones are similar but later performance of middle-class children is in advance of their working-class peers. The relative importance of genetic and environmental factors is still open to argument.

It is important to bear in mind when considering these influences, that while they often cause delay or advance in the maturation of spoken language, they must exist in extreme form to cause a speech disorder. Too often is a child's difficulty attributed in an off-hand way to the existence of one or more of these factors.   R.J. PURVIS

The Role of the Speech Therapist in Assessment

During an initial play period (p. 459) the speech therapist will be taking note of indications of understanding of speech and maturity of spontaneous vocalization.

Normally the child of 2 years has developed 'inner language' and shows this by understanding the symbolic nature of miniature objects. If he does so, even if there is no expressive language, the therapist can assume that he has some understanding of the world about him. By talking to the child and asking him to perform simple tasks it is generally possible to discover the extent of his comprehension of spoken language.

Frequently the child will produce spontaneous speech during the play session. This free conversation will give the therapist the opportunity to note gross deviations in articulation and sounds omitted and substituted. Multiple omissions and substitutions may be a warning sign that the child's hearing is defective even if previous tests did not show this. The therapist will watch for evidence of gesture, degree of eye-contact and attention span. Deficiencies in these skills are danger signals.

Once the right atmosphere has been created and the child is responding happily the paediatrician can join in and talk to the parents.

Following the initial visit a conference will be held involving all members of the assessment team. Before any form of speech therapy is begun further investigations may be needed and a more thorough assessment of language and speech.

The young child with a general developmental problem can be admitted to an activity group (p. 467) for on-going observation, assessment and treatment.

The child of 3 years or older with a mild developmental language problem may improve spontaneously following attendance at a preschool play group. However, a regular check is kept on the child's progress and further investigation may be indicated if behaviour problems occur, parental anxiety increases or there is not satisfactory progress in language development.

When the older child has a marked speech or language disorder a detailed assessment is necessary. Various formal tests may be used.

Reynell Developmental Language Scales (Reynell, 1969)
This test is particularly helpful in assessing children with language and speech delay who may or may not be retarded and those with neurological defects such as cerebral palsy. The test (p. 118) provides a comprehension age and expressive language age and frequently reveals weaknesses in the child's attempts to learn language structure. At the beginning of the Verbal Comprehension Scale A the child is asked to point to specific objects. In later sections the instructions become more complex, testing the child's ability to encode more than one idea at a time. Careful observation of the child's response to a double instruction may show that he fails to integrate two concepts successfully. Often

the mentally retarded child can only comprehend one idea, given verbally, at any one time. Presented with two instructions he becomes confused and is unable to respond correctly. The manner in which the child obeys the instructions may show if he fully understands prepositions such as in, on, upside-down and underneath.

The results of this test can provide the speech therapist with a basis for a programme to increase the child's comprehension of spoken language. If on the Reynell Scales comprehension is up to age but expression is not, the Expressive Language Scale can provide the basis for a programme to increase use of language.

Edinburgh Articulation Test (Anthony *et al.*, 1971)
The trained listener can identify marked articulation errors from the child's spontaneous speech but where a systematic record is needed, or a long-term record on which to assess progress, the Edinburgh Articulation Test is most useful. This was devised to test consonants in single word forms. The test consists of a book containing forty-one coloured pictures which are named spontaneously by the child or repeated after the examiner. Responses are recorded phonetically. Each test is scored in two ways, quantitatively and qualitatively. It is helpful to use a tape recorder because of the amount of transcription necessary. The handbook provides detailed information to help the therapist analyse findings. A comprehensive range of normal substitutions is given and also details of atypical articulatory characteristics. The quantitative sheet can be used as a record to monitor the child's progress.

Renfrew Picture Pointing Test (Renfrew, 1973)
Articulation errors occurring where there is good co-ordination of the oral and facial musculature may be attributable to poor auditory perception. The Renfrew Picture Pointing Screening Test for Auditory Discrimination gives a comprehensive method of testing auditory perception and allows for errors of vocabulary.

The test material consists of a picture book, instructions and scoring sheets. The pictures are designed to test phonetic sounds which are often confused by young speech-handicapped children. The child is allowed to scan the nine pictures on each page while the therapist points to each in turn, names it clearly and talks about it. The child then points to the pictures as they are named by the therapist. The results can be evaluated against possible discrimination errors, e.g. if a child of 5 years makes two or more discriminatory mistakes on any page, a course of auditory training based on these errors should be given.

The test is suitable for children of 5 years and older but by covering the last row of pictures on each page, children from $3\frac{1}{2}$ years can be tested. No ceiling for this test is given but it is found useful with children up to a mental age of 11 years where auditory difficulty is suspected.

Renfrew Action Picture Test (Renfrew, 1972)
This test is useful in assessing the child's capacity to comprehend syntactic rules.

It can be given to children from 3 years of age but the results are not standardized for those over 7 years. The test consists of nine action pictures, a scoring book and instruction manual. The therapist holds the pictures in her hand and shows each one in turn to the child. The question to be asked is printed on the side of the card facing the therapist. The answers are recorded exactly as spoken even if incorrect. Responses are scored separately for information and grammar. Discretion has to be exercised by the therapist to allow for unusual responses and dialectal differences but the detailed replies must be retained so that scoring will be consistent on any future test. The interpretation of the results may indicate several possibilities for the therapist to investigate, e.g. does the child know how to form plurals and indicate tenses; does he have a specific problem with grammatical construction of sentences?

Renfrew Word Finding Vocabulary Scale (Renfrew, 1972)
The scale is designed to assess the vocabulary of speech impaired children who are diffident about defining words. It tests the child's ability to find words from his memory bank rather than his ability to merely recognize words and can be helpful when the therapist suspects that the child has an expressive dysphasia. The use of nouns, verbs, adjectives and prepositions is tested. There are forty items which are presented to the child and pictures are provided to reduce errors from misunderstanding the questions about the last eleven items. The scale has been standardized on children between the ages of 3 years 6 months and 8 years 2 months. It is not recommended for those with suspected mental retardation because of the difficulty of some of the material.

The last two tests mentioned can be used to assess the language potential of a child who has bilingual parents and is showing a disturbed language pattern.

S. GOODWIN

References

ANTHONY A., BOYLE D., INGRAM T.T.S., MCISAAC M.W. (1971) *The Edinburgh Articulation Test*. Edinburgh: Churchill Livingstone.

BRAINE M.D.S. (1963) The ontogeny of phrase structure: the first phrase. *Language*, **39**, 1.

DAY E.J. (1932) The development of language in twins: II. *Child Development*, **3**, 179, 298.

INGRAM T.T.S. (1969) The development of speech in childhood. In *Planning for Better Learning. Clinics in Developmental Medicine No. 33*, eds, Wolff, P.H. and Mac Keith R. London: Heinemann.

MCCARTHY D. (1954) Language development in children. In *Manual of Child Psychology*, ed. Carmichael L., 2nd Ed. London: Chapman Hall.

MORLEY M.E. (1965) *The Development and Disorders of Speech in Childhood*, 2nd Ed. Edinburgh: Livingstone.

RENFREW C. (1972) *Word Finding Vocabulary Scale*. Revised Ed. Oxford: Renfrew.

RENFREW C. (1970) *Action Picture Test*. Oxford: Renfrew.

RENFREW C. (1973) *Picture Pointing Screening Test for Auditory Discrimination*. Oxford: Renfrew.

REYNELL J.K. (1969) *Reynell Developmental Language Scales*. London: National Foundation for Educational Research.

RUTTER M. and BAX M. (1972) The normal development of speech and language. In *The Child with Delayed Speech. Clinics in Developmental Medicine No. 43*. eds. Rutter M. and Martin J.A.M. London: Heinemann.

SMITH M.E. (1926) An investigation of the development of the sentence and the extent of the vocabulary in young children. *Studies in Child Welfare, University of Iowa*, **3**, 5.

TIZARD J. (1969) The role of social institutions in the causation, prevention and alleviation of mental retardation. In *Social-Cultural Aspects of Mental Retardation*, ed. Haywood H.C. New York: Appleton-Century Crofts.

TODD G.A. and PALMER B. (1968) Social reinforcement of infant babble. *Child Development*, **39**, 591.

Further Reading

BRITTON J. (1972) *Language and Learning*. Harmondsworth, Middlesex: Penguin Education.

HUTCHISON S. (1968) Some quantitative and qualitative criteria in articulation test scoring. *Journal of Disorders of Communication*, **3**, 36.

LURIA A.R. and LUDOVICH F.I (1971) *Speech and the Developments of Mental Processes in the Child*. Harmondsworth, Middlesex: Penguin Education.

O'CONNOR N. (1975) *Language, Cognitive Deficits and Retardation*. London: Butterworth.

RENFREW C. and MURPHY K., eds. (1964) *The Child Who Does Not Talk. Clinics in Developmental Medicine No. 13*. London: Heinemann.

REYNELL J. (1969) A developmental approach to language disorders. *British Journal of Disorders of Communication*, **4**, 33.

RUTTER M. (1970) *Language Retardation and Psychological Development*. London: Invalid Children's Aid Association.

RUTTER M. (1972) *Maternal Deprivation Reassessed*. Harmondsworth, Middlesex: Penguin Education.

RUTTER M. and MARTIN J.A.M. eds. (1972) *The Child with Delayed Speech. Clinics in Developmental Medicine No. 43*. London: Heinemann.

SECRETARY OF STATE FOR EDUCATION AND SCIENCE (1975). *Language for Life. Report of the Committee of Inquiry*, Chairman, Bullock A. London: Her Majesty's Stationery Office.

CHAPTER 10

Assessment of Gross and Fine Motor Function in Cerebral Palsy

Assessment is a prerequisite for any physical treatment. Assessments vary in depth and scope as well as content. Those required before treatment of any neurological disorder are among the most complex, and the assessment of cerebral palsy is probably the most comprehensive of all.

Physical assessment of the cerebral palsied child involves the systematic cataloguing, by observation and examination, of the child's present physical state and functional level; what he can do and, more important, what he cannot do that he should be able to do at his age. If he has physical inabilities, it is not enough merely to note them. Why is he unable to do these things? What is preventing him?

There are many possible reasons such as: disorders of muscle tone, tonic reflex activity, poor or absent postural control, inefficiency of muscles, extraneous movements, deformities, mobile or fixed and associated with soft tissue contractures, apraxia and agnosia.

If such deficits as these are insufficient to account for poor function, then the associated factors of motivation, intelligence and opportunity must be taken into account.

Physical assessment is an essential preliminary to any physical treatment, because the selection of techniques and the frequency and manner of their application cannot be decided until the patient's physical inabilities and their physical causes (as they appear at that time) have been identified.

A detailed physical assessment carried out at intervals of 4–6 months is one way of monitoring progress as well as the efficacy of treatment techniques. However, in cerebral palsy the maturing of an inherently abnormal nervous system poses different physical problems at different stages of development. Changes should be noted whenever they appear. Therefore assessment must also be a continuous process and changes in current status should be reflected in the treatment given.

In addition, physical assessment provides information about a child's level and quality of function that is useful to all disciplines united in providing his total management.

For a first assessment of a new patient to be truly objective, it is better that the physiotherapist should be unaware of the finer points of the diagnosis and those physical signs already recorded by the paediatrician or neurologist. Probably the only essential piece of prior information is the child's date of birth and his real age if he was born prematurely. If the therapist has not read the case notes, her findings cannot be influenced by preconceived ideas.

Perhaps some findings may seem to conflict. Perhaps the pattern that emerges will be one that cannot conveniently be given any of the accepted labels. This is preferable to the unconscious suppression of a definite physical sign. Everything of note should be faithfully recorded and any findings apparently at variance with the general presentation can be brought to the attention of the neurologist for confirmation and explanation. Few children with cerebral palsy fit exactly into any pigeonhole and what seems puzzling at one stage may appear entirely logical in retrospect.

The amount of information to be assembled makes it highly unlikely that the assessment can be completed in one session. Ideally, the child should be admitted as a daily patient to a special centre where he can be observed discreetly at length, can play with and get to know his therapist and be formally tested only after he has settled, when he is much more likely to present a true picture of himself. However, ideal conditions seldom prevail and assessment must often be done on an out-patient basis.

It is possible to establish immediate rapport with some infants and very young children and in such cases, two or three sessions may suffice. For those children who are wary of strangers, correspondingly more appointments will be needed, but preferably arranged fairly close together, in order that all aspects of assessment may be covered.

Every treatment centre has devised its own particular way of recording physical assessment, but while the manner of recording may vary, the content is unlikely to do so to any degree. This is because all physiotherapists working in the neurological field are united in the belief that only after a thorough assessment can the right techniques be selected and applied. What follows is not a method of assessment and recording identical to any other, but that employed at the Armitstead Child Development Centre, Dundee.

Children assessed there range in age from birth to 5 years. It therefore follows that not all sections are always relevant to every child. However, a standard format ensures that nothing that is of note is likely to be overlooked. The assessment form used at this Centre is shown in Table 10.1, and the composite sections of it are discussed below.

General Observations

Assessment begins as soon as one sees the child; whether he is carried into the room by his mother who then sits down and arranges him on her knee, or whether he is first observed lying flat, propped up, moving aimlessly about or playing purposefully in a nursery group. The following questions come immediately to mind:

Does he seem interested in his surroundings, or is he apathetic?

Is he making any movement and if so, does it appear to be wholly volitional, wholly involuntary, or a mixture of both?

TABLE 10.1. Form used to record findings on physical assessment of cerebral palsied children

Armitstead Child Development Centre
Physical Assessment

NAME———————————————— ADDRESS————————————————

D. of B.———————————— ————————————————

REAL AGE IF PREM.————————— ————————————————

PROBABLE GROSS MOTOR AGE————— PROBABLE FINE MOTOR AGE—————

GENERAL OBSERVATIONS

TONE   TONIC REFLEX ACTIVITY

Postural Reactions	P or A	N or Ab
PRIMARY REACTIONS		
1. Primary standing		
2. Primitive walking		
3. Placing reactions (a) upper limb		
(b) lower limb		
4. Moro reflex		
BASIC RIGHTING REACTIONS		
1. Neck righting reaction		
2. Body righting reaction on body		
ASSOCIATED RIGHTING REACTIONS		
1. Sideways protective extension of arms (parachute)		
2. Forward protective extension of arms (parachute)		
3. Landau reflex		
EQUILIBRIUM REACTIONS		
1. Prone		
2. Supine		
3. Sitting		
4. 'All fours'		
5. Standing		

MUSCLE INEFFICIENCY

TABLE 10.1.—*continued*

EXTRANEOUS MOVEMENTS

CONTRACTURES AND DEFORMITIES

PRESENT PHYSICAL ABILITIES

Gross Motor				*Fine Motor*	
Can	Rating	Can	Rating	Can	Rating

FURTHER COMMENTS

METHOD OF LOCOMOTION

TABLE 10.1.—*continued*

PRESENT PHYSICAL INABILITIES (FOR REAL AGE)		
Cannot	Cannot	Cannot

CORRELATION OF PHYSICAL DEFICITS AND INABILITIES

AIMS OF PHYSICAL TREATMENT

MANAGEMENT   EQUIPMENT

EXPLANATION OF CODES

Postural Reactions	*Present Physical Abilities*
Column 1—P or A = Present or absent	Rating
	D—Laboured, difficult
Column 2—N or Ab = Normal or abnormal	M—With moderate difficulty
(for real age)	E—Easily, but in an abnormal pattern of movement
	N—Normal performance

Is there anything about his posture or movements suggestive of tonic reflex activity, athetosis or ataxia?

If he is moving about the floor, is he doing so in a normal or an abnormal pattern of movement? Is his method of locomotion normal for a child of his real age?

If he is handling toys, how does he grasp them and what is he doing with them?

Such observations as these can be recorded before handling the child confirms and defines the problems more accurately. Later, his reaction to handling by a comparative stranger and the way he 'feels' in one's hands can also be recorded in this section.

Tone

The following questions should be considered:

Is there any variation from the norm and if so, is this increased or decreased tone general, or does it vary in degree from limb to limb, side to side or muscle group to muscle group?

Is any variation static, or is it affected by the position in which the child is placed?

Is the abnormality sufficiently marked to impose a definite limitation on function?

Abnormalities of muscle tone are further discussed on p. 277.

Tonic Reflex Activity

The most disabling reflexes in the young child are: asymmetrical tonic neck reflex, symmetrical tonic neck reflex and tonic labyrinthine reflex (p. 275).

The presence of the asymmetrical tonic neck reflex is normal in the very young child (Table 10.2), but its persistence after the age of 6 months is definitely abnormal. The symmetrical tonic neck reflex appears briefly in the normal child when he is beginning to crawl; the tonic labyrinthine reflex is always pathological.

The tonic neck reflexes arise in the proprioceptor organs of the neck muscles and the tonic labyrinthine reflex is evoked by stimulation of the otolith organs of the labyrinths. Thus all three are manifested in response to voluntary or involuntary changes in the position of the head.

Asymmetrical tonic neck reflex
When this reflex is present, turning the head to one side produces an extension of the limbs on that side, with flexion of the limbs on the other (p. 29). It is usually stronger on the right. Asymmetrical tonic neck reflexes can have a marked effect on motor function. If they are very strong, they take over completely, making it very difficult for the child to sit, to use his hands or to walk.

Symmetrical tonic neck reflex
Here, extension of the head stimulates extension of the arms and flexion of the legs, while flexion of the head induces flexion of the arms and extension of the legs. These reflexes are only rarely released in isolation, being usually present

TABLE 10.2. Normal development of postural reactions

Months:	1	2	3	4	5	6	7	8	9	10	11	12+
Moro	+	+	+	±	weak	very weak						
Placing reaction—limbs	+	+	+	+	+	+						
Asymmetric tonic neck reflex	±	+	+	±								
Primary standing	+	+										
Primitive walking	+	+										
Neck righting reaction	+	+	+	+	±	±	±	±	±	±	±	
Body righting reaction on body						+	+	+	+	+	+	±
Landau reflex			±	+	+	+	+	+	+	+	+	±
Protective sideways extension of arms						±	+	+	+	+	+	+
Protective forward extension of arms								±	+	+	+	+
Equilibrium reactions												
Prone						+	+	+	+	+	+	+
Supine							+	+	+	+	+	+
Sitting								+	+	+	+	+
Prone kneeling									+	+	+	+
Standing												±

with asymmetrical tonic neck reflexes. Strong symmetrical tonic neck reflexes make it virtually impossible for a child to maintain the prone kneeling position or to crawl.

Tonic labyrinthine reflex

Here, flexion of the head induces an overall increase in flexor tone and conversely, extension of the head is followed by an increase in extensor tone. Again, this reflex is rarely observed in isolation but usually in conjunction with tonic neck reflexes.

Either type of reflex may predominate and determine the type of abnormal motor response.

Other points to be remembered about these three reflexes are: the tonal changes induced by tonic reflexes are not instantaneous. There is a variable time lag and this must be taken into account; symmetrical tonic neck reflexes in particular exercise a more marked influence on the arms than on the legs; and reflex influence, while essentially geared to the position of the head, can also vary in degree according to the total position of the child.

Other relevant tonic reflexes are as follows.

Associated reactions
Here, strong use of one limb may induce an increase of hypertonus in others.

Positive supporting reaction
This is a normal response to weight-bearing which can be grossly exaggerated
in the spastic child, when contact between the forefoot and the ground, plus
weight-bearing, reinforces the typical pattern of extensor spasticity, i.e. extension,
adduction, medial rotation and plantar flexion (Fig. 10.1).

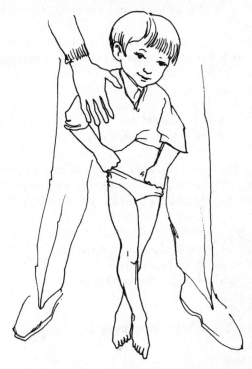

FIG. 10.1. Exaggerated positive supporting reaction in a spastic child aged 3½ years.

The assessment of tonic reflex activity is necessary for the following reasons:
it is an important indication of the severity of the child's motor handicap; if
marked, it places considerable limitation on both position and activity, and it is
an important factor influencing the choice of treatment techniques. An obvious
example of this would be the futility of attempting to teach a child to crawl
while he shows strong symmetrical tonic neck reflex activity. These reflexes
and reactions have been extensively described by the Bobaths (1966, 1971, 1975).

Postural Reactions

Normal postural reactions such as the righting and equilibrium reactions form
the automatic background of co-ordination for voluntary, skilled and learned
movements.

Normal postural reflex activity comprises automatic adjustments to changes of posture and antigravity action together with proximal fixation for the performance of distal movements. The gradual development of these righting reactions underlies and explains the sequence of normal motor development and therefore, their presence or absence at the wrong or right time has considerable significance in determining the cause of certain physical inabilities (Table 10.2).

The reactions selected at the Armitstead Child Development Centre as being of particular relevance to assessment and the methods of testing these are as follows.

When recording, it is customary to indicate whether the presence or absence of each reaction is normal or abnormal for the child's real age.

Primary reactions
Primary standing. The infant is held upright with the soles of the feet on a supporting surface. Then, by standing the child first on one leg and then on the other, an extensor response is elicited in the standing leg.

Primitive walking. The infant is placed on a table and supported in an upright standing position. The reaction of primitive walking is provoked by a slight forward inclination together with gentle forward propulsion.

Placing reactions of upper and lower limbs. The child is held vertically and the dorsum of the foot or back of the hand brushed against the edge of a plinth. This stimulates a response of flexion at hip and knee or elbow and then the plantar surface of the foot or palmar surface of the hand comes up to rest on the plinth.

Moro reflex. This reflex is described elsewhere (p. 36, 276).

Basic righting reactions
Neck righting reaction. With the child lying supine, the head is rotated to one side. There then follows a reflex rotation of the trunk to the same side (Fig. 10.2a and b). If the pelvis is fixed, the shoulder girdle and trunk follow the head. If the thorax is fixed, the pelvis rotates to the opposite side.

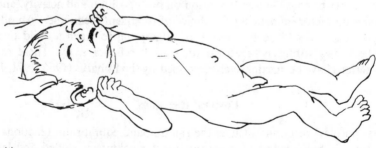

(a)

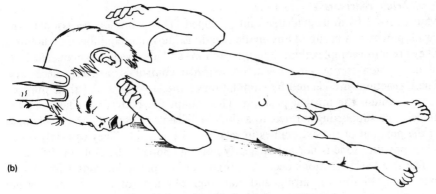

Fig. 10.2a and b. Neck righting reaction.

Body righting reaction on body. This is initiated as for the neck righting reaction, but the response is allowed to continue through side lying into prone. Therefore, there is a greater degree of rotation around the body axis.

Associated righting reactions
Protective sideways extension of arms (sideways parachute reaction). The child is supported at waist level in a sitting position and tipped to one side when the arm on that side should extend in a saving reaction, the hand opening with fingers extended and spread.

Protective forward extension of arms (forward parachute reaction). The child is turned into prone, held free in the air around the upper trunk and then moved quickly head first downwards when both arms should extend forwards in the saving reaction.

Landau reflex. The child is lifted prone, supported only by one hand under the chest. Positive response is shown in Fig. 10.3 (p. 138).

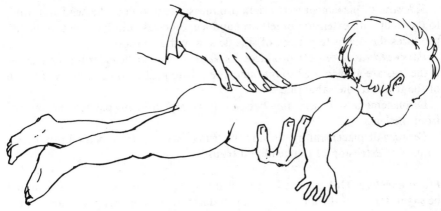

Fig. 10.3. Landau reflex.

Equilibrium reactions

Man evolved from a quadruped into a biped. This evolution necessitated the development of a group of automatic reactions known as equilibrium reactions. They are more complex than righting reactions and are specific to man. The level of integration is not yet known, but cortical control is probably necessary. These reactions are elicited by stimulation of the labyrinths and their purpose is to maintain the upright position. They adapt the body to a change in the angle of its supporting surface, to a shift in its centre of gravity and to changes in the position of the extremities in relation to the trunk. They can only occur when postural tone is normal or nearly normal (Bobath and Bobath, 1975).

The five basic reactions occur in prone, supine, prone kneeling with elbows extended ('all fours'), sitting and standing. Methods of testing and normal responses are as follows:

Prone. Test on a tilt board (Fig. 10.4). The normal reaction pattern is one of side flexion of head and trunk together with abduction of arm and leg on the raised side.

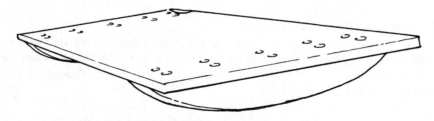

Fig. 10.4. Tilt board.

Supine. Test on a tilt board. The normal reaction pattern is again one of side flexion on the raised side.

Sitting. Testing is carried out on a static supporting surface with the feet un-supported.

Sideways displacement to the right produces side flexion of the head and trunk to the right with extension of left arm and leg. Sideways displacement to the left produces the opposite pattern of side flexion and extension.

Backward displacement produces forward flexion of head, trunk and arms. If the legs are also rotated to one side, then there is also compensatory rotation of the trunk to the same side.

Displacement sideways and backwards is procured by passive movements from the legs.

Forward displacement by pushing the trunk forwards from behind produces a pattern of extension of the head and trunk.

Prone kneeling. This is tested on a tilt board. On the raised side, there should be slight flexion of the limbs with a slight decrease in supporting tone and on the lowered side, a bracing of the limbs in extension and slight abduction. If the tilt is marked, then there should also be some side flexion of head and trunk to the raised side.

Standing. Standing is tested by passive movement at the hips. If displacement is to the right, then there will be slight side flexion of head and trunk to the left and abduction of the left arm and leg.

Muscle Inefficiency

Because a physiotherapist is concerned with movement and through movement, with muscles, an estimation of individual or group muscle weakness or strength forms an important part of most assessments. However, in cerebral palsy, such estimations are extremely difficult and to speak of weakness and strength at all can be misleading, since muscle performance is relative to muscle tone.

Abnormal muscle tone is the main factor influencing muscle action. This tonal abnormality may be variable and is frequently influenced by tonic reflex activity as well as by the position, segmental or total, in which any movement is attempted. Furthermore, abnormal muscle tone provokes certain peculiarities of muscle behaviour which should always be borne in mind when making any attempt to pinpoint the particular muscle group or groups preventing or distorting a specific functional activity, or contributing to a deformity.

These peculiarities are: inhibition in one action but not in another, difficulty initiating a contraction, difficulty maintaining a contraction, inability to work consistently through full range, poor endurance and early fatigue, difficulty in relaxing (a spastic muscle can more easily contract than relax).

These factors notwithstanding, there are certain circumstances in which it is necessary to attempt a more structured and measureable assessment of group muscle power; for example, before and after surgical intervention.

The Medical Research Council scale (1956) is used (Table 10.3), but should be modified. The steps from 3 to 4 and 4 to 5 are large ones and the use of plus and minus allows for greater accuracy.

TABLE 10.3. MRC Scale for evaluation of muscle power.

0	No contraction
1	Flicker or trace of contraction
2	Active movement with gravity eliminated
3	Active movement against gravity
4	Active movement against gravity and resistance
5	Normal power

Extraneous Movements

This is a convenient blanket term adopted to include the involuntary movements of athetosis and the disruption of voluntary movement of ataxia. A brief verbal description of the extraneous movements is required, including observations about frequency, severity, provoking circumstances and the degree of limitation such movements impose on useful function.

Contractures and Deformities

The term deformity is used here to mean a distortion of body shape obvious on inspection. Deformities in this age group are often mobile and usually secondary to disorders of tone. A contracture is a shortening of capsular, ligamentous or tendonous structures which prevents a full range of movement and produces a fixed deformity.

Physical Abilities

The child's gross and fine motor achievements are recorded here and also such static postural abilities as head control and balance in basic positions like sitting, since these static achievements are prerequisites of efficient movement. The manner of performance is also noted. In an attempt to restrict the volume of written recording that assessment entails, the following code is used: D laboured, difficult; M with moderate difficulty; E easily, but in an abnormal pattern of movement; N normal performance.

It is still sometimes necessary to add verbal comments if the exact nature and facility of a particular ability is to be satisfactorily indicated and space is reserved for this purpose. In addition, it is always desirable to have an explicit word picture of any mode of locomotion and space is also provided for this.

Physical Inabilities

A child's physical inabilities are all those postural, gross motor and fine motor abilities appropriate to a normal child of his real age which he does not possess.

Since there is some diversity of opinion about the appropriate ages for the achievement of some of these skills, it is highly desirable that there should be uniformity of opinion within any particular unit if confusion is to be avoided. A comprehensive list should be agreed upon and adhered to for check reference (Appendix 10.1).

Correlation of physical deficits and inabilities
Making the connection between cause and effect gives the physiotherapist her short-term aims of treatment, and consideration of the sum total of the information she has gathered will enable her to choose suitable positions for treatment and techniques which will be effective without reinforcing such adverse neurological manifestations as tonic reflex activity.

Under the heading of management, space is provided for a brief outline of special advice for all concerned with the child about handling, carrying and positioning. Space is also provided for itemizing the child's special requirements for furniture, foot wear, walking aids and transport (p. 307).

Armitstead Child Development Centre—Assessment of Upper Limb Function

TABLE 10.4. Form used to record assessment of upper limb function.

NAME..   ADDRESS..

D. of B...   ....

REAL AGE (IF PREM.)............................   PROBABLE FINE MOTOR AGE.....................

OPTIMUM FUNCTIONAL POSITION

ADVERSE LOCOMOTOR DEFICITS

DISTURBANCES OF SKIN SENSATION

Tactile	*Stereognostic*

ANY KNOWN VISUAL DEFECT

TEST OF MANIPULATION

TEST OBJECT	*Right Hand*			*Left Hand*		
	RATING	NORMAL	ABNORMAL	RATING	NORMAL	ABNORMAL
Rattle/ teething Ring						
Brick 2″						
1½″						
1″						
Beads large						
medium						
small						
Small sweets						
Pegs and board						
Posting box						
Shape board						
Screwpeg and nuts						
Pencil thick						
medium						
thin						
Ball throw						
catch						

TABLE 10.4.—*continued*

ADDITIONAL COMMENTS

CODE
E Efficient
A Slow/adequate
I   Slow/inadequate
X Unable

SELF-HELP SKILLS

Function	Grading	Code
Feeding Spoon		I Independent
Fork		
Cup		M Minimal assistance
Tooth brushing		
Face and hand washing		L Lot of assistance
Toiletting		
Dressing Socks and shoes		X Unable
Pants		
Trousers		
Dress		
Shirt		
Coat		
Pullover		
Hat		
Buttons		
Zips		

FURTHER COMMENTS

MAIN PROBLEMS

SUGGESTED ACTIVITIES

Assessment of Upper Limb Function

The presence of certain pathological manifestations of brain disorder prevents effective use of the hands on account of: strong asymmetrical tonic neck reflexes which make it impossible for the child to grasp an object while looking at it, or to keep his head in mid-line; retention of a strong Moro reflex with absent head control; severe athetoid movements which make it impossible to bring the hands forward into a functional position, and strong associated movements.

However, if a child without any such totally disabling deficits who is old enough to use his hands with purpose has difficulty in doing so, then analysis of his fine motor function is indicated. A general physical assessment will already have been carried out and some opinion formed of the level of his fine motor performance, but only as part of a general picture. A more detailed test of skill is necessary if all the facets of his poor function are to be revealed.

The form used for assessment of upper limb function at the Armitstead Child Development Centre is shown in Table 10.4.

Method of assessment
An optimum functional position for using the hands and any physical deficits likely to impair performance will already have been noted, e.g. patterns of spasticity in the arm, muscle 'weakness' and any restricted movement in the joints of shoulder, elbow, wrist or fingers. Such relevant observations as these form the first part of the assessment.

Any tactile or stereognostic disturbances of sensation in the hands should also be recorded and also any known visual defect.

Manipulative testing and suggested testing materials. A wide selection of test objects should be kept from which those most suited to a child's age can be chosen.

Rattle or teething ring demonstrate ability to grasp and release in a very young child.

Bricks of varying sizes demonstrate ability to grasp, retain and release with the smaller ones posing relatively greater problems. Used to build a tower, bricks also provide a test of co-ordination.

Beads of varying sizes, being round, are harder to pick up and retain than bricks. Both bricks and beads can be put into a container as a test of precision.

Small sweets provide an incentive as well as demonstrating the ability to pick up a tiny object and to retain grip while transferring to the mouth.

Small pegs and a board are used to test fine grip and precision.

Posting boxes and shape boards give some evidence of ability to recognize shapes as well as testing manipulative skill. Shape boards should have three or four basic geometrical shapes.

A screw peg and nuts require a certain sophistication of manipulation as well as testing the efficiency of pronation and supination.

Pencils and paper are used for testing dexterity, sustained control of a small object in use as well as copying ability. Pencils should be of varying thicknesses to accommodate varying strengths of grip.

Balls of several sizes for throwing and catching demonstrate hand–eye co-ordination as well as the ability to use both hands together.

Observation and recording of tests. The overall quality of performance is marked, giving each activity one of four gradings: E efficient; A slow/adequate; I slow/inadequate; X unable.

Next, the actual manipulation of the object is recorded as being normal or abnormal for real age. If it is abnormal, a short verbal description of the variant should follow. This is necessary, if the underlying physical cause is to be isolated and appropriate measures applied.

Children with problems of manual dexterity show a remarkable virtuosity of approach, but certain basic variants from the norm have been observed more frequently than others (Figs. 10.5a–d).

If a child has adequate mechano-motor equipment and is of a mental age to be able to copy or match straight lines and simple shapes, yet cannot do so, then he has either a disorder of perception (agnosia) or a disorder of performance (apraxia) and he requires a specific programme of sensori-motor stimulation (p. 326).

Self-help skills. The basic tests of manipulation are intended to do two things. To demonstrate how the child's way of using his hands differs from the normal and to highlight possible physical reasons for this, so that appropriate physical remedies can be sought. In addition, it is helpful to look at and grade certain

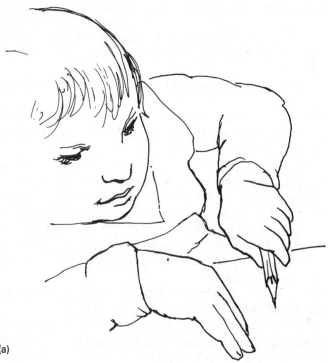

(a)

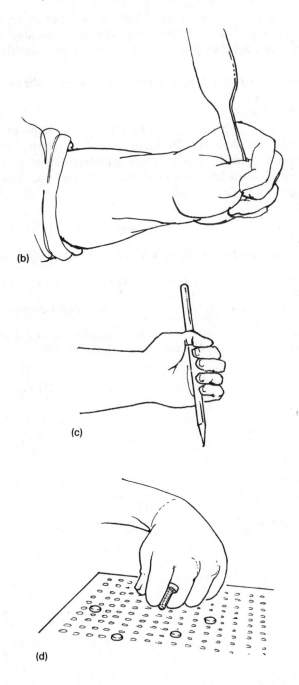

FIG. 10.5. Abnormal hand grips in cerebral palsied children of normal intelligence. (a) A diplegic child aged 4 years. (b) A diplegic child aged 3½ years. (c) An athetoid child aged 5 years. (d) A diplegic child with marked involvement of the upper limbs aged 3½ years.

basic self-help skills with which the child may or may not yet be familiar. Here, emphasis is on function and abilities are graded as independent, achieves with minimal assistance, achieves with a lot of assistance, or is unable.

Main problems. The main physical deficits contributing to the child's difficulties are listed here.

Suggested activities. Wherever possible, exercises to improve dexterity are converted into play activities. Positions should be chosen which combine optimum manual dexterity with adequate considerations of posture, tone and the prevention of deformity. Toys which have presented problems in testing are often the best ones to facilitate improvement.

References

BOBATH B. (1971) *Abnormal Postural Reflex Activity Caused by Brain Lesions*, 2nd Ed. London: Heinemann

BOBATH K. (1966) *The Motor Deficit in Patients with Cerebral Palsy. Clinics in Developmental Medicine No. 23.* London: Heinemann.

BOBATH B. and BOBATH K. (1975) *Motor Development in the Different Types of Cerebral Palsy.* London: Heinemann.

MEDICAL RESEARCH COUNCIL (1956) *Aids to the Investigation of Peripheral Nerve Injuries.* War Memorandum No. 7. London: Her Majesty's Stationery Office.

Appendix 10.1

Physical Abilities: Developmental Check List

Name _____ D.O.B. _____ Doctor _____

Diagnosis _____

4 weeks		Date						
Supine	(1) Asymmetrical posture predominates							
	(2) Intermittent part way roll							
Pull to sit	(3) Head lag marked, briefly erect at 90°							
Prone	(4) Turns head to side							
	(5) Intermittent crawling movements							
Standing	(6) Axillary support, reflex weight bears							

6 weeks								
Supine	(7) Asymmetrical posture still predominates							
	(8) Large jerky movements, limbs							
	(9) Intermittent part way roll							
Pull-to-sit	(10) Head lag marked, briefly in line 45°–90°							
Held sitting	(11) Erects head momentarily							
Prone	(12) Head briefly raised in mid-line							

8 weeks								
Supine	(13) More rhythmic movements, limbs							
Pull-to-sit	(14) Head lag lessening							
Held sitting	(15) Head raised and erect longer							
Prone	(16) Head mid-line, chin raised 1–2 in.							
	(17) Hips mainly extended							

Physical Abilities: Developmental Check List—*continued.*

12 weeks
Date

Supine — (18) Symmetric posture of head and arms

Pull-to-sit — (19) Still some head lag

Held sitting — (20) Back straighter, head thrust forward

Prone — (21) Face at 45° to couch

(22) Rests on forearms

(23) Can free arms from under chest

Standing — (24) Axillary support, bears some weight

16 weeks
Supine — (25) Symmetric posture, head mid-line

(26) Engages hands mid-line

(27) Smooth rhythmic movements, limbs

Pull-to-sit — (28) Questionable head lag, compensates well

Held sitting — (29) Back straight except lumbar curve

(30) Head set forward, steadily erect

Supported sitting — (31) Sits 10 mins+ cushions at sides/back

Prone — (32) Face at 90° to couch, rests forearms

(33) 'Swimming', whole weight on abdomen

Standing — (34) Axillary support, bears most of weight

20 weeks
Supine — (35) Smooth rhythmic movements of limbs

Pull-to-sit — (36) May lift head at beginning

(37) Sit, lie down, no head lag

Held sitting — (38) Head erect in line with trunk

Supported sitting — (39) Sits 10 mins+ cushions at back

Prone — (40) Chest raised, arms extended

(41) On verge of rolling to supine

Standing — (42) Axillary support, bears weight longer

Physical Abilities: Developmental Check List—*continued.*

24 weeks · *Date*

Supine and pull-to-sit	(43) Lifts head at beginning						
	(44) Arms assist in pull-to-sit						
Supported sitting	(45) Leans forward, re-erects						
Prone	(46) Legs and arms extended, weight on hands						
	(47) Rolls to supine R/L						
Standing	(49) Chest supported, bears almost all weight						

28 weeks

Supine	(50) Raises head, looks at feet						
	(51) Rolls to prone over R/L						
Pull-to-sit	(52) Head comes up in advance of trunk						
Sitting	(53) Sits briefly, hands forward for support						
Prone	(54) Bears weight on one hand						
	(55) Continuous roll to R/L						
Standing	(56) Chest support, takes all weight, bounces						

32 weeks

Supine	(57) Pull-to-sit on 2 fingers						
Sitting	(58) Sits erect, hands up for 30–60 secs						
Prone	(59) Pivots on abdomen through 45°						
Standing	(60) Stands briefly, hands held						

36 weeks

Supine	(61) Just pulling to sit on cot sides						
Sitting	(62) Sits steadily 10 mins.+						
Prone	(63) Creeps forward (amphibian)						
	(64) May get up to hands/knees						
Standing	(65) Placed standing holds with 2 hands						
	(66) Attempting pull up, gets to knees						

Physical Abilities: Developmental Check List—*continued*.

40 weeks		Date						
Supine	(67) Pulls to sit easily on cot sides							
Sitting	(68) Sits indefinitely							
	(69) Sitting to prone							
	(70) Prone to sitting							
	(71) Pivots using hands to assist							
Crawling	(72) Mixture hands/knees and creep							
	(73) May bottom shuffle							
Standing	(74) Pulls up to stand							

44 weeks							
Standing	(75) Holding on, lifts and replaces foot						
Crawling	(76) Hands/knees position						
	(77) Bottom shuffles						

48 weeks							
Supine	(78) Assumes sitting without aid						
Sitting	(79) Pivots on buttocks using feet						
Standing	(80) Cruises, sliding hands						
	(81) Walks 2 hands held						

52 weeks							
	(82) Lowers deliberately from standing						
	(83) 'Bear walk' hands/feet						
	(84) Cruises lifting hands						
	(85) Walks one hand held						

56 weeks							
	(86) Stands alone briefly						
	(87) May take 1–2 staggery steps						

15 months							
	(88) Beginning to kneel unsupported						
	(89) Gets up to stand from floor						
	(90) Can walk across room						

Physical Abilities: Developmental Check List—*continued.*

18 months

Date

(91) Walks well, feet slightly apart

(92) Kneels upright, balanced

(93) Runs stiffly and carefully

(94) Crawls upstairs

(95) Walks upstairs one hand held

(96) Backwards downstairs

(97) Seats self in child-size chair

21 months

(98) Runs more smoothly

(99) Walks backwards (imitating)

(100) Squats in play 5 mins+

(101) Stoops to retrieve toy

(102) Walks upstairs holding rail

(103) Walks downstairs one hand held

2 years

(104) Runs, knees flex, arms alternate

(105) Squats for long periods

(106) Rises without aid of hands

(107) Walks up/down stairs holding rail

0		3
1		4
2		5

0 = Impossible

1 = Can be held in position

2 = Can hold position after being placed

3 = Active but abnormal

4 = Near normal

5 = Normal

L/R — If the box opposite the particular ability is divided by a diagonal, it is then possible to indicate (L) or (R) sides.

D. M. ANDERSON

CHAPTER 11

Assessment of Family Problems

Severe developmental disorders of the kinds described in this book present society with major problems far beyond those of medical treatment. They primarily involve the family who face weighty problems every day. There are the practical difficulties of daily living, such as the need to carry an increasingly heavy child up and down stairs and those associated with social aspects, as in the case of a mentally retarded child who is too immature to play with his peers and too big to play with those of his own mental age, or the case of an intelligent spina bifida child with bowel and bladder incontinence. Problems of education will arise when physical handicaps, mental retardation, specific learning disorders or hyperactive behaviour make education difficult within the normal system. There will be later problems of employment, the prospect of which may worry parents when their handicapped child is still young. These are but some of the areas of difficulty. The whole nature of family life is likely to be altered, often to a major degree, by the need to give frequent or constant attention to the disabled child.

Some of these problems make steady drains on the time, physical and emotional energy and on the finances of the parents, particularly where the child is moderately or severely affected. Families are as much in need of help (and as entitled to help) with these problems as with the purely medical ones.

All parents, even those who are not usually articulate, are equally likely to have troubled and complex questions about the purpose and significance of this major event in their lives. Anyone involved with the parents of handicapped children will recognize the agonized question, spoken or silent, 'Why has this happened to us?' Associated questions arise, often fearful, irrational or angry ones, about the cause of the handicap, whether anyone is to blame, whether there might be similar risk to further children and about the effect of the handicap and parental strain on the siblings. At least one hopes the last question is asked in relation to siblings as, too often, they are expected to show an unrealistic selflessness and maturity far beyond their years. While the problems raised by these questions may seem different in character from the practical ones outlined above, they are at least as distressing to the parents and much help is needed for their resolution.

The social problems associated with handicap can have malignant aspects in that they tend to penetrate and invade the social milieu of the child. The family are most profoundly affected but the child's immediate community and the wider society are inevitably involved in attitudes, policies and the provision of resources, often major and expensive. Unless social treatment is early and sustained, the social consequences of handicap may become irreversible and may be more destructive in the long run than the precipitating condition. It is everyone's loss when, for want of early, adequate and continued help to parents, the unity of the marriage is destroyed, siblings develop behaviour disorders or vast sums are spent on institutional care, because society denies the parents the kind of resources that enable them to keep the child at home.

These considerations indicate that social help of various kinds should be available concurrently with medical treatment. Recent legislation has laid the groundwork for social work help to be available to those in need through Social Service Departments in England and Wales and Social Work Departments in Scotland. Such help should be increasingly available in the future as numbers of qualified staff increase in these departments and as systems for provision of social work support to the Health Services are developed.

However, it would be misleading to suggest that social workers are the only profession capable of understanding the problems and providing social support. All other professional people, such as doctors, nurses and therapists, who are involved with the care of the child with neurodevelopmental disorders, are in a position to affect the social prognosis profoundly. Because these professionals are in frequent and regular contact with the family they can develop the kind of relationships which encourage and enable parents to cope successfully. The key to making such relationships effective in social terms lies in recognizing parents as partners, indeed as principal partners. Parents are the main agents for the care and treatment of their handicapped child, giving 24-hour cover 7 days a week, often with inadequate resources.

Diagnosis of Handicap

Parents never start as willing agents; they find themselves thrust into the role without options at the traumatic time of first diagnosis. If this is at birth or in very early infancy, they will have had no time to form bonds of affection with the infant. That difficulty may be compounded if the infant requires transfer to a special unit, particularly one at a distance. These circumstances may contribute to rejection of the child. Efforts made to enable the mother and infant to be together, either by frequent visits (with special transport provided if necessary) or by mother living in at the hospital, may pay social dividends later.

If the diagnosis is made later its effect is particularly likely to be destructive to the marital relationship (Kirakowska, 1976). It is then equally important to ensure that both parents are involved in being told the diagnosis. Since fathers are less likely to attend clinics or out-patient departments later, than to be visiting hospital at the time of birth, it may be necessary to make special arrangements to involve them in the diagnosis and the treatment aims.

At whatever time the diagnosis is first discussed the occasion is crucial for the social prognosis. Helpful information given with understanding, with acceptance of and concern for the parents' distress, with ample time to allow them to assimilate the information and above all with assurance of continuing help, may strongly affect their future ability to deal with the total problem.

Parents describe their feelings at this time as a compound of shock, pain, numbness, incredulity, anger and helplessness. There is no ready social analgesic. The best help that they can be given is time and support while they cope with their reactions. Parents react in various ways. They may be distressed and tearful and need to be allowed to talk about their feelings. They may be angry and seek to blame or they may try to deny the diagnosis and wish to seek other opinions, in which cases they need explanations, reassurance and a kind of constant, understanding steadfastness. These reactions may seem negative but are not, or at least need not be, if they are accepted as natural and channelled into a co-operative partnership.

On the other hand, a primary reaction which appears to be quiet acceptance or even indifference may be a cause for more concern. Parents may react in this way because they have not understood and do not realize the implications of what is said; in this case the difficulties are only deferred. They may not have understood because the complexities of the condition are so esoteric; it is as likely that they are shocked into numbness and fail to take in more than the fact that there is something badly wrong.

Indeed for most parents there is probably a need for more than one discussion and more than one means of passing on the essential but often difficult to understand information, which they must have if they are to co-operate effectively in the child's management. The letter to the family doctor (copied to the community paediatrician and health visitor) should not only give the facts of the condition but outline what parents were told and how they seemed to react. This gives the opportunity of reinforcement from others who are familiar to them, who know their pattern of reaction in times of stress and their resources, and who can discuss some of the questions which parents were too confused or overwhelmed to ask at the initial interview. Many parent associations provide literature describing some of the main aspects of different disorders and their treatment and some parents find it helpful to have a written explanation which they can study later. Active members of local parents' groups may be prepared to offer friendship and support.

Parents will need the same kind of help when subsequent major decisions or changes arise, e.g. when surgical intervention is required, when new facets of the disorder are becoming manifest, when it becomes apparent that there will be special educational needs, when the child's condition is showing signs of deterioration and particularly when death is probable or certain. If throughout parents are offered attitudes of concern, support with practical difficulties, opportunities to ask questions and have the feeling that the professional staff are their allies, they will be enabled to act constructively.

Signs of Social Deterioration

Another way, in which those who have a long-term relationship with the families of handicapped children can work towards a healthy social outcome, is by being alert to signs of social deterioration and ensuring that direct social work help is then available. Such signs vary widely but include unusual tenseness in the parents or alternatively an apathetic response, apparent deterioration in the physical care of the child or in the appearance of the parents and indications of other disturbance in the family. Such deterioration is likely to be precipitated by extra stresses, e.g. when one parent is having to manage with very little support from the other, when one parent is absent (for reasons of employment, illness or desertion) or the father becoming unemployed. In these circumstances additional physical and emotional strain and possible financial difficulties will exacerbate the problems of management. Parents may feel that it is inappropriate to mention other troubles but they will usually respond appreciatively to general enquiries about how they are managing and more specific questions about siblings, finance, possibilities for leisure activities, baby-minding and so on.

Social Work Services for Handicapped Children and their Families

Social work departments now have responsibility for providing support to the Health Service. Two recent working party reports (Social Work Support for the Health Services, 1974 and Social Work Services in the Scottish Health Service, 1976) advise on the kind of arrangements that should be made with Health Boards to ensure an effective service. These will vary from area to area and will depend on geographical and other considerations.

Diagnosis and major decisions about treatment are likely to be made in a hospital setting. Continuing treatment will be supervised in hospital, assessment centre or local clinic and by the family practitioner. Paediatricians working in hospitals which employed social workers prior to reorganization will be accustomed to a referral system. This is unlikely to have altered in essence even if the structure is now different. Those hospitals which did not have the services of a social worker in the past, community services and family practitioners now have access to appropriate social work help through their local Social Work Department.

There are two main social work tasks. The first is to help families to come to realistic terms with those aspects of the disorder which cannot be altered and to plan their lives accordingly, taking all members into account. This requires knowledge of the medical condition, the stage it has reached and its implications, necessitating the closest co-operation and trust between medical staff and social workers. It also requires time, skill in communication and judgment in deciding when it is appropriate to encourage discussion of the painful, emotional aspects of the disorder. The social worker may work with a single member of a family, with the family as a unit or with groups of families with similar problems. He may also be engaged in trying to get the local community involved in accepting the problem helpfully.

The second task is that of mobilizing resources. This is complex and changing, requiring knowledge of a wide range of statutory and voluntary sources of help. The following are not placed in order of importance since needs will vary from one family to another and at different stages in the child's life.

Financial aspects

A number of studies have shown that the additional expense involved in rearing a moderately or severely handicapped child may be very much greater than is generally realized. For example, there may be considerable wear and tear on clothes (particularly shoes) from deviant walking patterns or from calipers; expense of many pounds per week may be incurred in visiting a child in hospital or in frequent outpatient attendances; there may be need for expensive equipment; there may be loss of parental earnings when a mother is unable to go out to work or when a father refuses more lucrative distant employment or overtime so that he can be available to help with the physical care of the child; there may be need for washing and drying machines where a child is incontinent and a family may have urgent need of a car (or a second car for the mother's use) because of the limitations on the whole family of the handicap of one member. Even when the income is good there may be financial strains, but when the income is moderate or poor the family's standard of living may be seriously affected.

Two statutory allowances, which can be claimed, are the Attendance Allowance and the Mobility Allowance. The first of these is a tax-free benefit for the severely disabled aged 2 years or older. There is a higher rate for those who need constant supervision by day and by night and a lower rate for those who need such attention by day or at night only. The Mobility Allowance is available from the age of 5 years for those who are unable (or virtually unable) to walk and are likely to remain so for at least 1 year. Leaflets giving fuller details of these allowances are available from Social Security offices. There are special needs grants for families whose incomes are at or below supplementary benefit level, e.g. for clothing, extra heating or special foods.

Additional help may be available from the Family Fund. This is financed by a government grant and administered by the Joseph Rowntree Trust. The fund was set up to provide aid for families caring for severely handicapped children under the age of 16 years. It is not intended to replace the statutory services oulined in the Chronically Sick and Disabled Persons Act (1970) but gives help which could not otherwise be provided. A grant from this fund might be given for or toward car purchase, driving lessons, alterations to houses, laundry equipment, special furniture, bedding and holiday expenses.

Aspects of practical management

In some instances parents may be less in need of direct financial help than of advice about existing services. Time is almost as important as money for families coping with handicap. This is particularly so when there are other children, for the handicapped child may unavoidably be seen as having priority and siblings may have to make do with what is left over. It may be possible to augment the time available to a mother by the provision of a home help (through the Social Work Department) particularly at times of special difficulty, such as during the later months of subsequent pregnancies or at times when siblings are ill. It may be necessary to relieve a mother of full time care of her handicapped child by admitting him to a nursery or play group. This has the additional advantage of helping the child socially and educationally.

As well as money and time, families need a suitable home in which to bring up a handicapped child, but houses (even the better ones) are not designed for the handicapped. Access outside and inside the house is important, particularly to toilet facilities, when there are problems of mobility or incontinence. Even one step is an obstacle for a child in a wheel-chair and stairs are a major hurdle for a child wearing calipers. It may be possible to carry an immobile 2-year-old child up and downstairs but, if at the age of 10, he is still not independently mobile, the house will by then have become unsuitable and potentially damaging to his physical and social development. Housing departments are often willing to rehouse families on medical grounds, but it is unreasonable to expect officials to be aware of the possible future implications of a medical diagnosis in housing terms. It is incumbent on the medical and social work staff to ensure that precise needs are stated on the medical certificate given for housing purposes and care should be taken to anticipate any future problems related to housing, although these may be surprisingly difficult to foresee. Occupational therapists from social work departments are now used by some local authorities to help in assessing housing needs before a house is offered. This seems an eminently suitable arrangement since the therapist is likely to be aware of probable future needs as well as present ones. As well as trying to ensure that housing is basically suited to needs, social work departments have powers to make such alterations and adaptations as are needed (e.g. provision of rails and ramps) to ensure maximum mobility. Medical staff and therapists are particularly well placed to judge when these aids are necessary.

Periods of family relief by admitting a child to hospital should be offered to parents before crises occur; usually a short break of up to 2 weeks is adequate. In some areas parents are encouraged to use this service by making arrangements directly with the secretary or nursing officer of the unit concerned rather than via a medical adviser. Special holiday arrangements may be made when problems of behaviour, incontinence or special diet make normal holidays difficult. Ideally this should be a holiday for the family as a whole rather than a further separation from the child, who may already have had frequent hospital admissions. However, on occasions, consideration of total family health suggests that the handicapped child should be admitted for that period to a hospital or holiday home, so that other members of the family can enjoy a complete change.

A wide range of practical aids is available including waterproof underclothing and incontinence pads, feeding aids, mobility aids and wheel chairs. Details about some aids and appliances are given in relevant National Health Service circulars and further information can be obtained from the Scottish Information Service for the Disabled and from the National Fund for Research into Crippling Diseases pamphlets entitled 'Equipment for the Disabled'.

Educational aspects
Elsewhere it is stressed (p. 322) that a child with disabilities, whether physical, mental or both, is in danger of being deprived because sensory and social experiences during the early, most formative years are abnormal. Many day nurseries, nursery schools and play groups are able to integrate handicapped

children into groups of normal children and give them special attention. Such facilities have great potential for compensating for deprivation and also for reducing the danger of over-dependency between parent and child. Social educ-tion of normal children in the group also benefits. In the past handicapped children were more often removed from the normal stream of society and thereafter found it difficult to become re-assimilated, since they and the normal world had never learned to live together.

The whole question of the child's education is one about which parents may need help and advice from a very early age. Even when it is not possible to give precise answers, because the progress of the disorder and future educational needs are uncertain, parents may need to talk over the possibilities and benefit from so doing, since too often they retain unrealistic expectations about eventual placement. From the age of 3 or 4 years parents should be brought into all discussions held with local education authorities and co-operate in decisions about the appropriate type of schooling for their child.

Voluntary Services

It is not only statutory services which have a role in aiding the families of children with neurodevelopmental disorders. Voluntary and self-help groups related to specific disorders are playing an increasingly significant part. Examples of national associations are the Spastics Society, the National Deaf Children's Society, the Spina Bifida Association, the Scottish Society for Mental Handicap and the National Toy Library Association. Such groups are generally run by and for families. Not every parent will choose to become a member but every parent should be given information about their local organizations. Many parents find great comfort in knowing that they are not alone and work enthusiastically with their associations. As well as mutual support the groups have a role in providing information. Some publish regular newsletters and information booklets which reinforce medical explanations. Some offer special holiday arrangements such as caravans or cottages to rent. They may also set up play groups, organize riding for the disabled and arrange loans of special equipment and suitable toys. Some raise money to sponsor specific research. These associations have a role in identifying major or acute social problems relating to different disorders and can concentrate on bringing pressure to bear on local and national government. A list of associations is given in Appendix 11.1.

Other less formal groups may be based on a local assessment centre or handi-capped nursery and include parents of children with a wide variety of disabilities. The existence of a parents' group within such a centre facilitates the involvement of parents in management and in continuing close relationships with professional staff.

Institutional Care

There will always be some instances where the severity of the condition or the limitation of the family's physical or emotional resources are such that no amount of supporting services could make care within their own family tolerable for the parents or reasonable for the child. In such instances, special measures of care may be necessary.

Where the main problem lies in the family's limited resources, the Social Work Departments may still be able to offer some care within the community. For example, some success has been achieved in fostering or adoption for handicapped children. Where the severity of the condition is the main problem, the proper solution may be good institutional care. An institution which is adequately staffed and which has resources of personnel and facilities to take the needs of the individual into account, may offer him more chance to develop his full potential than would a restricted home environment.

A decision to seek institutional care must never be imposed on the parents, since some constantly astonish by their resilience in coping with the apparently impossible. On the other hand, parents should not be denied institutional care for their child because they carry a clearly intolerable burden without complaint. Rather, as in all counselling of parents living with handicap, they should be encouraged to discuss and assess their feelings on the subject realistically, so that their decision is soundly based. They may need to be reminded that everyone in their family, the handicapped child, their other children and they themselves, have a right to a reasonable life.

References

DEPARTMENT OF HEALTH AND SOCIAL SECURITY AND WELSH OFFICE (1974) *Social Work Support for the Health Service*. London: Her Majesty's Stationery Office.

KIRAKOWSKA W. (1976) Counselling for special needs. *New Psychiatry*, **3**, 14.

SCOTTISH EDUCATION DEPARTMENT AND SCOTTISH HOME AND HEALTH DEPARTMENT (1976) Social Work Services in the Scottish Health Service: Edinburgh: Her Majesty's Stationery Office.

Further Reading

BLOOM F. (1974) *Our Deaf Children*. London: National Deaf Children's Society.

DEPARTMENT OF HEALTH AND SOCIAL SECURITY (1976) Help for Handicapped People (issued free by Social Security Offices and Social Work Departments).

FOX A.M. (1974) *They get this training but they don't know how you feel*. London: National Fund for Research into Crippling Diseases.

HEWITT S. (1970) *The Family and the Handicapped Child (Cerebral Palsy)*. London: Allen & Unwin.

NATIONAL BUREAU FOR CO-OPERATION IN CHILD CARE (1970) *Living with Handicap*. London: Longman.

WOODBURN M.F. (1974) *Social Aspects of Spina Bifida*. London: National Foundation for Educational Research.

Appendix 11.1

Information for Parents

PRACTICAL HELP FOR PARENTS OF A HANDICAPPED CHILD

Social Security benefits
The Department of Health and Social Security produces a comprehensive booklet containing details of all benefits available to families with a handicapped child.

The main benefits or allowances to remember are:

(1) Attendance Allowance
(2) Mobility Allowance
(3) Free prescriptions
(4) Hospital fares

Attendance allowance
For children aged 2 years and over who are severely disabled either physically or mentally and have needed a lot of looking after for 6 months or more. It is non-means tested and tax free. There are two rates:

(1) a higher rate for those who require attention by day *and* at night, and
(2) a lower rate for those who need attention either by day *or* by night.

Mobility allowance
A taxable weekly benefit to be introduced over a 3-year period from January 1976 for all adults under pension age and for children aged 5 or over who are unable, or virtually unable to walk.

Free prescriptions
For those with low incomes, children under 16, expectant mothers, mothers with children under one year and people with certain medical conditions. It is also possible to buy a 12 or 6 month prepayment certificate or season ticket if you need frequent prescriptions.

Hospital fares
Persons with a low income and having to attend hospital as a patient can get fares paid. If receiving supplementary benefit or family income supplement and able to use public transport, then fares to and from hospital can be refunded on production of order book or exemption certificate, when attending for treatment.

Other source of financial assistance

Family fund. A Government fund but administered by the Joseph Rowntree Memorial Trust, it aims to help families with children who are very severely handicapped. Help may take the form of goods, services or a grant of money for some definite purpose related to the care of the handicapped child. It is intended mainly to help in situations which are not at present covered by other services.

Address: The Secretary, The Family Fund, P.O. Box 50, York YO3 6RB.

Social work/social service departments
Services provided by social work departments for the physically and mentally handicapped and their families cover assistance with a wide range of practical and emotional problems associated with handicap. For detailed information contact local social work/social service departments, but a brief outline is given below:

(1) The personal services of a social worker assisting with practical and emotional problems.
(2) Domiciliary services: (a) home help
    (b) laundry service
    (c) telephone installation or rental
(3) Day centres and day nurseries
(4) Children's homes
(5) Holidays
(6) Recreational facilities
(7) Cheap travel and car sticker scheme
(8) Personal and domestic aids and home alterations

Frequently voluntary organizations and societies provide practical help of a specific nature relating to the type of handicap they cater for.

SOCIETIES AND ORGANIZATIONS

A very large number of societies and organizations exist which can offer help of a practical and/or supportive nature to a family with a handicapped child. Such societies can offer such help as holidays, equipment, advice, reading lists, and meetings with other parents.

For further information contact the society direct. Societies whose work covers the whole field of handicap are listed first, with those for a particular handicap under the name of that handicap.

General
British Red Cross Society,
9 Grosvenor Crescent,
London SW1X 7EJ.   Tel. 01 235 5454

Invalid Children's Aid Association (ICAA),
General Secretary,
126 Buckingham Palace Road,
London SW1.   Tel. 01 730 9891

National Association for the Welfare of Children in Hospital (NAWCH),
Exton House,
7 Exton Street,
London SE1 8VE.   Tel. 01 261 1783

The Family Fund,
P.O. Box 50,
York YO3 6RB.   Tel. 0904 29241

Disabled Living Foundation,
346 Kensington High Street,
London W14 8NS.   Tel. 01 602 2491/5

Scottish Information Service for the Disabled
13–19 Claremont Crescent
Edinburgh EH7 4HX   Tel. 031 556 3882

Autism
National Society for Autistic Children,
Mrs. M. Everard,
1a Golders Green Road,
London NW11.   Tel. 01 458 4375

Blind
Royal National Institute for the Blind,
224 Great Portland Street,
London W1N 6AA.   Tel. 01 387 5251

Research Centre for the Education of the Visually Handicapped,
M. J. Tobin,
School of Education,
University of Birmingham,
50 Wellington Road,
Edgbaston,
Birmingham.   Tel. 021 440 2450

Cerebral palsy
The Spastics Society,
16 Fitzroy Square
London W1P 5HQ   Tel. 01 387 9571

Scottish Council for the Care of Spastics,
22 Corstorphine Road,
Edinburgh EH12 6HP.   Tel. 031 337 2804

Western Cerebral Palsy Centre,
20 Wellington Road,
London NW8 9SP.   Tel. 01 722 9751

Deaf
National Deaf Children's Society,
31 Gloucester Place,
London W1H 4EA.   Tel. 01 486 3251

Breakthrough Trust (activities for deaf children and their families),
103 Ridgeway Drive,
Bromley,
Kent BR1 5DB.

National College of Teachers of the Deaf (books for parents and children),
Hon. Sec.,
Needwood School for the Partially Hearing,
Rangemore Hall,
Burton on Trent.   Tel. 028 371 2395

Royal National Institute for the Deaf,
105 Gower Street,
London WC1E 6AH   Tel. 01 387 8033

Deaf/blind
National Association for Deaf/Blind and Rubella Handicapped,
The Deaf Centre,
Hertford Place,
Queen's Road,
Coventry.   Tel. 0203 29680

Mental handicap
National Society for Mentally Handicapped Children,
Pembridge Hall,
17 Pembridge Square,
London W2 4EP.   Tel. 01 229 8941

Hester Adrian Research Centre,
The University,
Manchester M13 9PL.

Institute for Research into Mental and Multiple Handicap,
16 Fitzroy Square,
London W1P 5HQ.   Tel. 01 387 6066

National Association for Mental Health (MIND),
22 Harley Street,
London W1N 2ED.   Tel. 01 637 0741

Scottish Association for Mental Health,
57 Melville Street,
Edinburgh EH3 7HL.   Tel. 031 225 7632

Scottish Society for Mentally Handicapped Children,
69 West Regent Street,
Glasgow G2 2AN.   Tel. 041 331 1551/2

Dr. Barnardo's,
Tanners Lane,
Barkingside,
Ilford, Essex.   Tel. 01 550 8822

Mongolism
Down's Babies' Association,
c/o Chairman,
Quinbourne Community Centre,
Ridgeacre Road,
Birmingham B32 2TW.   Tel. 021 427 1374

Muscular dystrophy
Muscular Dystrophy Group,
26 Borough High Street,
London SE1   Tel. 01 407 5116

Speech impaired
Noah's Ark Trust (independent school and centre for children with severe
   communication difficulties)
31 Shaftesbury Road,
London N19 4QW.   Tel. 01 272 7230

British Dyslexia Association,
18 The Circus,
Bath,
Somerset BA1 2ET.   Tel. 0225 28880

Spina bifida
The Association for Spina Bifida and Hydrocephalus,
Devonshire Street House,
30 Devonshire Street,
London W1N 2EB.   Tel. 01 486 6100

Scottish Spina Bifida Association,
190 Queensferry Road,
Edinburgh EH4 2BW.   Tel. 031 332 0743

SPECIFIC NEEDS

Holidays
Break,
100 First Avenue,
Bush Hill Park,
Enfield,
Middlesex EN1 1BP.   Tel. 01 366 0253

Leisure
Pre-School Playgroups Association,
Alford House,
Aveline Street,
London SE11 5DJ.

Scottish Pre-School Playgroups Association,
7 Royal Terrace,
Glasgow G3.   Tel. 041 332 7310

Toy Libraries Association
Sunley House,
Gunthorpe Street,
London E1 7RW.   Tel. 01 247 1386

Riding for the Disabled,
National Equestrian Centre,
Kenilworth,
Warwickshire.   Tel. 0203 27192

National Association of Swimming Clubs for the Handicapped,
Mr. and Mrs. Edwards,
93 The Downs,
Harlow,
Essex.   Tel. 0279 25442

British Society for Music Therapy,
48 Lanchester Road,
London N6.   Tel. 01 833 1331

Family problems
National Marriage Guidance Council,
Herbert Gray College,
Little Church Street,
Rugby,
Warwickshire CV21 3AP.   Tel. Rugby 73241

Scottish Marriage Guidance Council,
58 Palmerston Place,
Edinburgh EH12 5AZ.   Tel. 031 225 5006

National Society for the Prevention of Cruelty to Children,
1 Riding House Street,
London W1P 8AA.   Tel. 01 580 8812

Further information on other Societies
This can be obtained from the following publications:
(1) The Sunday Times Self-Help Directory (1975), edited by Judith Chisholm and Oliver Gillie,
    published by The Times Newspapers Ltd.

(2) Handbook for Parents with a Handicapped Child (1972), by Judith Stone and Felicity Taylor, published by Home and School Publications.

(3) Services for the Young Handicapped Child (1972), published by the National Children's Bureau.

BOOK LIST FOR PARENTS OF HANDICAPPED CHILDREN

Autism

NATIONAL SOCIETY FOR AUTISTIC CHILDREN (1968) *Autistic children: innocents at risk.* £0.10

WING L. (1971) *Autistic Children: a guide for parents.* London: Constable. £2.00

Cerebral Palsy

FINNIE N.R. (1974) *Handling the Young Cerebral Palsied Child at Home.* London: Heinemann. £2.50

OSWIN M. (1967) *Behaviour Problems Amongst Children with Cerebral Palsy.* Bristol: J. Wright. £0.80

Deaf

EWING A. and EWING C. (1964) *Teaching Deaf Children to Talk.* Manchester: Manchester University Press. £2.75

Mental Handicap

KIRMAN B. (1968) *Mental Retardation.* Oxford: Pergamon. £0.40

DYBWAD C. (1973) *Mentally Handicapped Child under Five.* London: National Society for Mentally Handicapped Children. £0.15

CARLSON B.W. and GINGLAND R.R. (1962) *Play Activities for the Retarded Child.* London: Bailliere Tindall. £2.75

CLARKE A.M. and CLARKE A.D.B. (1959) *Practical Help for Parents of Retarded Children: some questions and answers.* Hull: Hull Society for Mentally Handicapped Children. £0.15

JACKSON C.H. (1970) *They Say My Child Is Backward: a guide for parents and educationalists.* London: National Society for Mentally Handicapped Children. £0.25

Mongolism

BRINKWORTH R. and COLLINS J. (1973) *Improving Mongol Babies and Introducing Them to School.* Belfast: National Society for Mentally Handicapped Children (Belfast). £0.50

VAN DER HOEVEN (1968) *Slant Eyed Angel: with a note on Down's syndrome.* London: C. Smythe. £1.50

Speech

CRAFT M. (1969) *Speech Delay: its treatment by speech play: a book for parents.* Bristol: J. Wright. £0.75

RENFREW C.E. (1972) *Speech Disorders in Children.* Oxford: Pergamon. £1.25

Spina Bifida (see p. 381)

FIELD A. (1970) *Challenge of Spina Bifida.* London: Heinemann Medical Books. £0.40

General Topics

PRINGLE M.L.K., DAVIE R., HANCOCK L.E., eds. (1969) *Directory of Voluntary Organisations concerned with Children.* National Bureau for Co-operation in Child Care. London: Longman. £5.00

ELWES N.D.B. (1973) *Aids for the Handicapped.* London: Spastics Society. £0.50

Note: Most organizations have book lists for parents.

E.C. GILCHRIST

CHAPTER 12

Examination of Infants and Young Children for Adoption

Adoption is a legal process whereby a child whose family is unable to care for him may achieve permanent and full family status in a substitute family. A basic knowledge of adoption law and of the processes involved enables doctors who are concerned with child adoption to be more effective in the reports they give and the advice they may offer to natural parents, the agency, the court, lawyers, the adopting parents or to the child himself.

The Adoption Act 1958 and the Children Act 1975 provide the present legal framework for adoption although other Acts, particularly the Children Act 1948 and the Children and Young Persons Acts 1963 and 1969, have some bearing on adoption practice (Appendix 12.1). The Children Act 1975 is being brought into practice gradually; some sections were implemented in 1976 and the rest will be introduced during the next 2 or 3 years as resources become available. A full adoption service will then be provided on a national scale, operated through local social work departments and approved voluntary adoption agencies.

Section 3 of the Children Act 1975 is of the utmost importance. It is a breakthrough in legal thinking that the child's interests come first in adoption proceedings and all future decisions in adoption practice must be made in the light of the following statement:

'*Duty to Promote the Welfare of Child*
3. In reaching any decision relating to the adoption of a child a court or adoption agency shall have regard to all the circumstances, *first consideration being given to the need to safeguard and promote the welfare of the child throughout his childhood*; and shall so far as practicable ascertain the wishes and feelings of the child regarding the decision and give due consideration to them having regard to his age and understanding' (author's italics)

Adoption has become an accepted feature of social life and when well managed is generally successful both for the adopting parents and for the child. Research in Britain and elsewhere has highlighted the value of adoption as a social service for children in need (McWhinnie, 1967; Seglow *et al.*, 1972; Fisch *et al.*, 1976; Bohman, 1972).

In Britain a total of about 23 000 decreasing to 21 000 Adoption Orders have been made each year in England and Wales in 1970–1975 and approximately one-tenth of this number in Scotland. About one-half of current adoptions are 'family adoptions', mainly by a mother and her new husband after a divorce. No medical examination is required in family adoptions and so the opportunity for counselling the mother on the complex relationships is missed. The Children Act 1975 suggests custodianship for such families (Grant, 1975).

It is not generally realized that healthy white babies are now seldom available for adoption, there having been a 75–80 per cent reduction in their numbers since 1968. There are, however, increasing numbers of other children who need homes. These include coloured children of all ages, children with mild handicaps requiring continued medical surveillance, children with more marked degrees of physical or mental handicaps who are now being offered for adoption, children with medical problems such as epilepsy and repeated urinary tract infections, and children with backgrounds of hereditary diseases or of psychopathy (especially schizophrenia and criminality), where the relative importance of genetic and environmental influences is unknown. The incidence of mental subnormality is high (up to 60 per cent in some series) in the offspring of incestuous relationships involving first degree relatives, usually father/daughter; other genetic conditions also have a significantly increased incidence. Some of these children may be offered for adoption. In addition there are older children who have usually spent several years in care or in foster homes and who may be over-sensitive, difficult or temperamental until well established in a warm accepting adoptive home. Sometimes two or three children in one family need to be placed together. It is encouraging that increasingly parents are being found who will provide loving homes for such children, previously considered difficult or impossible to place.

Early and repeated medical examinations are important for adoption purposes, in order that adopting parents do not unknowingly accept a handicapped child or, if willing to do so, that they fully understand the implications for the future of any handicap they feel able to accept. When abnormalities are found later, in children placed at an early age, some adopting parents are unable to accept the child fully and others are openly rejecting and unkind, although the handicapped child needs more understanding and acceptance than the normal child. It is for this reason that over the past 14 years the Medical Group of the Association of British Adoption and Fostering Agencies (ABAFA) has done its utmost to raise the standards of adoption medical practice by:

urging each adoption agency to appoint a competent medical adviser through whom medical information can be channelled and co-ordinated together with paediatric, child psychiatric, genetic and other consultant advisers;

ensuring that all babies and children for adoption are examined by competent doctors with knowledge and experience of child development and neurology;

producing medical report forms for both children and adopting parents which indicate what is needed and provide guide lines for the infant examination;

providing an advice service to doctors and others through the Association's headquarters, and by

providing educational facilities through the journal *Adoption and Fostering* (formerly *Child Adoption*), the publication of books and leaflets on various aspects of adoption and fostering, as well as by medical and social work meetings in various parts of the country to discuss the medical aspects of adoption.

The Processes of Adoption

It is necessary for doctors involved in adoption work to understand the various stages of what is a highly skilled and often lengthy social procedure. These processes can be summarized as follows:

the counselling of biological parents who wish to place their child for adoption;
a full assessment of the child and his potential;
the selection and preparation of adopters;
obtaining preliminary written consent to adoption from the natural parents or guardians of the child (under the 1975 Children Act there are alternatives, the parents may give their final agreement at any stage after the baby is 6 weeks old or a court may free the child for adoption without the parents' agreement in special circumstances;
the placement of the child in his new home and arranging for any special care or treatment he may need;
counselling for the adopters during the probationary period (this is at least 3 months by law);
the Court Hearing for making the Adoption Order;
registration of the child in the Adopted Children's Register; and
post-adoption counselling of natural parents and adopters when indicated and in some cases of the child later on.

At all stages it is the long-term welfare of the child which must be the first consideration for every worker involved, including medical personnel.

When the child is placed by a third party (most often by doctors and nurses) no pre-placement medical examination is required by law and very often there is totally inadequate assessment and preparation of the adoptive home. The court medical report is necessary before the Hearing and a conscientious doctor, seeing the child for the first time at this stage, may have misgivings about the placement but usually there is little he can do except discuss his concern with the guardian *ad litem*. When the Children Act 1975 is fully implemented third party placements will be prohibited.

The Purposes of the Medical Examination

The purposes of the medical examination of babies and children being placed for adoption are:

to ascertain the present medical and developmental status of the child;
to make a prognosis for his health and development;
to make recommendations for any special care or treatment which may be needed in the future;
to make reports for the agency, for the court and for the new family doctor.

It is *not* the purpose of the examination to 'pass' or 'fail' the child for adoption, although doctors have frequently acted in this way in the past. Theoretically no child is unadoptable if suitable parents can be found, although in practice some with severe mental or physical handicaps will not find a home.

Who Should Do the Examination?

The examination is a matter for a specialist who has training and experience in the development of young children and knowledge of normal emotional development and how this may be disturbed by family problems and by moving the child from one setting to another. Paediatricians, community child health doctors and some family practitioners have acquired the necessary expertise.

In cases where deviations from the normal are found, or where the child's condition or future needs are complicated in some way, it is important to discuss this with the medical adviser to the adoption agency, who will be responsible for informing the Case Committee of the implications of the medical reports. When the child is known to be handicapped, the paediatrician already caring for him will usually be the best person to make the reports. Careful plans must be made to link up the child's former medical care with specialists in the area in which he is being placed.

Increasingly, paediatricians are carrying out adoption medical examinations and advising agencies of children's future potential and special needs. When the medical condition is complicated it is even more important for a paediatrician with time and interest in the adoption field to be involved. Child psychiatrists are valuable colleagues when considering placements of some older children whose former existence may have led to serious emotional disturbance (Hersov, 1973). Psychologists have a part to play in the assessment of children past infancy and other specialists will be needed in particular cases. Geneticists can assist with increasingly accurate predictions on children with hereditary problems in their history and provide genetic counselling (Carter, 1969; Shields, 1975).

Medical Report Forms

The Adoption Agency Regulations require a child to be medically examined before he is placed with adopting parents and this examination and report is necessary to help the agency arrange a suitable placement. The Court Rules require the child to be examined before the Court Hearing and most Judges (or Sheriffs) prefer this to be done within the past month, at least in the case of infants. A statutory form is supplied by the court but this is most inadequate. When the Court Rules are re-drawn following full implementation of the Children Act 1975 new forms will be designed.

The Medical Group of ABAFA has designed medical report forms for use in the examination of infants and children being placed for adoption (Appendix 12.2). These are being used increasingly by adoption agencies throughout the country and it is hoped that they will become the statutory forms in the near future. The forms are intended to guide the examiners, to provide the agency's doctor with all the necessary information on which to assess the child's status, to help the social worker find the right home, and to ensure that the child's adopting parents and the new family doctor will have all the relevant medical information which they would have had if the child had been born to the family. This last may be important for the child as he grows older.

A knowledge of relevant social factors is desirable and social workers and doctors need to work closely with each other in the child's assessment.

Form A. The Parents' History
This concerns the biological mother and when possible the father. It is completed by the agency's case worker and incorporates information on the parents' physical and mental state, their medical history and the relevant medical and social histories of their families. The social worker confirms the details by enquiry from the family doctors involved.

Form B. The Perinatal Report
This is in two parts. Form B1 concerns the mother's obstetric history, the labour and the delivery. Form B2 records details of the physical state of the baby at birth and any abnormalities noted then or during his stay in the maternity unit.

Form C. Examination of the Child up to 2 years old
This is in three sections. The first refers to the history of the child and his natural parents obtained from Forms A, B1, and B2, and (from his current caretaker) social, medical, developmental and behavioural details since the neonatal period. The second section refers to the physical examination of the infant and the third to the developmental assessment; a developmental guide is provided for this last section. Finally the examiner is asked to state whether he found any mental or physical defect, whether further consideration of any matter is needed before placement and whether there is anything in the child's medical history or antecedents which should be discussed with the adopting parents.

Form D. Examination of the Child over 2 years old
This form includes the social, medical and neuro-psychiatric histories, examination of the child and the conclusions of the examiner on the child's physical, intellectual and emotional status.

Forms C and D are designed to cover the results of two examinations at intervals of at least 3 months. One will be made before placement and the other before the Court Hearing. Sometimes (e.g. when possible abnormality exists) intermediate examinations will be made and reports incorporated in the case records of the doctor concerned.

When Should the Examination be Carried Out?

The infant and toddler (0–2 years)
The earlier a child is placed with the adoptive family the better and delays for medical examinations must be avoided especially in infants and toddlers. If the pregnancy, labour and subsequent progress have been normal, there is no reason why a young infant, to be adopted soon after birth, should not be placed as soon as his mother is ready to make a firm decision. This may be in the first week or so of life if the mother is a stable girl who has had good support in pregnancy

and in the puerperium to help her come to her decisions. The child will be placed for fostering with the prospective family and at 6-weeks-old the probationary 3 months may begin, since at or after this age the mother may give her consent to adoption by law. This age was chosen to allow most mothers to recover fully from the effects of childbirth.

It is seldom wise to discourage a mother (especially of a first baby) from seeing and handling her infant even if briefly, because later on, and particularly when pregnant again, she may have considerable emotional turmoil with anxieties, fantasies and guilt about the relinquished first child. For example, she may wonder if it was *really* a normal baby and if she is 'able' to produce a 'good' baby. No compulsion should be used but a sensitive understanding of the mother's conflicts as she is working towards relinquishment should lead her attendants (doctor, midwife or social worker) intuitively to find the right moment for her to see this child who has caused so much anxiety for her. Some misguided obstetricians, especially in the private sector, prevent mothers from seeing their infants and this often results in deep unhappiness and regret later on. However, when the mother has already borne and nurtured a child or children, she may know that she would find relinquishment impossible if she handled this new baby. A glance at the child on the labour ward bed may be all that she can bear. Her wishes should be respected.

A few mothers may prefer to care for and even to suckle their babies before reaching a decision to place them for adoption. The attendants must realize that time may alter a mother's feelings which in any event often veer to and fro. It is important for the medical and nursing staff to be sensitive to all this and to discuss with the social worker, who is the mother's main counsellor and helper, the various plans and decisions reached at successive stages of pregnancy and in the puerperium. Flexible attitudes and sensitivity to the mother's changing emotions are crucial throughout this period.

If the child is to be placed in the first month of life the examination at birth (Form B2) together with the family and perinatal history (Forms A and B1) will constitute the major part of the medical assessment. A further examination a few days before placement will be concerned with the child's progress, behaviour and development, if no abnormalities have been detected thus far. A full medical report can then be made and recorded on Form C after the child has reached the age of 6–8 weeks and is in the adoptive home.

A difficult situation arises when there have been severe complications of pregnancy, labour, delivery or the neonatal period which might affect the baby's development (Davies, 1976; Brown *et al*, 1972). Situations that put the baby at significantly increased risk of later impairment are: maternal rubella; very low birth-weight ($\leqslant 1500$ g) and premature delivery (< 33 completed weeks of gestation), particularly if associated with a stormy postnatal period; prolonged sucking and swallowing difficulties, inappropriate for gestational age; hypertonia with irritability or, more importantly, hypotonia with apathy; convulsions other than simple biochemical fits; severe birth asphyxia and repeated apnoeic attacks, particularly if associated with frank neurological abnormality, and any infant reported as being 'severely ill' for a period of 2–3 weeks or longer.

However, there is a need to emphasis that exaggerated predictions of possible trouble have been greatly overdone in the past and have prevented many healthy children from finding homes (Forfar, 1969), as well as causing extra anxiety and tensions in and between adopters and adopted children. Nevertheless it may be wiser in these cases to defer adoption placement for 6–12 weeks until the infant's status can be ascertained with more confidence. An experienced foster mother is invaluable in assessing the child's behaviour during this time. There may be adopters, however, who prefer to accept the baby earlier and cope with whatever difficulties may arise, as they would have done if the child had been born to them. It must be made clear to them that most babies with abnormal neurological signs in the newborn period will lose them and become normal while others will show minor or even major handicap later on. Provided the adopters' ideas are realistic and it is judged that they are unlikely to reject the child if abnormality does present later, they should be allowed to have him whenever the mother is ready to place him. A careful appraisal of the child's progress will be needed in the immediate weeks after placement.

Older infants and toddlers, who may have stayed with their mothers or been in foster care or residential nursery before placement, vary very much in the security and care they have received. The examining doctor will need to take this into consideration during the developmental examination, as delays in growth or development or problems of behaviour may be due to changing or indifferent care and poor stimulation (Tizard, 1975; Wolkind, 1975).

When a child is at high risk of later handicap, or has a difficult background, it is probably wise to delay adoption placement for 8–12 weeks and observe development in an experienced and stimulating foster home. The full adoption may need to be delayed for 10–12 months, by which time most major developmental handicaps can be diagnosed.

After the 3 months probabionary period (which sometimes extends to 4 or 5 months) the Court will hear the adoption application and a second medical examination within a month of the Hearing is required on the prescribed Court Form. Because of the inadequacy of this, most responsible agencies arrange for a full assessment to be recorded on Form C for retention in their own records.

The preschool child (2–5 years) or older child

This examination should be made as soon as adoption placement is considered. It is strongly recommended that Form D should be completed for all children in long-term care of a local authority or voluntary child care agency. If adoption is planned later, the basic facts of the child's history and earlier status are then readily available and these, together with details of a fresh examination are recorded on another Form D.

After placement and before the Court Hearing, a further examination is needed as in the case of infants. When an older child is placed with adopters it is particularly important to monitor growth, development and behaviour during the probationary period as these are measures of happiness and well-being. A period of fostering before the adoption is completed is often desirable for older children, to give both child and adopters time to adjust and to be sure they want to finalize the adoption.

The Examination

In an ordinary family, regular developmental checks of babies and young children are undertaken to facilitate the early detection of handicap. In case of doubt an exact appraisal can often wait a while until the true picture becomes clearer. Before adoption of an infant or young child a very precise appraisal is needed, in order to forecast reasonably accurately what can be expected of his health and development in the future. This is not always possible and can be particularly difficult in the early weeks of life, especially when there is a history of perinatal problems (p. 219). Prognosis is also difficult in a toddler or pre-school child who has been neglected or deprived and may be functioning far below his potential. A period in sound foster care may help in the assessment of such a child. The abused child may increasingly be offered for adoption under the Children Act 1975, and Martin's work (1976) is outstanding in revealing the variety of disturbances and the child's need for treatment after living in an abusive home. It is important that both doctor and social worker on the one hand, and adopting parents on the other, realize what an examination of a young child can and cannot do. Illingworth has set this out in detail (1967, 1969).

The examination of health and development, including vision and hearing, will not differ from that prescribed in other chapters in this book but the doctor must realize the added importance of the adoption assessment, the need for thoroughness and the wisdom of assessing the influence of the social factors very carefully. A broad perspective of development is needed for all children but nowhere more than in the adoption field.

Since adopters are naturally anxious about the task ahead, optimism about indefinite hereditary factors is indicated. On the other hand when handicap *is* present, helping adopters towards a realistic appreciation of the future problems is essential.

The Hard-to-Place Child

This term has come into general use so it is mentioned here, but it is hoped that it will cease to be used once adoption agencies have broadened their view of adoption to include the placement of the disadvantaged or handicapped children mentioned earlier (p. 215). Such adoptions place an added strain on the over-worked agencies because they take longer to arrange and need more active follow-up care and counselling after placement. As yet in Britain there is much to be learnt about this type of placement, although a few agencies have done this work for many years.

Post-adoption counselling is often much welcomed by parents, especially those who take hard-to-place children and, when old enough, by the children themselves since they may believe that they were rejected by their natural parents because of handicap. For physically and mentally handicapped children the ordinary social work and other supports provided for all families with handicapped children will be available.

When older children (over 6 or 7 years) are placed, and sometimes at younger ages, the children need to be closely involved in placements by talking, drawing pictures or playing through the various processes to which they are being subjected, so that they can come to understand them and to believe all is done in their interests. At times painful decisions and partings may be needed and the child should be encouraged to feel that these are done to help him.

A new adoption agency, Parents for Children (Sawbridge, 1976) was set up in 1976 funded by the Department of Health and Social Security (DHSS) and other private sources. Its purpose is to explore all the facets of the placement for adoption of children with multiple handicaps or particular difficulties.

Subsidized adoptions

The Children Act 1975 allows the Secretary of State to authorize an agency to study the use of a subsidy for parents who take children for adoption. This will be particularly valuable for sibling groups in order to keep the children together.

Children in care

The important work of Rowe and Lambert (1973) indicated the need to re-examine criteria for care and placement of children who have to live away from their own families. Since paediatricians, community child health doctors and other medical personnel may be treating or supervising the progress of these children in care, it is important that they should be aware of their plight. In some cases a doctor might initiate discussions about the suitability of adoption for children whose parents have either ceased to take a proper interest in them or who have personalities, habits and modes of life, that make it unlikely that they can ever do so.

Access to Birth Records

Section 26 of the Children Act 1975, which came into force in 1976, made important changes in the law relating to access to birth records. It allows an adopted person over 18 years of age to see a copy of his original birth certificate. This has far-reaching implications for natural parents as well as the adopted person and his adopting parents. Guidance notes have been issued by the DHSS on this matter (1976). It is as well for doctors involved in original placements to be aware of this new procedure.

References

BOHMAN M. (1972) A study of adopted children: their background, environment and adjustment. *Acta Paediatrica Scandinavica*, **61**, 90.

BROWN J.K., COCKBURN F. and FORFAR J.O. (1972) Clinical and chemical correlates in convulsions of the newborn. *Lancet*, **1**, 135.

*CARTER C.A. (1969) Genetic considerations in adoption. *Medical Group Papers II, 32, 52*. London: Association of British Adoption and Fostering Agencies.

DAVIES P.A. (1976) Outlook for the low birthweight baby: then and now. *Archives of Disease in Childhood*, **51**, 817.

DEPARTMENT OF HEALTH AND SOCIAL SECURITY (1976). *Access to Birth Records. I. Information for Adopted People. II. Notes for Counsellors*. London: Her Majesty's Stationery Office.

FISCH R.O., BILEK M.K., DEINARD A.S. and CHANG P. (1976) Growth, behavioural and psychological measurements of adopted children. *Journal of Pediatrics*, **89**, 494.

FORFAR J.O. (1969) The role of the paediatrician in adoption medical practice. *Lancet*, **1**, 1201.

GRANT B. (1975) A proposed adoption by a mother and stepfather. *Child Adoption*, No. **81**, 15.

HERSOV L. (1973) The psychiatrist and modern adoption practice. *Child Adoption*, No. **71**, 17.

*ILLINGWORTH R.S. (1967) Assessment for adoption. *Medical Group Papers II, 56*. London: Association of British Adoption and Fostering Agencies.

ILLINGWORTH R.S. (1969) Assessment for adoption: a follow up study. *Acta Paediatrica Scandinavica*, **58**, 33.

MCWHINNIE A.M. (1967) *Adopted Children: how they grow up*. London: Routledge and Kegan Paul.

MARTIN H.P. and KEMPE C.H. (1976) *The Abused Child*. Cambridge, Mass: Ballinger Publishing Company.

*ROWE J. and LAMBERT L. (1973) *Children Who Wait*. London: Association of British Adoption and Fostering Agencies.

SAWBRIDGE P. and MacCLANAHAN W. (1976) Subsidised adoptions. *Child Adoption*, No. **84**, 15.

SEGLOW J., PRINGLE M.L.K. and WEDGE P. (1972) *Growing-up Adopted*. London: National Foundation for Educational Research.

SHIELDS J. (1975) Schizophrenia, genetics and adoption. *Child Adoption*, No. **80**, 19.

TIZARD B. (1975) The adoption of children from institutions after infancy. *Child Adoption*, No. **79**, 27.

WOLKIND S.H. (1975) Psychiatric disorders in children in institutions. *Child Adoption*, No. **81**, 34.

Further Reading

*ASSOCIATION OF BRITISH ADOPTION AND FOSTERING AGENCIES (1976) *Role of the Medical Adviser to an Adoption Agency*. London: Association of British Adoption and Fostering Agencies.

*COOPER C.E. (1968) Medical practice in adoption agencies. *Medical Group Papers I, 79*. London: Association of British Adoption and Fostering Agencies.

CRELLIN E., PRINGLE M.L.K. and WEDGE P. (1972) *Born Illegitimate: social and educational implications*. London: National Foundation for Educational Research.

*DONLEY K. (1975) *Opening Doors: finding families for older and handicapped children*. London: Association of British Adoption and Fostering Agencies.

FRANKLIN D.S. and MASSARIK F. (1969) Adoption of children with medical conditions. *Child Welfare*, No. **48**, 459, 533, 595.

GORDON R.R. (1975) Medical examination of the baby to be adopted. *British Medical Journal*, **1**, 31.

HOME OFFICE (1972) *Report of the Departmental Committee on the Adoption of Children (Houghton-Stockdale Report)*. London: Her Majesty's Stationery Office.

HOME OFFICE AND SOCIAL WORK SERVICES GROUP, Scotland, Advisory Councils in Child Care (1976) *A Guide to Adoption Practice*. London: Her Majesty's Stationery Office.

JACKA A.A. (1973) *Adoption in Brief: an annotated bibliography*. London: National Foundation for Educational Research.

KADUSHIN A. (1970) *Adopting Older Children*. New York: Columbia University Press.

KELLY J.B. and WALLERSTEIN J.S. (1976) The effects of parental divorce. *American Journal of Orthopsychiatry*, **46**, 21, 257.

KORNITZER M. (1968) *Adoption and Family Life*. London: Putnam.
MEADOW R. (1975) The paediatricians role in the adoption of children with special needs. *Child Adoption*, No. **80,** 11.
PRINGLE M.L.K. (1967) *Adoption Facts and Fallacies: a review of research in USA, Canada and Britain 1948–1965*. London: Longmans.
Rowe J. (1966) *Parents, Children and Adoption*. London: Routledge and Kegan Paul.
*RUTTER M. (1969) *Psychological development: predictions from infancy*. *Medical Group Papers II, 37, 52*. London: Association of British Adoption and Fostering Agencies.

* Obtainable from ABAFA, 4 Southampton Row, London, WC1B 4AA.

Appendix 12.1

Acts, Regulations and Rules
(obtainable from HMSO)

England and Wales
The Children Act (1948)
The Adoption Act (1958)
Children and Young Persons' Act (1963)

Children and Young Persons' Act (1969)
   Part I. A Guide for Courts and Practitioners
Children Act (1975)
Adoption Agencies Regulations (1976)
Adoption (High Court) Rules (1976)
Adoption (County Court) Rules (1976)
Adoption (Magistrate's Court) Rules (1976)

Scotland
The Children Act (1975) (as above)

The Adoption Act (1958)
Adoption Agencies (Scotland) Regulations (1967)

Appendix 12.2

Sample Medical Report Forms
(other forms obtainable from ABAFA)

CONFIDENTIAL
FORM A (MOTHER OR FATHER)

NAME OF AGENCY ....Telephone no. ....

ADDRESS ....

....

MEDICO-SOCIAL REPORT ON MOTHER OR FATHER OF CHILD

To be completed by the social worker concerned from information given by
close relatives of child and parent's family doctor

Name of child (surname underlined) ....

Date of birth of child ....

1.	Age of mother/father (and year of birth)	
2.	Skin colour	
3.	Eye colour	
4.	Hair colour and texture	
5.	Racial origin	
6.	Height	
7.	Weight or build	
8.	Any particularly noticeable physical characteristics?	
9.	Estimated intelligence (IQ if known and date)	
10.	Social and educational record, jobs, special interests	
11.	Occupation	
12.	Occupation of her/his father and mother	
13.	Present state of health	
14.	Sex and ages of all other children of mother/father and state of health and development	

15. Is there a history of, or evidence of, mental handicap or illness, unstable personality, epilepsy, allergy, diabetes, hereditary defects, degenerative disorders, renal disease, congenital defects or any other disease in the mother/ father? Please give details.

16. If history inadequate, please state so

17. Are any of the conditions mentioned above or any familial disorders present among near relatives (e.g. parents, children, siblings, grandparents, aunts, uncles, first cousins)? If details not available please state so

18. Particulars of any circumstances or conditions not mentioned above which may assist medical assessor or about which adopters may require to be informed

19. Has mother cared for the child? If so, for how long?

20. Has the father seen or is he maintaining the child?

21. From whom was the information on this form obtained? State relationship, if any, to mother

22. Name and address of doctors from whom further information can be obtained (state whether mother's/father's G.P. or other doctor)

Signature of social worker ....
   (*print in capitals after*)

Agency ....

Address ....

....

Date ....   Telephone no. ....

For use of agency medical adviser

NAME OF AGENCY .... Telephone no. ....

ADDRESS ....

....

MEDICAL REPORT ON CHILD EXAMINED FOR ADOPTION

OR RECEIVED INTO AGENCY CARE

Please do not complete this form until you have been given Form A (medico-social history),
Form B.1 (obstetric history) and Form B.2 (neonatal history)

Reference can also be made to the ABAA—Brief Guide to the Screening of Development

Name (surname underlined) ....Sex ....

Other name by which known ....

Date of birth ....

FIRST EXAMINATION: Date ....Age ....

Persons accompanying child   ....

SECOND EXAMINATION: Date ....Age ....

Persons accompanying child   ....

HISTORY

The information in questions 1 to 9 is also for the benefit of the child's new family doctor

1. History of biological mother relevant to child's future (please read Forms A and B.1)	
2. History of biological father relevant to child's future (please read Form A)	
3. History of siblings relevant to child's future (please read Forms A, B.1 & 2).	
4. Estimated gestation in weeks (please read Form B.2)	

5. Birth history (please read Forms B.1 and B.2)	
6. Birth weight (please read Form B.2)	
7. Length at birth (please read From B.2)	
8. Head circumference at birth (please read Form B.2.)	
9. Post-natal history (please read Forms A, B.1 and B.2). Please use separate sheet if necessary	
(a) Details of care since birth (please indicate all changes of care)	
(b) Duration of breast feeding	
(c) Details of present feeding	
(d) Details of any feeding difficulty (e.g. poor sucking, difficulty in swallowing or slow feeding)	
(e) Details of any illness or operation since birth, (e.g. infection, skin trouble, accidents, convulsions, fainting or cyanotic attacks, allergic upsets, respiratory disorders) or any other health problems	
(f) Details of any hospital admission or attendance at out-patient or special clinic (other than child health clinic)	
(g) Reports of any unusual behaviour (e.g. apathy, too quiet, restlessness)	
(h) Evidence of hearing reported by person caring for child	
(i) Evidence of seeing reported by person caring for child	

(j) Immunization (with dates)	Diph	Polio
	Tetanus	Measles
	Pertussis	BCG
	Smallpox	Others

(k) Care since birth (Please give details of all moves and reasons)	

EXAMINATION
PART 1—PHYSICAL ASSESSMENT

	1st examination (date:)	2nd examination (date:)
10. Weight		
11. Length or height		
12. Skull (abnormality in shape, size, ossification, fontanelle or sutures) Head circumference		
13. Facies (e.g. mongolism)		
14. Eyes and vision (N.B. squint, cataract, nystagmus) Ophthalmoscopic examination		
15. Mouth (e.g. cleft palate, number & state of teeth)		
16. Ears and hearing (N.B. deformity of pinna) Auroscopic examination		
17. Skin (e.g. naevi, rash, jaundice, unusual pigmentation)		
18. Neuromuscular system:		
(a) Posture		
(b) Degree of alertness (e.g. interest in surroundings, concentration, response to examiner)		
(c) General activity and vigour		
(d) Muscle tone (e.g. hypotonia, asymmetrical tone, hypertonia, clench fist)		
(e) Primitive reflexes, please tick if present:		
Rooting reflex		
Grasp reflex		
Moro reflex		
Asymmetrical tonic neck reflex		
(f) Tendon reflexes:		
Knee jerks		
Ankle jerks		

	1st examination (date:)	2nd examination (date:)
(g) Plantar response (extensor or flexor?)		
(h) Abdominal reflexes		
(i) Any evidence of cerebral palsy (e.g. hemiplegia, adductor spasm, shortened hamstrings or tendo Achilles, limited supination of hand, wasting)		
19. Spine, joints and limbs, (e.g. talipes or other musculo-skeletal deformity). Screening test for dislocation or subluxation of hip (Barlow's or Ortolani's test)		
20. Abdomen (e.g. distension, palpable liver, spleen, kidney or other mass, hernia)		
21. Genito-urinary system (e.g. hypospadias, undescended testes or vulval anomalies)		
22. Cardio-vascular system (e.g. dyspnoea, tachypnoea, cyanosis, or abnormal praecordial pulsation, femoral pulses, cardiac murmurs)		
23. Respiratory system (e.g. dyspnoea, movement, rate, wheeze, chest deformity)		
24. Special tests:		
(a) Urine: albumin: reducing substance:		
(b) Phenylketonuria:		
Guthrie test		
Phenistix		
Other		
(c) Serological test for syphilis (if required): Tests		
Result		
Date		
(d) Sickling test (where relevant)		
(e) Other tests (please specify)		

PART 2—DEVELOPMENT ASSESSMENT

Please note stages reached: (key to stages of development enclosed)

	1st examination (date:)	2nd examination (date:)
25. (a) Posture, gross motor and loco-motion		
(b) Vision and manipulation		
(c) Hearing and speech		
(d) Social behaviour and play		

CONCLUSIONS

26. Do you think that the child has any significant defect? (specify): (a) Physical (b) Mental		
27. Do you think that there are any medical circumstances which: (a) Require further consideration before placement? (b) Indicate the need for further examination (specify time)? (c) Should be communicated and explained to adoptive parents?		
28. Any other observations: (please use separate sheet if necessary)		

Signature (*print in capitals after*) ....

Qualifications ....

Address..

....

Date .... Telephone no. ....

For use of agency medical adviser

CHAPTER 13

Mental Retardation

Definition and Classification

The definition of mental retardation accepted by the American Association for Mental Deficiency (AAMD) (Grossman, 1973) is that it 'refers to significantly subaverage general intellectual functioning existing concurrently with deficits in adaptive behaviour and manifested during the developmental period'. Classification may be based on measures of degree of disability or on aetiology of the condition.

Classification by degree of disability (intellectual functioning; adaptive behaviour) Although intelligence tests provide objective measures of performance in a range of standardized test situations, their interpretation is fraught with difficulty (Chapter 6). They are not only a measure of innate ability but are dependent also on experience and teaching and reflect performance in a particular test situation at a particular time, results being influenced by examiner, environment and current well-being. Study of a subject's performance on sub-sections of intelligence tests is often more informative than overall scores and is of particular value in planning remedial measures. An added complication is the difference in standard deviation of different intelligence tests, and for this reason the classification adopted by the AAMD defines groups on the basis of standard deviations (Table 13.1).

TABLE 13.1. Intellectual Functioning in Mental Retardation (After Grossman, 1973)

Level of mental retardation	Intelligence quotient	
	Standard deviation units	Stanford Binet Scale (S.D. 16)
Mild	2.01 to 3.00	52–67
Moderate	3.01 to 4.00	36–51
Severe	4.01 to 5.00	20–35
Profound	5.01–	–19

The 'borderline' category (IQ 65–85) which is included in the current International Classification of Diseases (WHO, 1965) has been dropped by the AAMD.

Intelligence tests are used from the age of 2 years but are not applicable to younger children when it is difficult to measure reasoning and problem-solving capacity, Developmental tests are used below this age and the predictive value of these is discussed elsewhere (p. 44). Particularly in the lesser degrees of developmental delay, considerable caution must be exercised in the interpretation to parents of developmental assessment tests; performance can deteriorate or improve, and discussion should be orientated towards present achievement and proposed therapy rather than long-term prognosis.

Intellectual level alone does not determine an individual's performance in the community; this is dependent on many factors including personality, behaviour, cultural background and social opportunity. Some individuals of low normal intelligence require considerable support and guidance while many mildly subnormal persons lead successful independent lives. For this reason classifications based on adaptive behaviour as opposed to measured intelligence have been in common use for many years. The older legal definitions of idiots, imbeciles and feeble-minded persons were based on criteria such as the ability to guard against common dangers or to live an independent life. Such classifications are a measure of social competence and conformity, and have the advantage of indicating need for services, i.e. 'administrative' prevalence.

In the infant and young child adaptive behaviour is judged on sensori-motor development, communication, self-help skills and interaction with other persons. Later in childhood the criteria are largely educational and social, and in the adult they are based on employment capability and performance in home, family and society.

Classification according to aetiology
Several aetiological classifications of mental deficiency have been proposed dependent on genetic background, pathological findings, sociological factors or timing of causative influence. The following sub-divisions of mental retardation are used in the International Classification of Diseases (1965) and in the 1973 revision of the Manual on Terminology and Classification in Mental Retardation (Grossman, 1973):

> following infection and intoxications;
> following trauma or physical agents;
> with disorders of metabolism, growth or nutrition;
> associated with gross brain disease (postnatal);
> associated with diseases and conditions due to (unknown) prenatal influences;
> with chromosomal abnormalities;
> associated with prematurity;
> following major psychiatric disorder;
> with psycho-social (environmental) deprivation;
> other and unspecified.

The following simple classification which indicates genetic or non-genetic aetiology as well as timing of environmental damage is used here to provide groupings convenient for subsequent consideration of the prevention of mental handicap:

> *Genetic:* chromosomal; single gene
> *Environmental*: antenatal; perinatal; postnatal

Multifactorial: particularly subcultural mental defect due to a combination of poor genetic endowment plus adverse pre-, peri- or postnatal influences. Also includes common congenital malformations such as neural tube defects which may be complicated by mental handicap.

Mental handicap arising from purely genetic cause or from environmental damage is often severe and frequently accompanied by other abnormalities such as cerebral palsy, epilepsy and congenital defects. Subcultural mental defect, of multifactorial aetiology, is more often mild and is associated with low social class and poor home environment.

Incidence and Prevalence

The incidence of mental defect at birth is unknown since only a few of the more severe forms can be distinguished clinically, biochemically or cytogenetically at this age.

Incidence of recognizable conditions varies geographically and racially, while in the case of some of the less common syndromes, insufficient data are available for final conclusions about incidence. The figures given in Table 13.2 represent values taken from a variety of sources.

TABLE 13.2. Incidence of specific conditions associated with mental retardation.

Chromosomal disorders	
*Trisomy 21	1/600 –1/1400
*Trisomy 13	1/5000 –1/15000
*Trisomy 18	1/2000 –1/7500
Cri-du-chat (5p–)	1/50000–1/100000
Metabolic disorders	
Phenylketonuria	1/4000 –1/20000 (UK)
Homocystinuria	1/20000–1/250000
Galactosaemia	1/40000–1/70000
Maple Syrup Urine Disease	1/60000
Hurler's Syndrome	1/10000–1/40000
Hunter's Syndrome	1/40000–1/200000
Miscellaneous	
Epiloia	1/30000–1/50000
De Lange's Syndrome	1/30000–1/40000
Apert's Syndrome	1/166000

* From chromosome studies on over 46 000 newborn infants: Trisomy 21: 1/981; Trisomy 18: 1/7500; Trisomy 13: 1/15383—Hamerton *et al.*, 1975.

In the case of inborn errors of metabolism, screening programmes have shown that some disorders are more common than was originally thought. For example, the incidence of phenylketonuria, which was considered to be comparatively rare occurring only once in 40 000–50 000 births, has now been shown to range from 1 in 4000 births in Southern Ireland and Western Scotland to 1 in 60 000 in Japan (Sorsby, 1973).

Similarly, more accurate information about the incidence of Down's syndrome has been provided by chromosome studies on consecutive births. The mean incidence from six such studies involving over 46 000 infants was 1 per 981 live births, with a range from 1.5 per 1000 in Edinburgh, Scotland, to 0.7 per 1000 in New Haven, Connecticut, USA (Jacobs *et al.*, 1974; Hamerton *et al.*, 1975). Spontaneous abortions show a higher frequency of trisomy 21 and about three of every four affected fetuses do not reach term.

Antenatal infections contribute significantly to the incidence of mental handicap. Stern *et al.* (1969) suggested that rubella and toxoplasmosis might together be responsible for 2 to 3 per cent of all cases of mental deficiency. Positive tests for toxoplasmosis are found in approximately one-third of adults in Britain and there is about a 1 in 200 chance of mothers acquiring the infection some time during pregnancy. About one-third of the fetuses of these mothers are infected and one-third of infected fetuses develop clinical disease.

Approximately half the adult population of this country have serological evidence of past infection with cytomegalovirus. In a prospective study of pregnant women in London, Stern and Tucker (1973) showed that almost one-half of the infants of mothers who experienced primary cytomegalovirus infection were congenitally infected; in follow-up studies one in five of the infected infants was mentally retarded. The authors estimated that in England and Wales 400 infants annually out of a birth population of 830 000 would have severe brain damage caused by cytomegalovirus.

By prevalence of mental deficiency we mean the number of cases identified at a particular age. True prevalence refers to the absolute number identified whereas administrative prevalence indicates the number requiring services or assistance. At all ages mild mental handicap is more common than severe defect and more males than females are affected.

Recognized prevalence of mental deficiency is heavily dependent on the criteria of definition. When these are related largely to school performance in mid and late childhood the peak prevalence of about 1 per cent is found. Under the age of about 7 years estimates of prevalence must be interpreted with caution. Kushlick and Cox (1973) found that the reported prevalence of all grades of subnormality for the age group 0–4 years ranged from 0.7 to 12.5 per 1000. The figures for severe subnormality were more in agreement ranging from 0.53 to 0.91 per 1000 but were much lower than in older age groups, suggesting that the majority of young affected children were not included in the statistics. While a proportion of children recognized as mentally retarded during school years may have deteriorated in function from dull and backward to mentally deficient because of an adverse socioeconomic environment, the lack of cases reported in preschool years is probably due mainly to non-recognition of milder defect and to understandable caution in labelling a child mentally defective.

In preschool years development of a child's potential is dependent entirely on his home environment and immediate surroundings. Hindley (1962) showed that performance in developmental and intellectual tests improved over the period 6 months to 5 years in social classes 1 and 2, remained approximately the same in class 3 and deteriorated in classes 4 and 5. Similarly, Heber *et al*

(1972) found a falling performance during early years in children selected for study because of the low intelligence of their mothers.

Environment and social class have been shown by a number of authors to exert a marked effect during school years when there is increasing divergence in attainment between children of different social class. It has been suggested that a proportion of the mental handicap recognized at school entry in children from poorer homes may arise from bias in a number of formal intellectual tests towards middle class and from the limited use of language in poorer homes, with resultant inability of the children to express themselves. However, the disadvantaged child from very inadequate surroundings has not only different, but lesser stores of knowledge, with retardation particularly in language development and reasoning skills, important ingredients for academic success.

Aetiology and Prevention

Aetiology of mental retardation and other handicapping conditions is also discussed elsewhere (Chapter 1). Where the cause of mental retardation is known or suspected it may be possible to implement preventive measures. Unfortunately however, the cause of retardation remains obscure in a substantial proportion of patients, especially in the mild handicap range.

Genetic causes
Chromosomal. Trisomy 21 is the main chromosomal defect causing mental retardation, being responsible for about 5 to 10 per cent of all mental defect. Prevention of conception in high-risk situations can be supplemented by a programme of antenatal screening by amniocentesis, with a view to termination of affected pregnancies. Aminocentesis should be recommended when one parent carries a balanced translocation for mongolism. However, this is found in only about 1.3 per cent of mongol births and in most of these the parental chromosome abnormality will not be detected until one infant with Down's syndrome has been born. Older mothers comprise a second high risk group and amniocentesis can justifiably be offered to mothers over 35 years. Also, since the birth of two mongol children in a family can cause major emotional and management problems, amniocentesis should be offered to any mother who has had a mongol child even if she is young and the risk of recurrence is low. Other chromosome defects can be recognized at the same time and tests can routinely be carried out for open neural tube defects by estimation of alpha fetoprotein in the amniotic fluid.

Single gene disorders. In the majority of single gene disorders responsible for mental defect, genetic counselling *per se* (p. 249) is unlikely to reduce the incidence significantly. Among conditions inherited as autosomal dominants, the more serious disorders such as epiloia arise as mutations in a high percentage of cases. In autosomal recessive inheritance, first affected children in a family account for about five out of six cases, limiting prevention by counselling unless simple reliable tests for the heterozygote become available or are available as in Tay-Sach's disease, for which preventive programmes are in use in high risk groups. In X-linked recessive inheritance also, most affected children are first cases in the family and frequently prevention by counselling must await the birth of the first affected child.

Antenatal diagnosis by amniocentesis may permit termination of a pregnancy when the fetus is affected by an inborn error of metabolism. However, although such tests have been shown to be reliable for several metabolic errors and are potentially available for many more, they are highly specific. They are of considerable benefit to the individual family but do not lead to a significant overall reduction in the incidence of mental defect. At present the principal method of reducing mental deficiency due to inborn errors of metabolism is by a screening programme at birth followed by dietary or other appropriate treatment.

Environmental causes
An increasing number of agents are recognized as potentially damaging to the fetus and a further proportion of mental handicap, particularly in the severe defect range, may be due to unrecognized antenatal hazards. The extent of the problem is unknown, but it may be substantial as suggested by Drillien's (1968) observation in children of IQ below 55 that half 'exhibited congenital anomalies which must have arisen at an early stage of gestation'. Since preventive measures may be possible in many instances, this is an important field for further research.

Physical agents, drugs and chemicals. These are discussed in Chapter 1.

Infections. The danger to the fetus of rubella during pregnancy is well established, and although infection during the first trimester is responsible for the most severe effects, lesser degrees of damage may result from later infection. Active immunization is used in the UK to confer immunity on girls below child-bearing years and in the US is applied to both sexes at a lower age in an attempt to reduce the reservoir of infection in the population. Immunization is valuable also in selected populations such as staff in maternity and children's hospitals and nurseries. Mothers exposed to rubella at any time during pregnancy must be investigated for evidence of recent infection. When serological tests show either a rising maternal antibody titre or specific IgM antibodies, termination of pregnancy is justifiable; use of γ globulin in these circumstances is of little or no value (Public Health Laboratory Service, 1970).

In view of the importance of cytomegalovirus infection as a cause of mental handicap, attempts are being made to produce an effective and safe vaccine (Elek and Stern, 1974). Toxoplasmosis is not preventable by immunization, but epidemiological studies have shown the domestic cat to be the most common vector of the disease and it would seem reasonable that young married couples should be discouraged from keeping cats as pets until their families are complete.

Maternal phenylketonuria. Mental deficiency in the offspring occurs with untreated maternal phenylketonuria, although not with non-phenylketonuric hyperphenylalaninaemia when the level of blood phenylalanine is below 15 mg/

100 ml (Hsia, 1970). Girls who have been treated from birth for phenylketonuria are now approaching child-bearing years and it is important that they are identified so that appropriate diet can be re-commenced early in pregnancy. It is possible that other congenital metabolic errors in the mother could damage the fetus by a similar mechanism and research into this possibility is being carried out.

Nutrition and mental retardation. Nutrition of the infant before and after birth is important for normal development and harmful effects of under-nutrition on brain development have been demonstrated both in the experimental animal and the human. The critical period for brain growth in the human extends from the second trimester to the third or fourth postnatal year, during which time under-nutrition can give rise to retardation in all the main fields of psycho-motor development, particularly in language. A proportion of light for date infants have been malnourished before birth. Delayed feeding of low birth-weight infants was common practice until a few years ago and may have been responsible for a proportion of the mentally handicapped children found in earlier follow-up studies. Later postnatal undernutrition arising from a variety of causes has been shown to be associated with developmental delay. It has been difficult, however, to distinguish between the effects of malnutrition and those of other adverse environmental factors which often coexist.

Complications of pregnancy and perinatal period. Pregnancy and perinatal complications, particularly when associated with low birth-weight and premature delivery, make a significant contribution to the incidence of mental retardation combined with neurological defects (p. 8). They are of much less importance in the aetiology of isolated mental handicap (Drillien, 1969).

Postnatal environment. The postnatal causes of mental defect include many common illnesses and their complications (p. 11). Mental deficiency resulting from accidents is increasing but is a potentially preventable cause of handicap. Equally important is the prevention of non-accidental injury or child abuse (Chapter 20). Although the occurrence of mental deficiency following lead poisoning is clearly recognized, the contribution of lesser degrees of lead exposure to the prevalence of mental deficiency is uncertain. Raised concentrations of lead are more common in mentally retarded children than in controls and increased body lead has been found also in hyperactive children. It is not always clear, however, whether the lead is responsible for the mental symptoms or whether (as seems likely in most cases) the findings result from pica and pro-longed floor play of retardation, or because of a more contaminated environment associated with social deprivation or handicap. In some areas of the US lead poisoning is sufficiently common to warrant screening programmes.

Multifactorial causes
Subcultural (familial) mental retardation. The relative importance of genetic and environmental factors in the aetiology of subcultural defect is debatable.

Attempts to reduce its frequency by sterilization in some states of the US were based on fallacies, and there are a number of reasons why children of mentally defective parents might be expected to have higher intelligence than their parents. For example, the parent may be mentally subnormal as a result of acquired cerebral damage from disease or injury, or as a consequence of adverse socio-economic factors in early life. In these circumstances the genetic endowment of the offspring will not be affected, although the parental performance in the work situation and at home may perpetuate the problem by failing to provide the child with an environment adequate for full expression of his potential. The idea that there exists a static pool of low social class, low intelligence individuals perpetuating subcultural mental defect indefinitely has been countered by Birch *et al.* (1970) in their study 'Mental Subnormality in the Community'.

Adverse environmental influences which may be important in the aetiology of subcultural defect include pregnancy and perinatal factors and postnatal illnesses. Both pregnancy complications and premature births are more common in mothers of poor social class. In the postnatal period the infant from an adverse home environment is more likely to have illnesses and hospital admissions with separation from parents in his first years of life.

The further adverse influence of the materially poor unstimulating home is well recognized. Children from poor homes adopted into a better environment develop faster than expected from their background. The improvement in short-term performance of individuals removed from a particularly barren institution was demonstrated by Skeels and Dye (1939) and their much better long-term status by Skodak (1968). There is a clear difference especially in language development between children with severe defect (such as Down's syndrome) remaining in their own homes, provided these are good ones, and those admitted to institutions. However, it is important to remember that good institutional care can provide at least short-term gains compared with adverse home circumstances, although there may be unwanted long-term effects on behaviour, social competence, ability to be a good parent and ability to develop ties and affection.

Presentation of Mental Retardation

Early weeks
Some conditions which are regularly associated with mental retardation, such as Down's syndrome, microcephaly and phenylketonuria can be recognized in early postnatal life from physical findings or by biochemical screening. Other infants are considered to be 'at risk' because of features in the family history, less gross physical stigmata or perinatal complications.

Later infancy
In later infancy developmental delay can be recognized during routine developmental screening of all or of 'at risk' infants, or from the observations of mother or medical and nursing attendants. The mother has the advantage of long and close observation of her own child whom she can compare with siblings and other children, and she deserves sympathetic hearing of any anxieties with a

view to accurate assessment of the child's well-being. Gross motor delay is the most easily recognized facet of retarded development, but many retarded children show much better progress in this than in other fields of development. The 'too good' infant should always arouse suspicion as should the one who has frequent and persistent screaming for no apparent reason. Although delay in acquisition of language can arise for many reasons, the most frequent cause of severe delay is mental retardation. However, mental retardation should not be diagnosed from delay in one field of development alone or without comprehensive evaluation of the whole child and his environment.

Early childhood
From the second year of life onwards the retarded child shows increasing failure to develop social relationships, this being aggravated by impaired ability to communicate. Behaviour problems such as temper tantrums, screaming, destructive play and aimless hyperactivity may become evident and may be the reasons for referral to paediatrician or child psychiatrist. The child may present also with eye defects or in the audiometry clinic with suspected deafness and an increasing proportion of children are referred from such clinics for full assessment. A detailed history of early development should differentiate between progressive and non-progressive retardation.

Later childhood
Less severe mental retardation may not be evident until near school age or after the start of formal education, particularly when the cultural background is deficient and the child blends with his surroundings. However, some of the most acute parental distress is seen when no suspicion has arisen that a child is retarded until he fails to progress in the normal class.

Laboratory Investigations

Screening tests in early infancy
Guthrie test is a microbiological test for phenylketonuria carried out on blood collected on thick filter paper from a capillary puncture. A small disc of the blood-soaked paper is placed on a special agar culture plate and raised serum phenylalanine levels permit growth around the disc of a bacterium which has been seeded on the culture medium. The test is reliable and can be extended to cover at least 16 different metabolic errors although used mainly to detect raised levels of phenylalanine, galactose, histidine, methionine, tyrosine, valine and leucine.

Partition chromatography of blood amino acids using paper or thin layer methods provides an equally satisfactory screening procedure which can be carried out on whole blood collected on filter paper as above or on serum obtained from blood collected in capillary tubes. These methods permit the detection of a range of different metabolic errors involving amino acids and can be extended to cover disorders of sugars, organic acids, phenolic acids and indoles. One-dimensional chromatography of urinary amino acids has also been utilized for screening purposes.

Other methods. Less frequently used screening tests include automated fluorometric assay of blood phenylalanine, automated chemical assay of tyrosine and an enzymatic method for the detection of galactosaemia.

Congenital hypothyroidism can be detected in the neonatal period by assay of either thyroxine or thyroid-stimulating hormone in dried blood spotted on filter paper (Dussault *et al.*, 1975; Irie *et al.*, 1975). Screening by these methods suggests that congenital hypothyroidism is at least as common as phenylketonuria and since early treatment is important a good case can be made for their routine use.

Investigation of the mentally retarded child
The same care should be taken in investigating and prescribing treatment for the mentally retarded as is taken with physically ill patients of normal intelligence, and detailed investigation reduces the proportion of cases in which no aetiological diagnosis is made. It could be argued that as the likelihood of finding specific aetiological factors decreases with rising intelligence, it would be reasonable to concentrate diagnostic resources on the more severely handicapped. However, mild subnormality may be found in specific pathological conditions, e.g. epiloia and mosaic mongolism, so that any decision to limit investigation should not be based on the intellectual level alone.

The mildly retarded child with intelligent parents and a good home is more likely to have a specific recognizable cause for his retardation than the equally retarded child of backward parents from a poor home. In research studies, detailed laboratory investigations may be required in all children recognized as mentally retarded, but in clinical situations consideration of cost effectiveness will encourage selectivity in the field of mild subcultural defect. In any child specific features of case history or physical examination may indicate a need for comprehensive investigation or for specific tests. Accurate aetiological diagnosis is occasionally important for treatment and frequently important to parents for genetic counselling and to dispel uncertainties and doubts.

Urine tests. A range of urine tests, most of them capable of being performed in smaller laboratories, is available for the study of mental retardation and programmes suitable for the detection of a large number of metabolic errors have been prepared (Carson *et al.*, 1962; Berry *et al.*, 1968; Buist, 1968). Minimal urine investigation of any retarded child should include the following:
 Odour, e.g. of maple syrup in maple syrup urine disease or of sweaty feet in isovaleric acidaemia (the child may also have an unusual body odour, Mace *et al.*, 1976).
 Sulphosalicylic acid test for protein
 Reducing substances, e.g. Clinitest for any reducing substance and Clinistix® or Testape® for glucose.

Ferric chloride. In addition to the blue-green colour in phenylketonuria, ferric chloride may give colour changes in other metabolic errors or with excreted drugs and chemicals.

Cyanide-nitroprusside test for sulphur-containing amino acids cystine and homocystine.

Tests for mucopolysaccharides (glucosaminoglycans), e.g. Alcian Blue test.

Rothera's test for ketones.

Dinitrophenylhydrazine test for keto acids.

Ehrlich's aldehyde test for porphobilinogen.

Partition chromatography (paper or thin layer) for the study of amino acid excretion pattern.

Selectively used urine tests include examination for metachromatic material, culture for cytomegalovirus and special chromatographic procedures such as ion exchange column chromatography for the study of amino acids and gas chromatography for organic acids.

Chromosome studies. Chromosome studies are necessary in any child with severe mental retardation of unknown causation. They are indicated also in the more gross clinically recognizable syndromes (p. 246), suspected mongol mosaicism with 'mongoloid' traits, abnormalities involving multiple systems of the body and in the presence of minor abnormalities commonly seen in chromosome disorders (p. 246).

X-rays and tomography. Skull radiographs may be used to confirm the presence of craniostenosis or for the demonstration of intracranial calcification in congenital toxoplasmosis, congenital cytomegalovirus infection and Sturge–Weber syndrome, and may show typical changes in a few other conditions such as Hurler's syndrome. X-rays of the long bones may assist in the diagnosis of mucopolysaccharidoses, lipidoses and mucolipidoses. In the vast majority of mentally retarded individulas no specific changes are demonstrated by conventional radiography.

However, the introduction of computerized transaxial tomography has provided a safe, painless technique for investigation of the child with developmental delay. It has reduced greatly the need for contrast techniques using air or radio-opaque material. It can be used to demonstrate excess fluid in ventricles, subarachnoid space or porencephalic cysts. The large ventricles associated with Sotos' syndrome are readily shown and developing or treated hydrocephalus can be monitored. Characteristic changes in the white matter are seen in progressive leukodystrophies, and the cerebral changes of epiloia are evident by this technique before calcification is visible on routine x-rays and before the skin manifestations occur. The interested reader is referred to Gomez and Reese (1976) and Kazner *et al.* (1976).

Serology for antenatal infections (rubella, cytomegalovirus, toxoplasmosis, syphilis)

In infants who are suspected at birth of having acquired an infection *in utero* raised IgM and sometimes IgA in the cord serum may support the diagnosis; IgM antibody specific for the infecting organism indicates that the antibody is of fetal origin. Maternal antibody levels should also be investigated. In the slightly older child interpretation of serological tests may be difficult, raised titres may be due to postnatal infection and low titres may represent the natural decline of antibody. Studies of cytomegalovirus infection (Melish and Hanshaw, 1973) indicate that antibody titres would be of little value by 3 to 4 years for the diagnosis of antenatally acquired infections.

Other tests. Estimation of serum electrolytes and urea may be helpful in the recognition of renal diabetes insipidus, Lowe's syndrome and hypo-adrenalism with mental deficiency. Uric acid concentration should be measured in suspected Lesch Nyhan syndrome. Blood lead estimation should be used freely since early treatment could be important. Thyroid function tests, blood ammonia and serum calcium are used in appropriate patients and metachromatic inclusions in cultured fibroblasts and in lymphocytes may be searched for in suspected mucopolysaccharidosis. High blood lactate and pyruvate and high serum alanine levels may indicate Leigh's encephalomyelopathy. Serum amino acid chromatography is readily performed and is complementary to urine chromatography. A considerable number of individual enzymes can be quantitated in leucocytes or cultured fibroblasts, and estimations of these carried out in experienced laboratories should be used to confirm individual metabolic errors. Electroencephalograms are seldom of value in undifferentiated mental defect, but may be used on clinical indications such as infantile spasms or degenerative neurological disorders. Nerve, or less frequently, brain biopsy may also be helpful in progressive disease (Brett and Lake, 1975).

Clinical Conditions

Inborn errors of metabolism
A large number of inborn errors of metabolism are associated with mental deficiency, usually of severe degree. In many cases no specific clinical features are recognizable but some show signs and symptoms which may suggest the diagnosis. A few of the better known disorders are summarized in Table 13.3.

Chromosomal abnormalities
The more gross abnormalities of the chromosomes, such as trisomy 21, involve many genetic loci so that defects of several systems of the body, including abnormality of the brain with mental deficiency, are common associates. Improved laboratory methods, particularly the introduction of banding techniques, have facilitated recognition of individual chromosomes and definition of lesser defects. Several new syndromes, many of which are characterized by mental retardation, have been described and are reviewed by Lewandowski and Yunis (1975). Some minor abnormalities are common to several of these syndromes and a selection of stigmata from the following list indicates the need for chromosome studies:

TABLE 13.3. Selected inborn errors of metabolism associated with mental retardation.

Group of disorder	Condition	Principal clinical features (AR = Autosomal recessive; XL = X linked, R = recessive, D = dominant)
Amino acids	Phenylketonuria (PKU)	AR. Fair hair, blue eyes, mousy odour, eczema and mental retardation. Classical picture now rare. Atypical forms may be unresponsive to low phenylalanine diet. Differential diagnosis: other hyperphenylalaninaemias.
	Homocystinuria	AR. Best known variety arises from cystathionine synthase deficiency. Fair complexion malar flush, arachnodactyly and skeletal abnormalities (kyphoscoliosis; genu valgum). Eye defects, including dislocation of lens from age 2–3 years. Liable to venous and arterial thromboses.
	Branched-chain ketoaciduria (Maple syrup urine disease: MSUD)	AR. Classical form shows progressive deterioration from birth, with spasticity and convulsions. Milder intermittent variant causes neurological symptoms, including coma, during acute infections.
	Isovalericaciduria	AR. Severe metabolic acidaemia and neurological symptoms such as lethargy, convulsions and coma in early weeks. Offensive, sweaty feet odour.
	Hyperglycinaemia (a) Ketotic	AR. Includes propionicacidaemia and methylmalonicaciduria. Severe acidosis, often fatal, from soon after birth.
	(b) Non-ketotic	AR. Early and severe retardation.
	Argininosuccinicaciduria	AR. Friable hair, episodic vomiting, ataxia, convulsions. Severe mental defect.
	Hyperammonaemia (a) Ornithine transcarbamylase deficiency	XLD. Males die soon after birth with vomiting, convulsions, coma. Females may have episodic symptoms related to protein intake or intercurrent infection.
	(b) Carbamyl phosphate synthetase deficiency	Inheritance uncertain. One of several hyperammonaemias which may cause intermittent vomiting, dehydration, convulsions and coma.

Carbohydrates	Galactosaemia	AR. Early hepatosplenomegaly, jaundice, vomiting, failure to thrive. Postnatal cataracts
	Mucopolysaccharidoses	
	Hurler's syndrome (MPS 1 H)	AR. Most common type. Early progressive mental and physical deterioration. Coarse facial features, apathetic expression, corneal clouding, deafness. Kyphosis. Hepatosplenomegaly. Claw hand.
	Scheie's syndrome (MPS 1 S)	AR. Moderate somatic changes, corneal clouding. Normal intelligence.
	Hunter's syndrome (MPS 2)	XLR. Milder Hurler-like picture. No corneal clouding. Deafness more common.
	Sanfilippo's syndrome (MPS 3)	AR. Severe mental deterioration. Mild physical changes.
	Leigh's encephalomyelopathy	AR. Early progressive weakness, hypotonia and mental deterioration. Ataxia, tremors, optic atrophy, nystagmus or bizarre eye movements.
Lipids		
(a) without marked visceromegaly	Tay-Sachs disease (GM2 gangliosidosis)	AR. Severe progressive mental deterioration from 4–7 months. Cherry red spot at macula.
	Metachromatic leukodystrophy (late infantile form)	AR. Onset in second year. Progressive difficulties in walking, hand function and speech. Mental deterioration and sometimes convulsions appear later.
(b) with marked visceromegaly	Generalized gangliosidosis (GM1)	AR. Hurler-like features and progressive deterioration.
	Infantile Gaucher's disease	AR. Progressive neurological symptoms in early months.

Severe mental retardation. Impaired growth.

Skull: microcephaly; abnormalities of shape, sutures, fontanelle.

Facies: mid-face hypoplasia; abnormalities of nose, lips, palate, micrognathia.

Skin and hair: mid-line scalp defect, dimples, frizzy hair, hypoplastic nails.

Eyes: slanting eyes and microphthalmia, hypertelorism, strabismus, coloboma.

Ears: low-set ears, malformed or simple pinnae; pre-auricular dimples, pits or tags.

Hands: ulnar deviation, hypoplastic or absent thumb, syndactyly, simian creases, unusual dermatoglyphic pattern, e.g. multiple whorls.

A variety of major malformations may be present, such as congenital heart disease or imperforate anus.

Trisomy 21 (Down's syndrome). Down's syndrome is the most common autosomal abnormality associated with mental defect. Mongol mosaicism accounts for 1–2 per cent of clinically recognized mongols, but may be found also in the presence of minimal clinical signs. The mosaic mongol may develop from either a normal or trisomic zygote, probably mostly from the latter. On the basis of maternal dermatoglyphics Penrose (1965) estimated that about 10 per cent of mothers of mongols might be mosaics and a number of such cases have been confirmed by chromosome studies.

Trisomy 13 (Patau's syndrome). About half of these grossly abnormal infants die within the first month of life and practically all within the first year. The main diagnostic features are moderately low birth-weight, microphthalmia, cleft lip and palate, low abnormal ears, congenital heart disease, polydactyly and capillary haemangiomata especially over the forehead.

Trisomy 18 (Edwards' syndrome). These infants have a mortality rate in the first year similar to that for trisomy 13. They show fewer gross external changes but, apart from the first impression of a rather small rather feeble infant with low malformed ears, small mouth, micrognathia and narrow palpebral fissures, the clinician should be alerted by the tightly clenched hands with index and fifth fingers overlapping the second and third fingers and by the 'rocker bottom' feet

Cri du chat syndrome (deletion of short arm of chromosome no. 5 (5p–)) This is the only chromosome anomaly recognized primarily by the typical cry of the infant and secondly by his physical appearance. The cry which has been likened to that of a kitten or a shrieking owl is fairly strong, sharp and plaintive and is confined to the expiratory phase. It becomes less typical after the first year. The larynx is small and rudimentary and liable to obstruction during respiratory infection. Both pre- and postnatal growth are retarded, birth-weight at term being around 2500 g. The head is small and the face round. Downward outward slanting palpebral fissures and widely spaced eyes with epicanthic folds are reliable clinical features, while micrognathia and low placed ears are usually found. Mental deficiency is invariably present. Although the majority of affected infants fail to thrive and die in childhood, a few survive to adult life by which time the typical cry has gone and the face is long and narrow.

Antenatal infections

Rubella syndrome. Early descriptions of the rubella syndrome stressed the classical symptom triad of blindness, deafness and congenital heart disease, but it is now evident that there can be widespread involvement of the body organs. The affected infant is characteristically light for date and in the neonatal period may show hepatomegaly, jaundice and thrombocytopenia. Lung and bone changes may be seen on x-ray. Cataracts are common and pigmentary retinopathy may be present. A macular skin rash may persist for weeks or months after birth. Microcephaly and mental retardation are evidence of neurological involvement. In infants exposed to rubella at any stage of pregnancy, cord serum should be tested at birth (p. 451). Even in the absence of clinical signs, sero-positive cases should be carefully followed up.

Cytomegalovirus infection. The clinical manifestations of cytomegalovirus infection in the newborn infant are primarily a reflection of duration of infection, with the most severe CNS damage occurring with infection early in fetal life. The majority of newborn infants excreting cytomegalovirus are apparently well but others show hepatosplenomegaly, jaundice, purpura, respiratory symptoms or failure to thrive. Mental deficiency may occur in both groups and may be accompanied by microcephaly and intracranial calcification.

Toxoplasmosis. Infection of the fetus may occur at any stage of pregnancy. Abortion or stillbirth may result. At birth the infant may show evidence of prolonged infection with hydrocephalus, choroidoretinitis and intracranial calcification, or of more recent infection with jaundice, haemolytic disease and purpura. Later mental deficiency is common.

Antenatal drugs and chemicals

Three examples are given from the growing list of drugs which may damage the fetus.

Hydantoin is associated with poor prenatal growth, cranio-facial anomalies, nail and digital hypoplasia and mental deficiency (Hanson and Smith, 1975).

Trimethadione causes a syndrome characterized by developmental delay, V-shaped eyebrows, epicanthus, palatal abnormality and low-set malformed ears (Zackai *et al.*, 1975).

Alcoholism of the mother causes pre- and postnatal growth deficiency and developmental delay. Characteristic cranio-facial abnormalities include microcephaly, short palpebral fissures, epicanthic folds, maxillary hypoplasia, micrognathus and sometimes cleft palate (Jones and Smith, 1975).

Neuro-cutaneous syndromes

The neuro-cutaneous disorders characterized by abnormality of skin and nervous system are a reminder of the embryonic derivation of both tissues from the ectoderm.

Epiloia (tuberose sclerosis). This autosomal dominant condition shows marked variability of expression and is frequently missed both in its milder forms in the adult and in its early stages in the child. The fully developed picture in the adult shows the characteristic rash of adenoma sebaceum involving the butterfly area of the face, the shagreen patch of the back, sub- or peri-ungual fibromata, phakomata of the retina, intracranial calcification and often involvement of other tissue such as kidney and lung.

Less obvious forms in the adult are important to the paediatrician who has to decide whether epiloia in the child results from a mutation or has been inherited. Careful physical examination of the parents for minimal signs and if necessary skull x-rays should precede genetic counselling. About 80 per cent of cases arise as mutations.

The earliest clinical sign is irregular, usually oval, depigmented areas of the skin, sometimes described as shaped like the mountain ash or rowan leaf. These areas are lighter than the surrounding skin but not white like vitiligo. Their presence may suggest the diagnosis in the infant with infantile spasms. Adenoma sebaceum appears between 2 and 5 years but intracranial calcification may be demonstrated earlier.

Sturge–Weber syndrome (cerebral angiomatosis, encephalo-trigeminal angiomatosis). This condition occurs in only about one per 100 000 of the population. It is characterized by a port-wine vascular naevus on the face in the distribution of one division, especially the first, of the trigeminal nerve, accompanied by generalized or focal convulsions and intracranial calcification which often shows 'tram-lines' distribution. Hemiparesis may be present and about two-thirds of affected persons are mentally retarded.

Ataxic telangiectasia. This presents about the second year of life with progressive cerebellar signs in the form of ataxia, intention tremor and speech difficulty. The telangiectasia, which is most typically conjunctival but may also involve the butterfly area of the face, the pinnae and the anticubital and popliteal fossae, usually appears 2–3 years later. A low concentration of serum IgA is a useful diagnostic finding and probably explains the susceptibility of affected children to respiratory infections. Increasing physical handicap is accompanied by some impairment of mental development. Inheritance is an autosomal recessive.

Miscellaneous syndromes associated with mental retardation
An increasing number of syndromes which may be, or regularly are, associated with mental retardation are being recognized and the reader is referred to standard texts such as those of Smith (1970), Gellis and Feingold (1968), and Birth Defects Atlas published by the National Foundation, March of Dimes (Bergsma, 1973). The National Foundation also publishes the journal Syndrome Identification giving individual case reports of new syndromes or variants of old ones. The

identification of a syndrome may be important when there are genetic implications.

Management

Mental retardation requires a multi-disciplinary approach for both diagnosis and management (Chapter 2). Education plays an increasing role as the child nears school age and the Education (Handicapped Children) Act 1970 for England and Wales and corresponding legislation for Scotland make education departments responsible for the education of all children of compulsory school age irrespective of the presence of handicap or of its nature or degree. The seriously handicapped child is no longer ineducable: he attends school and is supervised by teachers.

The ways in which the presence of a handicapped child affects the family and the practical advice and help required are discussed in Chapter 11.

Genetic advice

Genetic advice is seldom requested but is frequently desired and required. Parents often have fallacious ideas about the aetiology of handicap, the contribution of heredity, the relative contribution from maternal and paternal family trees and the possible significance of other abnormalities in relatives. An active policy of offering advice must be pursued and, even when there is a high-risk inheritance pattern, knowledge of the risks can be preferable to fear of the unknown. In the case of autosomal recessive inheritance it is helpful to explain the contribution from both parents and to stress that all persons carry a number of harmful recessive genes.

A simple classification on which the genetic counsellor can base his advice is as follows.

Environmental aetiology. In the majority of instances, as in the rubella syndrome, recurrence in subsequent pregnancies is unlikely and parents can be reassured.

Genetic aetiology. Chromosome studies can be carried out on the child and his parents and high-risk situations identified. Antenatal diagnosis by amniocentesis may be recommended in selected circumstances (p. 236). With single gene abnormalities precise recurrence risks can usually be calculated and are high, unless the previous child was affected by a fresh mutation. In a number of inborn errors of metabolism antenatal diagnosis is possible (p. 236).

Multifactorial aetiology (with genetic and environmental influences). Recurrence risks are calculated from population surveys and tend to be moderately low, mostly in the 1/20 to 1/50 range, following the birth of one affected child.

For detailed consideration of the genetics of mental retardation the reader is referred to Slater and Cowie (1971) and Bundey and Carter (1974).

Specific treatment

Specific treatment is available for few conditions causing mental handicap.

Hypothyroidism should be treated as soon as the diagnosis is made and endemic cretinism can be prevented by administration of iodide to the mother before conception. Several inherited disorders of metabolism causing mental defect can be treated successfully when early diagnosis is made. The most common form of treatment is dietary restriction, reducing intake of the dietary constituent which cannot be metabolized; e.g. phenylalanine in phenylketonuria, galactose in galactosaemia, methionine in homocystinuria. In some disorders large doses of a vitamin which is the precursor of the appropriate coenzyme may be successful in treatment; e.g. pyridoxine controls a proportion of cases of homocystinuria and biotin some cases of propionicacidaemia. Methods of direct enzyme replacement are under study for a number of these disorders but are not clinically available.

Associated abnormalities and handicaps
Mental handicap, whether severe or mild, rarely occurs alone. Associated physical defects are more common in the severely retarded children, and behavioural problems in the milder, but there is no hard and fast division.

Eye defects. The importance of routine ophthalmic and orthoptic examination of all mentally handicapped children referred for comprehensive assessment was recently stressed by Bankes (1974) who found only 39 out of 171 such children to be ophthalmically normal. A significant refractive error was found in 52 per cent of the children and strabismus in 40 per cent. Bankes provides useful references to previous studies, all showing a high incidence of abnormalities even in the minimally handicapped. Early recognition and management of ocular abnormalities are important to both the child and his parents as, apart from visual acuity, the aesthetic importance of correcting strabismus (even in the severely handicapped child) should not be underestimated.

Ear defects. Hearing impairment is common in non-specific mental deficiency as in specific conditions such as cerebral palsy (p. 284), trisomy 21, mucopolysaccharidoses, congenital rubella syndrome, congenital syphilis and hydrocephalus. Some degree of hearing impairment is estimated to occur in 30–50 per cent of severely subnormal children. It is important to emphasize that hearing defects may develop at any time and may be a cause of deteriorating performance. For example, the mongol child who has frequent upper respiratory infections may become deaf from chronic middle ear infection. Therefore hearing tests should be carried out both at the initial assessment and at regular intervals thereafter in all children known to be handicapped. These tests must cover different frequencies since normal speech development requires hearing over the complete range. Parental observations about the child's hearing are valuable both at the initial interview and after the parents have been alerted to observe the child's reactions in domestic situations.

Dental disorders. The incidence of caries in mentally handicapped children is high. Conservative dental treatment should be encouraged and in the severely handicapped child this may require supervision by a hospital dentist who is interested and experienced in the field. General anaesthesia may be necessary for dental fillings. Fluoride administration should be encouraged as well as tooth and gum hygiene, preferably using electric toothbrushes.

Convulsions. Convulsive disorders are very frequently associated with mental handicap (Kirman, 1975). This subject is discussed fully in Chapter 17.

Behaviour problems. Early recognition of handicap provides an opportunity to prevent or treat the behavioural problems which are frequently encountered in in the mentally handicapped child. These can add greatly to the family difficulties and in later childhood or early adult life may lead to institutional care. The term 'bizarre behaviour' is sometimes applied but, at least in the early stages, the behavioural problems of retarded children are the same as those seen in normal children. They are magnified and aggravated by the discrepancy between chronological age and behavioural pattern, prolonged by inappropriate management and modified by the concomitant emotional overtones within the family. Some habits of the mentally retarded child are socially undesirable or may be disturbing to their parents. These include self-stimulation by head banging, rocking, masturbation and the eye kneading of the blind, aggression towards others by nipping, biting, kicking and spitting, inappropriate affection by hugging and kissing of strangers and sometimes a desire for pleasurable sensory inputs as from feeling smooth fabrics such as ladies' clothing. Unfortunately, parents may welcome and encourage bad behaviour in its early stages as evidence of progress. Moreover, the child soon learns to use such behaviour as a means of gaining the attention he does not acquire in other ways. His parents are already emotionally upset by the primary handicap and they may have doubts about their own competence and ability to cope. The common-sense approach, which allows most parents of normal children to deal successfully with early behaviour problems, seems too simple and parents of a handicapped child often expect that special methods of management outwith their knowledge will be necessary. Frequently they fail to apply the discipline which is as necessary for him as for the normal child.

It is comparatively easy to modify the behaviour of a child in the setting of a day clinic or hospital, and staff must guard against claiming or accepting credit for a child's good behaviour in such a setting. Therapists and psychologists should be encouraged to visit the family home to determine the causes of behavioural problems and to decide the best method for their elimination. Operant conditioning techniques are of proven value in both the normal and the handicapped child and are applicable even in the presence of severe mental defect. Basic behaviour modification techniques should be taught to parents who can employ them in the home for the management of bad habits and also for the teaching of language and other skills. As a consequence, the self-confidence of the parents is restored and they feel less dependent on advisers when fresh problems arise.

Before advice is given the behaviour pattern must be analysed in some detail with regard to timing of the undesirable trait, concomitant events, possible precipitating factors and methods of management tried by the parents. Positive reinforcement of desirable behaviour is often easier and more successful than punishment for undesirable habits, but both may be used. The programme must be tailored to the individual circumstances and, in the case of extinction of unwanted behaviour, parents should be warned that there may be an initial period of aggravation of the problem when the benefit a child receives from his habit is withdrawn. It is helpful to reassure parents that the advice given will be 'common sense' but that it is often difficult for those closely involved in a situation to analyse it, and much easier for the therapist or psychologist to take a detached view. Video recordings can be used to analyse in detail events preceding and following a particular behaviour pattern and for demonstrating these to parents.

A simple example of behaviour modification is the management of a child with temper tantrums. Analysis of this situation revealed that these occurred initially at the time he came home from nursery school, at which point he screamed and kicked unless his mother gave him sweets. She achieved temporary respite by giving in to his demands but the success the boy achieved soon led him to use the same device in other situations. The mother was advised to withdraw the reward (sweets); she was also instructed to isolate him in the corridor until he behaved since it would have been difficult for her to ignore the ensuing tantrum and any attention she gave would have acted as a reinforcer for tantrums. After an initial increase in the frequency of the tantrums, as the boy tried harder than ever to achieve his desired goal, the habit was steadily extinguished so that within a month only an occasional 'reminder' was required. By this time it was possible to offer the child the opportunity of indulging in alternative and acceptable behaviour which would earn him rewards in the form of praise and affection.

Hyperactivity. Hyperactivity in normal children of average intelligence is considered in Chapter 25. Other children with overt neurological damage or disease such as mental retardation, cerebral palsy or epilepsy may also exhibit overactive behaviour. The problems of parents of coping continuously with a severely hyperactive child will be obvious to all who have had such a child in their consulting room for 5 minutes. Treatment clearly depends on causation, and environmental stress should be sought and if possible alleviated. Even when the environment is not of direct aetiological importance, the provision of adequate space and absence of restrictive features can be beneficial. The clinical psychologist can play a useful part in modification of the child's behaviour and counselling of the parents. Epilepsy in the hyperactive child should be treated with drugs other than barbiturates which may exacerbate the overactivity. Primidone, which is chemically related to phenobarbitone, can cause similar problems and is best avoided. In the presence of EEG abnormality without convulsions the role of anticonvulsant therapy is not well-defined.

The CNS stimulant drugs (p. 486) are of more value in the so-called developmental hyperkinetic syndrome than when more overt cerebral damage is present and they are seldom of benefit in mental deficiency. Various tranquillizers are helpful in hyperkinetic children, e.g. the 5-year-old child may be tried on diazepam (2·5–5 mg three times per day) but may require major tranquilisers such as chlorpromazine (10–20 mg) or thioridazine (10–15 mg). These drugs are first choice in the mentally retarded child and their early use can be of considerable benefit by breaking the cycle whereby hyperactivity leads to increasing family tension and aggravation of the hyperkinesis.

Sleep problems. Sleep disturbances are common in all children. In the normal child a sleep routine is established with the help of firm but loving parental handling of the common bedtime difficulties and nocturnal waking. In the mentally handicapped child the majority of such problems are similar in causation, clinical pattern and management to those in the normal but they are often more severe and difficult to manage by the time advice is sought. Very much less common is the child who 'turns night into day' as a direct consequence of cerebral pathology. Problems arise in the mentally handicapped child from a variety of causes but the rapid disappearance of symptoms if the child is admitted to hospital emphasizes the importance of environmental influences. Admission of both mother and child may have greater long-term benefit than admission of the child alone. The nocturnal screaming and crying of a defective child can soon exhaust parents and disturb neighbours; in the short-term it can lead to child abuse and in the longer term to increasing family tension and eventual rejection of the child. When treatment is supervised in the home advice will usually require to be accompanied by more immediate relief using a sedative such as nitrazepam or trimeprazine, often in quite large dosage. Mothers should be instructed to repeat the dose when it is clearly ineffective after an hour or more.

Language and communication. One of the most obvious and incapacitating handicaps accompanying mental defect is speech delay. Use of verbal language is frequently more retarded than development in other fields and, although gestures are used more than in the normal child, parents often complain that the mentally handicapped child is frustrated by inability to make his needs or wishes known. Understanding of speech tends to be more in line with the overall developmental level and, although some parents claim that their child 'understands everything that is said to him', analysis of the level of understanding shows that only a limited number of common words or phrases provoke appropriate reactions. Indeed, parents tend to limit the vocabulary they use in speaking to the child to well tried items, consciously or unconsciously adding appropriate gesture, so that it is difficulty to decide from the history whether the child responds to speech or to the overall situation.

The reasons for delay in language development are varied. Undoubtedly a major factor is the complexity of language comprehension and expression which requires a basic level of intelligence and conceptual thinking. Opportunity for learning may be lacking for the handicapped child with absence of the normal feedback between parent and child so that parents are discouraged and speak little to the child, perhaps replacing speech with gesture. The lower verbal skills of the child in a non-stimulating environment such as some institutions are well-known. However, many children's homes can provide better opportunity for language development than the child's own home. In both the institutional and

and domestic situation emotional factors are important. Speech delay may result from deafness (p. 462) as in the mentally normal child.

Management of the language problems of the mentally deficient child should begin early in the home with more conscious 'teaching' than in the normal child, with frequent repetition and with positive reinforcement of appropriate responses. In the teaching of single words, care must be taken that the correct association is learned by the child, e.g. 'cup' and 'drink' may readily be confused. Later, continued stress on teaching single words can inhibit learning of word combinations.

The level of the child's language development should be discussed with the parents, explaining the normal sequence of progress, which is the same as in the non-handicapped child, and setting appropriate targets. In the early stages advice will usually be necessary on methods of gaining the child's attention and suppressing unwanted behaviour. Parents should be advised to guard against laying undue stress on accurate word formation when early speech is appearing or correct grammar when early phrases are produced.

Non-verbal communication is both a precursor of and an alternative to speech and its early use by both parent and child as the sole or main means of communication is a possible cause of poor progress in speech development. However, the combination of speech and sign language may well be beneficial. In some schools for the deaf Paget Gorman sign language is combined with the use of speech, with the intention of establishing maximum communication and in the hope that one form of communication may reinforce the other. A similar approach to the young mentally handicapped child is worthy of consideration, and the advantages of early communication may not be accompanied by delay in acquisition of language, provided speech and sign language are used concurrently. Later non-verbal communication can be dropped if adequate speech develops, or retained and amplified if it does not.

Preschool education and intensive stimulation programmes
The factors which influence the acquisition of language, perceptual skills and conceptual thinking in the young child of average intelligence are complex. The home environment plays a major role both because of the close ties within the family and because of the time available for learning. However, individual homes and social classes differ considerably, particularly in usage of language. Children in middle-class homes are talked to more than in working-class homes and are asked more questions intended to extend deductive and constructive thinking and increase the child's familiarity with language.

The home background is likely to be of particular importance to the mentally handicapped child who may not learn spontaneously from his environment, but may have to be taught even simple motor and sensory skills and self-care techniques such as feeding, toiletting and dressing. However, even severely mentally retarded individuals can benefit from appropriate teaching, and studies of learning abilities and methods of teaching in this group have shown a need for breakdown of tasks into simple steps and for repeated 'overlearning' until the skill becomes almost automatic. Operant conditioning techniques can be used both to increase the child's attention span and for the teaching of individual skills.

When learned, many skills will be carried out equally well by the moderate retardate as by the normal person. Neither the well-equipped home alone nor the ordinary nursery school is adequate for the moderately retarded child. He requires programmed teaching, initiated and directed by trained staff and continued by the mother, to take advantage of the maximum possible learning time and the mother–child relationship. Tizard (1974) has calculated that a child who attends half-days at nursery school from his third to his fifth birthday will have spent only about 4 per cent of the waking hours of the first 5 years of his life at school.

Research studies have demonstrated the short-term benefit of intensive stimulation programmes in specific groups of children. These include specific types of mental defect such as mongolism, but the group which has received most attention in recent years, which is the largest and where long-term gains could be greatest and most worth while, is that comprising children with sub-cultural mental retardation. Criteria of selection have varied so that it is difficult to compare separate programmes. The Head Start programmes in the US were directed broadly towards disadvantaged and deprived children. However, it could be more profitable to consider which individual factors in the child's environment are most important in preventing development of his full potential. Among the children studied in the National Survey for the Plowden Report (Central Advisory Council for Education, 1967) parental attitude was found to be one of the most important factors influencing primary school achievement whereas Heber and his associates (1972) considered low IQ of the mother to be the best single predictor of poor intellectual performance by the child and they selected children for further study on this basis.

The Head Start programmes in the US produced some benefit to the child but have been criticized as being of far too short duration, lacking reinforcement and narrowly based. They were directed largely towards the child alone, with little involvement of the parents or consideration of the home environment, and they offered opportunity to learn rather than a structured teaching programme. In contrast, Heber and his colleagues intervened early when the child was 3 months old avoiding the need to 'catch up' and attempting to obtain maximal use of the child's genetic endowment. Emphasis was laid on language development and cognitive skills with intensive individual tuition for the child, initially on a one-to-one basis. A parallel rehabilitation programme for the mother provided instruction mainly in the fields of child rearing and household management. At 5½ years of age the experimental group of children were clearly superior to the controls in measures of intelligence, language and, to a lesser extent, learning ability. In drawing conclusions, however, Heber is cautious and emphasizes the need for prolonged follow-up.

A number of other intensive stimulation programmes have been used and the reader is referred to a review by Clarke (1973) of their application to sub-cultural mental deficiency. In a comprehensive review of preschool education in the UK, Tizard (1974) discusses current research concerned with early education of socially disadvantaged children, indicating that the greater part of nursery school teaching in this country is of unproven and doubtful value to this group. Its limitations are similar to those of the Head Start programmes.

Obviously, educational resources should be concentrated on those children most likely to show long-term benefit but, even assuming that programmes can be of lasting value, there is no general agreement about which children should be selected, at what age the programme should commence, its content, intensity, duration, or the best method of involving parents. Some children from a poor environment 'rise above' their background while others fail to do so and it is important to identify the factors responsible for this difference; intelligence, personality, initiative, perseverance, parental attitude, educational opportunity and so on. The potential long-term gains both to the individual child and to the next generation make continued research in these fields essential.

References

BANKS J.L.K. (1974) Eye defects of mentally handicapped children. *British Medical Journal* **2**, 533.

BERGSMA D., ed. (1973) *Birth Defects Atlas and Compendium*. Baltimore: National Foundation, March of Dimes and Williams and Wilkins.

BERRY H.K., LEONARD C., PETERS H., GRANGER M. and CHUNEKAMRAI (1968) Detection of metabolic errors; chromatographic procedures and interpretation of results. *Clinical Chemistry*, **14**, 1033.

BIRCH H.G., RICHARDSON S.A., BAIRD D., HOROBIN G. and ILLSLEY R. (1970) *Mental Subnormality in the Community. A clinical and epidemiological study*. Baltimore: Williams and Wilkins.

BRETT E.M. and LAKE B.D. (1975) Reassessment of rectal approach to neuropathology in childhood. Review of 307 biopsies over 11 years. *Archives of Disease in Childhood*, **50**, 753.

BUIST N.R.M. (1968) Set of simple side-room urine tests for detection of inborn errors of metabolism. *British Medical Journal*, **2**, 745.

BUNDEY S. and CARTER C.O. (1974) Recurrence risks in severe undiagnosed mental deficiency. *Journal of Mental Deficiency Research*, **18**, 115.

CARSON N.A.J. and NEILL D.W. (1962) Metabolic abnormalities detected in a survey of mentally backward individuals in Northern Ireland. *Archives of Disease in Childhood*, **37**, 505.

CENTRAL ADVISORY COUNCIL FOR EDUCATION (ENGLAND) (1967) *Children and their Primary Schools*, Vol. 1, p. 32; Vol. 2, p. 181. London: Her Majesty's Stationery Office.

CLARKE A.D.B. (1973) The prevention of subcultural subnormality: problems and prospects. *British Journal of Mental Subnormality*, **19**, 1.

DRILLIEN C.M. (1968) Studies in mental handicap. II. Some obstetric factors of possible aetiological significance. *Archives of Disease in Childhood*, **43**, 283.

DRILLIEN C.M. (1969). Complications of pregnancy and delivery. *Mental Retardation*, **1**, 280.

DUSSAULT J.H., COULOMBE P., LABERGE C., LETARTE J., GUYDA H. and KHOURY K. (1975) Preliminary report on a mass screening program for neonatal hypothyroidism. *Journal of Pediatrics*, **86**, 670.

ELEK S.D. and STERN H. (1974) Development of a vaccine against mental retardation caused by cytomegalovirus infection *in utero. Lancet*, **i**, 1.

GELLIS S.S. and FEINGOLD M. (1968) *Atlas of Mental Retardation Syndromes. Visual diagnosis of facies and physical findings*. Washington: U.S. Department of Health, Education and Welfare.

GOMEZ M.R. and REESE D.F. (1976) *Computed Tomography of the Head in Infants and Children. Pediatric Clinics of North America*, Vol. 23, p. 3. Philadelphia: W.B. Saunders.

GROSSMAN H.J. (1973) *Manual on Terminology and Classification of Mental Deficiency. Special Publications*, No. 2. Washington, D.C.: American Association for Mental Deficiency.

HAMERTON J.L., CANNING N., RAY M. and SMITH S. (1975) A cytogenetic survey of 14,069 newborn infants. I. Incidence of chromosome abnormalities. *Clinical Genetics*, **8**, 223.

HANSON J.W. and SMITH D.W. (1975) The fetal hydantoin syndrome. *Journal of Pediatrics*, **87**, 285.

HEBER R., GARBER H., HARRINGTON S., HOFFMAN C., FALENDER C. (1972) Rehabilitation of families at risk for mental retardation. *December, 1972, Progress Report. Rehabilitation Research and Training Center in Mental Retardation*. Madison, Wisconsin: University of Wisconsin.

HINDLEY C.B. (1962) Social class influence on the development of ability in the first five years. In *Child and Education. Proceedings of the XIV International Congress of Applied Psychology*, ed. Nielsen, G.S. *Vol. 3*, Copenhagen: Munksgaard.

HSAI D.Y.Y. (1970) Phenylketonuria and its variants. *Progress in Medical Genetics*, **7**, 29.

IRIE M., ENOMOTO K. and NARUSE H. (1975) Measurement of thyroid-stimulating hormone in dried blood spot. *Lancet*, **ii**, 1233.

JACOBS P.A., MELVILLE M., RATCLIFFE S., KEAY A.J. and SYME J. (1974) A cytogenetic survey of 11,680 newborn infants. *Annals of Human Genetics*, **37**, 359.

JONES K.L. and SMITH D.W. (1975) The fetal alcohol syndrome. *Teratology*, **12**, 1.

KAZNER E., LANKSCH W. and STEINHOFF H. (1976) Cranial computerised tomography in the diagnosis of brain disorders in infants and children. *Neuropädiatrie*, **7**, 136.

KIRMAN B. (1975) The backward baby: treatment and counselling. In *Mental Handicap*, eds. Kirman B. and Bicknell J., p. 270. Edinburgh: Churchill Livingstone.

KUSHLICK A. and COX G.R. (1973) The epidemiology of mental handicap. *Developmental Medicine and Child Neurology*, **15**, 748.

LEWANDOWSKI R.C., JR. and YUNIS J.J. (1975) New chromosomal syndromes. *American Journal of Diseases of Children*, **129**, 515.

MACE J.W., GOODMAN S.I., CENTERWALL W.R. and CHINNOCK R.F. (1976) The child with an unusual odor. *Clinical Pediatrics*, **15**, 57.

MELISH M.E. and HANSHAW J.B. (1973) Congenital cytomegalovirus infection. Developmental progress of infants detected by routine screening. *American Journal of Diseases of Children*, **126**, 190.

PENROSE L.S. (1965) Dermatoglyphics in mosaic mongolism and allied conditions. In *Genetics Today, Proceedings of the XI International Congress of Genetics*, ed. Geerts S.J. Vol. 3, p. 973. London: Pergamon Press.

PUBLIC HEALTH LABORATORY SERVICE: WORKING PARTY ON RUBELLA (1970) Studies of the effect of immunoglobulin on rubella in pregnancy. *British Medical Journal*, **2**, 497.

SKEELS H.M. and DYE H.B. (1939) A study of the effects of differential stimulation on mentally retarded children. *Proceedings of the American Association on Mental Deficiency*, **44**, 114.

SKODAK M. (1968) Adult status of individuals who experienced early intervention. In *Proceedings of the First Congress of the International Association for the Scientific Study of Mental Deficiency*, ed. Richards B.W., Reigate, England: Michael Jackson.

SLATER E.T.O. and COWIE V. (1971) *The Genetics of Mental Disorders*. London: Oxford University Press.

SMITH D.W. (1970) Recognizable patterns of human malformations. Genetic, embryologic and clinical aspects. *Major Problems in Clinical Pediatrics*, Vol. 7. Philadelphia: W.B. Saunders.

SORSBY A. (1973) *Clinical Genetics*, 2nd Ed., p. 86. London: Butterworth.

STERN H., ELEK S.D., BOOTH J.C. and FLECK D.G. (1969) Microbial causes of mental retardation. The role of the prenatal infections with cytomegalovirus, rubella virus and toxoplasma. *Lancet*, **2**, 443.

STERN H. and TUCKER S.M. (1973) Prospective study of cytomegalovirus infection in pregnancy. *British Medical Journal*, **2**, 268.

TIZARD B. (1974) *Early Childhood Education. A review and discussion of research in Britain*. London: National Foundation for Educational Research.

WORLD HEALTH ORGANIZATION (1965) *International Classification of Diseases*. London: Her Majesty's Stationery Office.

ZACKAI E.H., MELLMAN W.J. and NEIDERER B. (1975) The fetal trimethadione syndrome. *Journal of Pediatrics*, **87**, 280.

Further Reading

BEREITER C. and ENGELMANN S. (1966) *Teaching Disadvantaged Children in the Pre-School.* Englewood Cliffs, New Jersey: Prentice-Hall.

CLARKE A.D.B. (1969) *Recent Advances in the Study of Subnormality*, Revised edition. London: National Association for Mental Health.

DAVIE R., BUTLER N. and GOLDSTEIN H. (1972) *Studies in Child Development. From Birth to Seven.* London: Longman.

DOUGLAS J.W.B. (1964) *The Home and the School.* London: MacGibbon and Kee.

DOUGLAS J.W.B., ROSS J.M., MAXWELL S.M.M. and WALKER D.A. (1966) Differences in test score and in the gaining of selective places for Scottish children and those in England and Wales. *British Journal of Educational Psychology*, **36**, 150.

FORREST A., RITSON B. and ZEALLEY A. (1973) *New Perspectives in Mental Handicap.* Edinburgh: Churchill Livingstone.

GRIFFITHS M.I. (1973) *The Young Retarded Child. Medical Aspects of Care.* Edinburgh: Churchill Livingstone.

PRINGLE M.L.K., BUTLER N.R. and DAVIE R. (1966) *Studies in Child Development. 11,000 seven-year-olds.* London: Longman.

KIRMAN B. and BICKNELL J. (1975) *Mental Handicap.* Edinburgh: Churchill Livingstone.

MACKAY R.I. (1976) *Mental Handicap in Child Health Practice.* London: Butterworth.

TIZARD J., SINCLAIR I., CLARKE R.V.G. (1975) *Varieties of Residential Experience.* London: Routledge and Kegan Paul.

CHAPTER 14

Cerebral Palsy

Aetiology

Cerebral palsy has been defined as 'a disorder of movement and posture due to a defect or lesion of the immature brain' (Bax, 1964). Its chronicity and non-progression are implicit in this and the nearly similar definitions of other expert groups or individuals. Degenerative diseases of the central nervous system are excluded, together with disorders of movement and posture which are due only to mental defect. Cerebral palsy is not a single entity but a heterogeneous complex whose aetiology is diverse, changing and still too often unknown or imprecisely identified. A classification framework makes the discussion of aetiology easier, but neurologists and others have been engaged for well over a century on such diverse constructions (see Ingram's historical review, 1964) that choice becomes a daunting prospect for the clinician. One akin to Ingram's own, and that used by Hagberg and his colleagues (1975a, b), is favoured here.

TABLE 14.1. Types of cerebral palsy and their relative frequency in a Swedish series. From Hagberg B., Hagberg G. and Olow I. (1975b) *Acta Paediatrica Scandinavica*, **64**, 193.

Type	Number	%
Hemiplegia	200	36
Tetraplegia	19	3
Spastic diplegia	186	33
Ataxic diplegia	31	5
Congenital ataxia	44	8
Athetosis	20	4
Dystonic forms	60	11
TOTAL	560	100

The relative frequency of the various types of cerebral palsy in a recent large unselected series from one well-defined Swedish region is shown in Table 14.1 (Hagberg *et al.*, 1975b). The authors have grouped possible causative factors under four headings: prenatal, perinatal, postnatal and unknown. Their estimates for cerebral palsy as a whole, and for each of the various types, are shown in Table 14.2.

It is easy to understand how known harmful influences during the period of organ development (included under prenatal) may lead to cerebral palsy by alteration of the form of the brain. After the first trimester is over, assigning such causes becomes less easy. The growing brain's constantly changing water and electrolyte content, its developing hormonal influences, its growth spurts,

TABLE 14.2. Presumed aetiology of various types of cerebral palsy in a Swedish series. From Hagberg B., Hagberg G., and Olow I. (1975b) *Acta Paediatrica Scandinavica*, **64**, 193.

| Type of cerebral palsy | No. | Presumed Cause | | | | |
		Prenatal (%)	Perinatal (%)	Postnatal (%)	Unknown (%)	Total (%)
Hemiplegia	200	23	41	6	30	100
Tetraplegia	19	42	37	11	10	100
Spastic diplegia	186	25	57	3	15	100
Ataxic diplegia	31	45	39	3	13	100
Congenital ataxia	44	25	18	16	41	100
Athetosis	20	5	85	0	10	100
Dystonic forms	60	26	65	7	2	100
Total	560	27	49	7	17	100

first of neuronal cells and then of glial cells with accompanying increases in dendrites and synapses, mean that the same injurious factor could have very different effects at 20, 30 or 40 weeks of intrauterine life. The two most important influences at any time after the first trimester are likely to be the metabolic consequences of either a diminished amount of oxygen reaching the brain, or impaired cerebral perfusion. Some of the factors which are associated with such hypoxia and ischaemia in the second and third trimesters of pregnancy and the first week of life are shown in Table 14.3. After the perinatal period, the postnatal causative factors are usually easier to identify, and include most importantly infections and trauma.

TABLE 14.3. Some factors associated with cerebral palsy

| Prenatal | | Perinatal | Postnatal |
First trimester	Later pregnancy		
Congenital malformation	Threatened abortion	Toxaemia	Infection
Genetically determined disorder	Chronic maternal illness	Antepartum haemorrhage Other placental and/or	Injury Cerebrovascular
Intrauterine infection	Toxaemia	cord conditions leading	accidents
Threatened abortion	Intrauterine growth retardation	to fetal hypoxia and/or ischaemia	Epilepsy
	Intrauterine infection	Birth trauma Severe birth asphyxia Infection Pre-term birth Intrauterine growth retardation Hypoglycaemia Hyperbilirubinaemia Shock, due e.g. to haemorrhage	

Note: The prenatal period as defined here corresponds approximately to the first two trimesters of pregnancy. The perinatal period includes the third trimester, the most important part of which may be the period immediately before, during and after birth, and the first week of life. Postnatal is defined for purposes of this Table to mean after the first week of life.

Some generalizations can be made before commenting briefly on aetiological factors in the different types of cerebral palsy. Low birth-weight has always been disproportionately represented, approximately 40 per cent of children weighing 2500 g or less in most series. Retarded intrauterine growth after the 35th week of gestation is frequent (Hagberg *et al.*, 1976). Abnormalities of pregnancy and the perinatal period are significantly increased, a fact first appreciated by William Little (1862). This is to some extent explained by the relatively high proportion of low weight babies involved, for their mothers tend to have more complicated pregnancies. Multiple pregnancy is over represented (Griffiths, 1967) and this cannot be explained solely by the high incidence of low birth-weight (Illingworth and Woods, 1960). Males are more frequently affected than females.

Aetiological factors associated with different types of cerebral palsy.
Hemiplegia. Aetiology is unknown in about one-third (Ingram, 1964; Hagberg *et al.*, 1975b). In these cases suspicion falls on genetic cause or some prenatal event such as infection or vascular occlusion, occurring sufficiently long before birth to allow the fetus to recover, and without clinically recognizable illness in the mother. Just over one-half of those destined to be hemiplegics seem to have had some insult early in gestation (see Table 14.2). In two-fifths perinatal factors such as birth injury, leading to subdural or other intracranial haemorrhage, and severe hypoxia seem to predominate, though a few cases (8 per cent) are associated with exchange transfusion (Hagberg, *et al.*, 1975b) which might suggest an embolic cause. Among postnatal events which account for the remainder, well-documented aetiological factors are viral and bacterial meningitides or encephalitides, head injury, epilepsy and cerebrovascular accidents (Brandt, 1962; Isler, 1971). On the basis of arteriographic studies, an inflammatory carotid arteritis, in association with acute tonsillitis, has been postulated as a causative factor by Bickerstaff (1964).
Tetraplegia (synonymous with Ingram's double hemiplegia). Prenatal factors such as growth retardation and maternal illness or severe hypoxia during the perinatal period are reported in the majority of these cases. Developmental abnormalities, including malformations of the brain, implicate adverse factors in early gestation in some congenital cases. In the minority of patients with postnatally determined tetraplegia, the causes are as for acquired hemiplegia, including severe head injury.

Spastic diplegia. Several authors have pointed to a bimodal birth-weight distribution (Evans, 1948; Childs and Evans, 1954) and a highly significant correlation with immaturity is well established. The aetiology in the low birth-weight group has been widely discussed but remains uncertain apart from the common factor of pre-term birth. A review of the literature does not suggest consistent support for serious neonatal illness as a cause; indeed other forms of cerebral palsy seem as common amongst the most seriously ill, very low birth-weight infants who now survive with mechanical ventilation (Fitzhardinge *et al.*, 1976; Marriage and Davies, 1977).

Hydrocephalus could selectively damage corticospinal fibres involving legs more than arms and some degree of ventricular dilatation is relatively common in infants dying in the early neonatal period, whether or not they have intraventricular haemorrhage (Jacobi, *et al.*, 1974; Davies and Tizard, 1975). In very immature infants who survive, ventricular dilatation can be present without increased head size (Korobkin, 1975). The findings of a lower haematocrit on the second day of life in those destined to be diplegics compared with non-diplegics of similar weight and gestation has suggested haemorrhage into body tissue, particularly the brain (Churchill *et al.*, 1974). However it is difficult to reconcile the recent decrease in spastic diplegia (Davies and Tizard, 1975; Hagberg *et al.*, 1975a) with a relative increase in intraventricular haemorrhage (Machin, 1975), the latter possibly associated with injudicious alkali therapy (Simmons *et al.*, 1974; Wigglesworth *et al.*, 1976), if the two conditions are causally related.

No one has yet confirmed or denied Griffiths' (1967) observation that spastic diplegia is significantly more common in first than second born twins; she suggested that birth injury might be the cause as the head of the first twin would be the principal dilator of the cervical canal. Episiotomy appears to have become more commonly practised as spastic diplegia has decreased (Davies and Tizard, 1975). It is possible that subarachnoid haemorrhage, which may lead to hydrocephalus, is now occurring less frequently in those infants, whose birth-weight is above the mean (Hagberg *et al.*, 1976).

Compared with mothers of pre-term diplegics and of normal children, mothers of mature diplegics tend to marry later and be older. They tend to be generally subfertile and in particular relatively infertile immediately before the birth of a diplegic patient (Drillien *et al.*, 1962; 1964). These authors suggested that in some cases children were retarded and diplegic in whole or part because of factors which were damaging to them in early fetal life. In some others harmful perinatal factors appeared to cause additional damage.

Ataxic diplegia. The majority of cases are associated with pre- or perinatal factors. Those of very low birth-weight who have this form of cerebral palsy may be survivors of neonatal intraventricular haemorrhage. In general aetiological factors are more closely allied to those for spastic diplegia than for congenital ataxia. Postnatally acquired and congenital hydrocephalus (Hagberg *et al.*, 1975b) are characteristically followed by ataxic diplegia. Genetic factors predominate in a small number of mature infants without hydrocephalus.

Congenital ataxia. The aetiology differs from other cerebral palsy syndromes in that not infrequently it may be genetically determined and inherited as an autosomal recessive disorder (Gustavson *et al.*, 1969). Brain malformations particularly of the cerebellum and cerebellar connections, are common. Postnatal cases are associated with viral infections and hydrocephalus in particular.

Athetoid and dystonic forms (dyskinetic cerebral palsy). Perinatal factors far outweigh others in importance. There are two outstanding and well-documented causes, hyperbilirubinaemia and severe birth asphyxia (Gerrard, 1952; Churchill and Colfelt, 1963; Griffiths and Barrett, 1967).

Autopsy evidence

Neuropathological studies in the human have been able to offer only a limited contribution to our understanding of aetiology, for the often normal life span of the cerebral palsied patient means that reparative processes in the brain may obscure the original lesion. There is nevertheless much interesting reading in the monograph by Christensen and Melchior (1967) which describes a prospectively followed series.

The lesions of periventricular leucomalacia, so named by Banker and Larroche (1962) but first described over a century ago, were considered by these authors (and many others since) to be the cause of spastic diplegia, because they could interrupt the course of corticospinal fibres. Periventricular leucomalacia is most commonly considered to consist of areas of infarction resulting from perfusion failure in circulatory border zones. It is obviously difficult to know if this could be so. More recent examinations of the brains of immature infants, some of whom had undergone prolonged mechanical ventilation, have shown these lesions to varying degrees (Brand and Bignami, 1969; Armstrong and Norman, 1974; Grunnet *et al.*, 1974; Smith *et al.*, 1974; Schneider *et al.*, 1975).

Terplan (1967) noted that neurones in the cortex of the immature infant were significantly less frequently affected than those of mature infants under comparable conditions of hypoxia. Clinical experience suggests that following similar conditions of hypoxia, pre-term infants less often show obvious neurological abnormality later than do mature infants (Scott, 1976).

Hemsath (1934) drew attention to a little publicized injury of the occipital bone most commonly seen in breech delivery; this still happens. A synchondrosis occurs between the squamous and basal parts of the occipital bone and is liable to cause gross traumatic injury to the cerebellum.

Experimental evidence

Work on the animal fetus and newborn may help us to understand the situation in the human, though the precision with which the intensity and duration of any insult to the animal can be measured bears little relation to the relative uncertainty of human perinatal events. Furthermore, experiments are rarely conducted with immature animals and uncritical extrapolation is unjustified. However, the work of Myers and his group in recent years is of interest and some aspects have been summarized recently (Myers, 1975). In the fetal Rhesus monkey, total asphyxia leads to brain stem damage with hemispheres spared. Partial asphyxia with ensuing acidosis predominantly damages the cortex and brain oedema occurs. Hypoxic insults without acidosis (presumably less severe) produce lesions in the white matter and these may include focal areas of periventricular leucomalacia. A combination of hypoxia with acidosis and a period of superimposed total anoxia leads principally to damage of the basal ganglia; this is the area of the brain damaged in the human with athetoid and dystonic forms of cerebral palsy. Ischaemic insults are thought to exert their harmful effects through hypoxia and acidosis occurring either during the period of insult or in the recovery period (Gamache and Myers, 1975).

Prevention

Prevention of disease depends on avoidance or modification of its cause (Wynn and Wynn, 1976). As we have seen, there are still wide gaps in our knowledge of the causation of cerebral palsy. During the period of the Swedish survey (1954–70) there was a significant decrease in the total incidence of cerebral palsy from 2.2 per cent in the first 4 years to 1.3 per cent in the last 4 years (Hagberg *et al.*, 1975a). The decrease was most significant for the syndromes of spastic and ataxic diplegia associated with low birth-weight and for all types of cerebral palsy due to perinatal causes. A similar reduction in the incidence of spastic diplegia among those weighing 1500 g or less, born 1961–70, was noted by Davies and Tizard (1975). Since mortality rates are slowly but steadily decreasing for all weight groups this suggests that intensive perinatal care *has* been important in prevention.

On balance it seems likely that improved social well-being and obstetric care have been and will continue to be of more importance than advances in neonatal care; although improvements in neonatal resuscitation and nutrition, and the prevention of hypothermia, hypoglycaemia and as far as possible, hypoxia have probably all played a minor part. However, paediatricians can claim to have made it possible to virtually abolish dyskinetic forms of cerebral palsy secondary to Rhesus haemolytic disease by avoiding hyperbilirubinaemia, though this is made easier as isoimmunization itself becomes modified or prevented by appropriate anti-D immunoglobulin treatment of the mother. Kernicterus is occasionally reported at autopsy in severely hypoxic and acidotic infants of very low birth-weight when bilirubin levels have been low (Gartner *et al.*, 1970), and it is possible that mechanical ventilation of such infants (introduced in the mid-1960s) could be salvaging a small number who will be severely handicapped (Fitzhardinge *et al.*, 1976; Marriage and Davies, 1977).

The detection of impaired fetal well-being by a variety of tests is now becoming possible (see review by Symonds, 1976). Their wider application should lead to a further reduction in the incidence of those types of cerebral palsy which appear to be most common in infants with intrauterine growth retardation and other evidence of fetal deprivation (Hagberg *et al.*, 1976). The oft quoted 'continuum of reproductive casualty' concept advanced by Lilienfeld, Pasamanick and Rogers (1955) finds support in Drillien's (1972) work, and again in the Swedish series. If fetal hypoxia and consequent acidosis can be minimized and severe birth asphyxia intensively treated, the outlook should be favourable (Steiner and Neligan, 1975; Scott, 1976) unless serious prenatal damage has already occurred.

At present one must be somewhat less hopeful about prevention of cerebral palsy due to prenatal conditions with so many of them still unknown. Ill-defined socioeconomic disadvantage plays some part in an increased incidence and measures (equally hard to define) to relieve this are clearly desirable. The risk of infection, greatest in this group of poor mothers, may be prevented in the future to some extent by immunization (e.g. against cytomegalovirus) if the safety of vaccines can be assured. Women showing serological conversion for *Toxoplasma gondii* infection are said to show a significantly lower incidence of congenitally infected infants when treated with spiramycin compared with untreated controls (Desmonts and Couvreur, 1974), but it is unlikely that screening programmes to detect pregnancy sero-conversion could be envisaged at present.

It is generally agreed that cerebral palsy due to most postnatal causes has been reduced by improvements in social care as much as anything. However, child abuse seems to be increasing and here again social intervention among those at greatest risk is likely to be the single most rewarding measure. Other contributory factors to the reduction in acquired cerebral palsy are the lowered incidence of gastroenteritis with prevention or improved treatment of hypernatraemia and the earlier diagnosis and better treatment of bacterial meningitis.

P.A. DAVIES

Classification

The usefulness of a classification of the cerebral palsy syndromes is limited by the fact that in the early years of life the final picture may be by no means clear and because mixed types and presentations that do not fit easily into any of the conventional categories are more common than is usually recognized. In addition, there is a grey area between what is clearly a mild degree of cerebral palsy and minor abnormal neurological signs which may largely resolve or become more obvious with the passage of time. The varying incidence and severity of associated disorders in patients with similar types of motor and movement disturbances also make comparisons difficult. Nevertheless, certain syndromes are seen sufficiently often to merit a classification framework for the purpose of identifying aetiology (and hence ways of prevention), for comparing the efficacy of different methods of treatment and to facilitate communication.

Classification by clinical findings
Patients can be classified by clinical presentation as follows.

Hemiplegia, a unilateral spastic paresis affecting the arm more than the leg.

Bilateral hemiplegia, a spastic paresis (often asymmetrical) affecting all four limbs, with more marked involvement of arms than legs. This type of cerebral palsy is also called spastic tetraplegia or quadriplegia. Some writers reserve tetraplegia for the commoner manifestation with marked bulbar paresis and quadriplegia for cases with less severe or absent bulbar involvement.

Diplegia, paresis affecting all four limbs but much more marked in the legs than in the arms. Diplegia is subdivided into hypotonic (atonic), dystonic and spastic stages. Commonly the infant and young child progresses through all these stages but occasionally remains for a prolonged period (or permanently) in the hypotonic or dystonic phase.

Ataxic cerebral palsies subdivided into, cerebellar ataxia, characterized by hypotonia, inco-ordination of voluntary movements and impairment of balance; *ataxic diplegia*, in which spasticity of diplegic distribution is superimposed on ataxia, and the *dysequilibrium syndrome*, characterized by pronounced difficulty in maintaining an upright body posture and in experiencing the position of the body in space.

Dyskinetic cerebral palsy, characterized by involuntary movements and disorderly changes of tone affecting the bulbar musculature, the face, trunk and all four limbs.

Mixed and unclassifiable.

Classification by severity
A classification by severity is useful in monitoring progress and assessing the efficacy of therapy. Ingram (1964) suggested the following terminology based on functional impairment. This must be considered in relation to mental age.

Hemiplegia. Mild, the affected hand is used independently for everyday activities.
Moderate, the affected hand is used only to assist the unaffected hand.
Severe, the affected hand has no useful function except perhaps as a prop or support.

Bilateral hemiplegia. Mild, some use of the upper limbs is retained.
Moderate, some use of the lower limbs is retained.
Severe, there is no use of the limbs.

Diplegia, gait by 4–5 years. Mild, gait is clumsy rather than disabled.
Moderate, the child is unsteady when walking and cannot run.
Severe, at best assisted walking only is possible.

Ataxic and dyskinetic syndromes, by 4–5 years. Mild, without significant functional loss in everyday activities though the child is abnormally clumsy, independent walking is achieved.
Moderate, the child needs some assistance in everyday activities and may need some support for walking.
Severe, the child needs total assistance in all but the simplest everyday activities and cannot walk even with support.

Clinical presentations
As would be expected from the diffuse and differing nature of the underlying pathology, clinical findings in individual patients also vary widely. However, the clinical presentations seen most often are as follows.

Hemiplegia. In congenital cases no abnormality may be noted in the first few months but if the infant is examined (possibly because of a hemisyndrome noted is the newborn period) the affected arm is seen to lie alongside the body with forearm pronated, palm facing down and thumb adducted. Poverty of movement is noted in arm and leg and tone and tendon reflexes are reduced. Increasing tone, with tendon reflexes becoming brisker than on the unaffected side, becomes obvious after 3 months or so, with the hand characteristically clenched, thumb in palm. Marked hand preference instead of normal ambidexterity is evident, when at 5–6 months, the infant is reaching for toys. Athetoid movements of hand and fingers may be seen later.

In acquired hemiplegia more obvious paresis affecting face and limbs is immediately apparent. The hypotonic phase is brief and is superseded by hypertonicity within 1–2 months.

Dwarfing of the affected limbs and vasomotor disturbance (the hand and foot feeling cold) are common. Epilepsy occurs in one-third to one-half, being more common in acquired hemiplegics. Mental retardation is present in about one-third of patients.

Bilateral hemiplegia. In congenital cases severe brain damage is usually apparent from birth. Severe feeding difficulties occur due to bulbar involvement. The infant shows poverty of movement with increasing hypertonicity in all four limbs. Physical disability is marked, epilepsy is common and mental retardation usual.

Diplegia. The characteristic findings of an established cerebral diplegia may take many months to emerge, and initial presentation is variable. Most often the infant shows some poverty of movement, delayed motor development, hypotonicity, reduced tendon reflexes and exaggeration of primitive reflexes. In the dystonic phase tone is unexceptional at rest but there is an increase in extensor tone on handling and positioning, particularly when the child is held in vertical suspension (p. 137). Primitive reflexes, especially the ATNR, placing and walking are retained well past the normal age. Finally flexor hypertonous takes over with the risk of contractures.

Although involvement of the upper limbs may be minimal, careful examination reveals some abnormality in virtually all cases. Involuntary movements may be seen especially in the hands. Bulbar paresis (less marked than in bilateral hemiplegia) occurs most often when the arms are obviously affected.

Dwarfing of pelvis and lower limbs is found in established cases. Epilepsy occurs in about one-third and mental retardation in up to one-half. Physical disability is more pronounced with prolongation of the hypotonic or dystonic stages.

Ataxia

Congenital ataxia presents in infancy with hypotonia (which may be very marked and cause diagnostic difficulties), hyperextensibility at joints, reduced or absent tendon reflexes, poverty of movement and considerable delay in gross motor development.

When the infant starts reaching for objects, movements are abnormally clumsy for age and intention tremor becomes obvious later when finer hand movements are attempted. Truncal ataxia may become evident on sitting and standing. Support for walking may be needed for a long time and when independent walking is achieved, it is characteristically 'drunken', on a wide base, flat-footed and with arms up for balance. Epilepsy is rare. About one-third of patients are mentally retarded.

Ataxic diplegia. Initially infants present with the signs described above although these are usually less marked. By 3–6 months hypotonia is giving way to increased tone and knee and ankle jerks become easily elicitable. Spasticity is usually mild or moderate.

Gait is unsteady but less wide based than in ataxia and there is a tendency for the child to walk on toes or on the inner borders of the feet (as in diplegia). Intention tremor is apparent when fine motor actions are attempted. Epilepsy is quite frequent and mental retardation more common than in pure ataxia.

Dysequilibrium syndrome. Hypotonia with markedly defective postural function, pronounced motor delay, severe language delay and mental retardation was described by Hagberg *et al.* (1972). In a significant proportion of cases an autosomal recessive mode of inheritance is postulated.

Dyskinetic cerebral palsy. Most infants who present later with this type show frank neurological abnormality in the neonatal period which gradually resolves though, if such an infant is kept under surveillance, he is noted to become generally hypotonic with motor delay. Feeding difficulties are common and persist. Later chewing and swallowing difficulties are exacerbated by involuntary movements of the feeding musculature. Primitive reflexes are exaggerated and maintained beyond the normal age. An oblitary ATNR at 6 months is a significant sign. Restriction of upwards gaze is characteristic of kernicterus.

Head, neck and limb control remains poor. Involuntary movements appear gradually. At first these may take the form of mass movements of trunk and limbs on handling or attempted voluntary movement, the child being thrown into extension. More discreet involuntary movements of face and limbs, whenever the child attempts an action, are most usually obvious after the age of 2 years though minor manifestations (especially in fingers and toes) may be seen earlier. Epilepsy is rare. Patients are frequently within the normal range of intelligence. Hearing loss is a common association.

Mixed types and unclassifiable. Many patients exhibit characteristics of more than one type of cerebral palsy although usually one type predominates. In other instances the pattern of neurological abnormality does not fit readily into any of the accepted categories and indeed it may be difficult to decide whether or not the child should be classified as having a cerebral palsy. It often seems that these difficult to classify patients suffer from developmental malformation rather than from damage to an initially normal central nervous system. As cerebral palsy due to perinatal damage decreases, the relative importance of brain malformation will increase. It is expected that computer assisted tomography will contribute significantly to the diagnosis of these cases in future.

C.M. DRILLIEN

Physical Aspects

This section is written with the premise that the spinal cord and brain stem are, in the normal human, fully programmed for antigravity support and automatic stepping; that the integrative action of the basal ganglia and cerebellum add to these brain stem reactions the functions of equipoise and locomotion; and that the voluntary system acts upon this co-ordinated moving base. It is concerned therefore with the symptoms resulting from the disorganization of systems, rather than with reflexes.

Cerebral palsy was aptly defined by the Little Club (1959) as 'a persistent *but not unchanging* disorder of movement and posture, appearing in the early years of life and due to a non-progressive disorder of the brain, the result of interference during its development. Persistence of the infantile type of motor control, such as may be seen in intellectually handicapped children, is not considered to be cerebral palsy.' This definition, arrived at after much debate, holds good today. Anybody who has followed such cases for even a few years will recognize that cerebral palsy, though due to a static lesion, changes a great deal in the course of time. Pathological studies have shown that in almost all cases the responsible lesions are diffusely scattered in the nervous system, although hyperbilirubinaemia selectively affects the basal ganglia and anoxia may also do so.

The accepted categories of cerebral palsy are described (p. 265). Although most cases fit fairly well into one or other of these groups there are many that do not, and it is more important to analyse the functional deficit than to categorize the patient. Since the lesion is usually diffuse it is common to get mixtures of physical disabilities, e.g. a child with a spastic quadriparesis may show some involuntary movements or ataxia, so that even if the spasticity is remedied to some degree by treatment it may be found that he still cannot walk because of impairment of balance. The accepted categories or 'diagnoses' are only rough descriptive terms and are in fact of very little practical value because they give scant indication of the child's actual state. For example, it is of little consequence whether paresis is accompanied by spasticity or rigidity; similarly the term ataxia fails to distinguish cases with inco-ordination of the limbs from those with truncal instability.

In a personal series of 863 cases the frequency of different types of cerebral palsy was hemiplegia 16 per cent, diplegia/quadriplegia 46 per cent, ataxia 11 per cent and dyskinetic syndromes 26 per cent (of these 8 per cent were cases of pure athetosis). The changing frequency and incidence of the various types is well shown in the Swedish study of Hagberg *et al.* (1975) (Table 14.4).

TABLE 14.4. Relative frequency of different types of cerebral palsy and population incidence by date of birth (Adapted from Hagberg *et al.*, 1975)

	1959–62 (%)	1963–66 (%)	1967–70 (%)
Hemiplegia	28	38	41
Quadriplegia	4	1	5
Diplegia/ataxic diplegia	46	35	31
Ataxia	6	8	12
Dyskinetic syndromes	16	18	11
Total	100	100	100
No. cases	172	182	141
Incidence per 1000 live births	1.89	1.67	1.34

If one is to understand the actual disabilities suffered by patients, it is necessary to ask what the phenomena encountered in cerebral palsy actually mean. These can be divided into two main groups: the principal motor disorders and the associated disorders (p. 282). The principal motor disorders are those disorders of movement and posture which manifestly separate these cases from cases of mental subnormality without motor abnormality, which merit special attention if the child is ever to attain even limited independence and which justify our saying that a given child has 'cerebral palsy'. The associated disorders are disorders of other cerebral functions, attributable to the diffuse nature of the lesions and which, though common, are not essential to the diagnosis. Examples are perceptual and speech disorders, epilepsy and mental subnormality. Thus a child with cerebral palsy may have none or all of these and still be categorized as cerebral palsied because he is disabled from the point of view of posture and movement while another child with fits and a language disorder may show minor neurological abnormality such as extensor plantar responses, but is not accepted as having cerebral palsy in the ordinary sense. In a given case of cerebral palsy one or other of the associated disorders may be more important than the primary motor disorder in determining management; but in general the associated disorders are less important than the main motor disability.

THE PRINCIPAL MOTOR DISORDERS

These are:
  disorders of postural fixation;
  failure of suppression of crude postural reflexes centred in the brain stem;
  disorders of tone due to involvement of the brain stem facilitatory and
    inhibitory mechanisms;
  paralysis and disorders of the pattern of voluntary movements;
  involuntary movements, and
  failure of development of cortical reactions.

Disorders of postural fixation

Defective postural fixation, as seen in inability to maintain the head or trunk erect, is the most important and obvious defect in all cases of cerebral palsy except the mildest of hemiplegias. The basic head/trunk-erecting mechanisms fail to work when they should and the infant fails to pass the motor milestones of head-raising, sitting with rounded back, sitting with a hollow lumbar curve, and so on. Concomitant with this motor delay there may or may not be hypertonus of the limbs. If the limbs are spastic one has the paradox of the child who is stiff in his limbs but floppy in his trunk. The *'floppiness' of the trunk is not hypotonia in the ordinary sense* (p. 277) but is due to absence of the normal postural reflexes responsible for trunk erection (the bracing of part on part) and equipoise.

In order to understand the many disorders of the postural reactions encountered in cerebral palsy it is necessary to revise and simplify one's concept of the nervous system. The scheme outlined here is based on the classical studies of André-Thomas and colleagues (1952, 1960), who dealt with infant development, and of Purdon Martin (1967), who dealt with postural reflexes and the basal ganglia in adults. All disorders of the basal ganglia are accompanied by disorders of posture. The basis of this principle is quite simple: the spinal cord and brain stem are fully programmed for antigravity support of the lower limbs and for automatic stepping. Thus the movements of the neonate are basically the same as those of the anencephalic who survives more than a few days. Evidence for this is to be seen in films made by Gamper (1925/6)* on the anencephalic and by Graham Brown in 1939 (Lundberg and Phillips, 1973) on the movements of decerebrate cats. The latter shows that the acutely decerebrate cat, provided with balance, can adjust its step accurately to the speed of a treadmill and can produce smooth and perfectly co-ordinated movements of walking, trotting and cantering: it is by no means the spastic decerebrate caricature of the physiological textbooks. However, these three 'brain stem preparations', the neonate, the anencephalic and the properly handled acutely decerebrate cat are devoid of three important functions, viz. equipoise, the power to initiate locomotion, and voluntary activity. The first two are provided by the basal ganglia while voluntary activity acts upon the combined brain stem–basal ganglia system which functions as a continuously co-ordinated 'moving base': the cortex chooses the moment, the moving base provides the pattern. All the reflexes required for equipoise pass through the basal ganglia and are integrated there. They are, therefore, disturbed by lesions of these ganglia. Since the lesion causing cerebral palsy is either diffuse or in some cases confined to the basal ganglia, it follows that in the majority of patients disorders of basic postural reactions will be found, quite irrespective of any disorder of voluntary movement or of tone. However, it is important to recognize that (1) in early life the disorders of postural fixation will be most evident because voluntary movement has not developed at that time, and (2) a *normal* voluntary movement cannot occur on a background of abnormal postural fixation. Such a movement is

---

* Film: A Human Mid-Brain Preparation, as described by Eduard Gamper (translated by J.A.V. Bates) obtainable from Spastics Society, Fitzroy Square, London W1P 5HQ.

bound to be rendered abnormal by instability of posture, just as naval or tank gunfire is bound to be inaccurate if the turret's orientation is not continuously adapted to the motion of the vehicle.

The principal postural reactions are summarized in Table 14.5. They are not as difficult to remember as one might fear, for they are commonplaces of daily life. One has only to bear in mind that *any* movement of head or limb must be accompanied by an automatic counter-movement of the trunk if balance is to be preserved. These reactions are developed in the first 2 years of life. They furnish all our automatic activities of sitting, rising, standing, turning and walking, and when they begin to fade, senescence has begun.

It is important to recognize that each postural reaction is specific and has a pattern of its own. One of them can be absent while the rest are present, though more commonly several, or most, are absent. As examples: the tilting reaction

TABLE 14.5. Principal Postural Reflexes (Adapted from Purdon Martin, J.,
The Basal Ganglia and Posture)

Reaction	*Main 'centre'*
Antigravity mechanisms	
Antigravity support by the limbs (positive supporting reactions) and automatic stepping	Proprioceptive, via brain stem but subject to cortical inhibition; insufficient for equilibrium
Mechanisms for postural fixation	
Head and trunk erecting mechanisms	
Counterpoise reactions: reactions sustaining balance and resisting forces tending to make the body fall by rotation about its pivot, i.e. during limb and head movements	Proprioceptive via the basal ganglia
Tilting reactions to instability of the base (whether in sitting, standing, all-fours or lying)	
(1) head and trunk	Labyrinths, via basal ganglia
(2) limbs	Proprioceptive via basal ganglia
Protective reactions	
Protecting the upright posture *after* displacement by a horizontal force, i.e. after 'overbalancing'	Proprioceptive, via basal ganglia
Reaction to falling (parachute reaction)	Probably cortical
Righting (rising) reactions	
Enabling the body to regain the sitting or standing posture, and preserve its balance in the process	Proprioceptive via the basal ganglia
Locomotive reactions	
By shift of the centre of gravity:	
(1) tilt, to start and stop	
(2) sway, to continue walking	Caudate nuclei
(3) controlled lateral fall for turning	
Visual postural reactions	
Aiding labyrinthine righting, head elevation, but using same final common path	Visual cortex

may be absent in one direction yet present in others; protective stepping may be absent to one side but present to the other; the initiation of locomotion may be present when its reverse, stopping, is not possible (this after all is seen in the toddler who can only stop by running into something or somebody) and automatic, tireless head elevation may be lacking though voluntary head raising to command is present, but transient. The examiner must, therefore, learn to detect these defects in postural adjustments and, for example, distinguish between voluntary stepping (making steps to order), automatic stepping (stepping movements when 'frog-marched'), and protective stepping (stepping when pushed out of balance). This is of more than theoretical importance, for the protective step is vital to euqipoise: without it the child shows what is termed 'felled-pine ataxia' and is in danger of injury. After a few unprotected falls he may be reluctant to attempt walking again, preferring to widen his base and crawl bear-wise or not move at all.

The postural problems confronting the infant can be put simply as follows: he emerges at birth from a capsule in which he has been weightless (though nevertheless orientated by his otolith organs in relation to gravity) into an environment in which his trunk and limbs are suddenly subjected to the full force of gravity. He must resist gravity or be splayed out, and then, with the help of his labyrinthine righting reflexes, oppose gravity and ensure that his head is up and his eyes are parallel with the horizon. Next he must elevate his trunk with his head up on it, utilizing the body-righting reflexes acting on the neck, and learn to counterpoise a moving limb or his head, automatically, in order to prevent overturning on any attempted movement. To be safe he must develop protective reactions in his arms and later in his legs. The next major problem is that of balancing the trunk on the narrow base of the feet, and only after this has been achieved will it be possible for him to utilize his automatic stepping mechanism by a controlled forward tilt of the trunk. At this stage he still has difficulty counterpoising a leg by shifting his trunk automatically to the opposite side, and so he will tend to fall upon the rising leg, with a resultant short step and wide base. Finally he achieves automatic counterpoising of the rising leg and thus is able to step over an obstacle, kick a ball, or walk upstairs; when at the age of 3 he can do this last, without holding on, he has perfected his counterpoising mechanism. Disorders of these mechanisms are almost all of the negative sort (failure to brace part on part for trunk erection, or failure to prevent overturning); thus in the early years the treatment of cerebral palsy is mainly concerned with the stimulation and reinforcing of reactions which a normal young child masters in his first 2 years. Absence of a postural reaction at the appropriate age does not necessarily mean that the pathway for it is totally destroyed: if a patient is found to be sitting after 20 years the necessary pathways must have been present from the start, at least in part.

Ataxia exemplifies a number of disorders of the postural reactions. It can be divided into limb ataxia and truncal ataxia. Both kinds of ataxia are associated with hypotonia in the true sense because the normal cerebellum activates the muscle-spindle facilitatory system of the brain stem (p. 277). The grossest form of limb ataxia is intention tremor, clearly an impairment of postural fixation at the proximal joints resulting in rhythmical alternation. This is common in congenital cerebellar ataxia. Truncal ataxia is of greater frequency and importance in infancy. Here there is failure to maintain the centre of gravity over the base.

Failure of suppression of primitive brain stem reflexes

Movements can be regarded as evolving from simple, invariable, spinal reflexes to more elaborate patterns governed by higher centres. The most lowly, such as withdrawal from pain, are the most rigidly organized in the sense that a given stimulus can only result in a given response. The higher motor functions are less 'organized' in that they leave open the possibility of a *choice of reactions:* thus if a protective side step with one foot is prevented, the other will come across to give an almost equally effective alternative. When the motor system is damaged complex movements tend to suffer first, leaving the cruder or less complex. This process involves a reduction of choice and the severely damaged child may be able to react only by means of certain crude reactions centred in the brain stem.

In their pure form these reactions appear in a transitory fashion in infancy (Table 14.6). The 'brain stem reflexes' are quickly absorbed into much more elaborate movement patterns imposed by the basal ganglia and eventually supervised by the cortex; in the fully developed system we cannot discern separate reflexes, all we see is a smooth and efficient movement. Damage disorganizes the system from above, in order of complexity, downwards. When the spinal cord is cut off from the brain only spinal reflexes are seen; when the

TABLE 14.6. Evolution of infantile reflexes.

Moro	Present from birth to 4 months
Placing	Present from birth onwards
Positive supporting	Present from birth to 2 months, reappearing when the foot-grasp goes
Hand-grasp	Present from birth to 3 months
Foot-grasp	Present from birth to 8 months
Asymmetrical tonic neck	Variable at birth; present at 1 to 4 months; never powerful
Symmetrical tonic neck	Absent at birth; appear briefly at 6–8 months for the first crawl
Tonic labyrinthine	Feeble at birth, quickly overcome by labyrinthine head righting reflex
Labyrinthine head-righting	Appears at 2 months; powerful by 3 months
Body-on-head righting	Present from 4 months, seen on pull up to sit
Body-on-body	Present from 3–8 months: (abolition of fetal curve)
Body rotative	Present from 9 months; the beginning of rising, struggles when supine
Protective arm reactions (Lateral before forward and backward)	Appear from 4–9 months; necessary before safe sitting
Tilting (Forward, backward and lateral)	Appear from 5–12 months; needed for sitting and walking on uneven surfaces

brain stem is functionally separated from the hemispheres only brain stem reflexes and postures are seen. In many cases of severe cerebral palsy most of the movements of which the child is capable can be analysed in terms of reflexes whose 'centre' is known to be in the brain stem, and which have been released as positive signs by damage to higher centres. Although termed reflexes these patterns may to some extent be under voluntary control. They may in fact constitute the whole repertoire of the child's movements, each movement being performed in a stereotyped fashion.

Brain stem reflexes act upon the distribution of postural tone. The reflexes principally concerned are the tonic labyrinthine reflex and the labyrinthine righting reflexes, the tonic neck reflexes, the neck and body righting reflexes and the startle (Moro) reaction. These all interact with one another in normal development and they also interact with other complex movement patterns which are not definitely localized within the brain stem.

The tonic labyrinthine reflex affects tone diffusely. The sensor is the otolith organs which provide continuous information about the position of the head in relation to gravity. As a result of the action of this reflex extensor tone is maximal when the individual is supine, while flexor tone is maximal in the prone position. If this reflex is disinhibited the characteristic result in the supine position is retraction of the head with retraction of the shoulders and adduction of the externally rotated arms, which are flexed at the elbows so that the fists are up by the ears. This posture may also be dominant in the erect position. At the same time there is extension and adduction of the legs, which are often crossed. In the prone position, increase in flexor tone is marked, especially at the hips and knees, while the flexor hypertonus in the neck may prevent elevation of the head. The grossest exaggeration of this reflex in the supine position, approximating to the tonic or decerebrate fit, is seen in the form of violent total extension spasms to which both quadriplegic and athetoid children are subject, making feeding, bathing and dressing almost impossible. They are sometimes to some extent under voluntary control, constituting the child's only mode of expression or resistance. Protrusion of the tongue is commonly seen during the spasms but is probably an unrelated phenomenon and, though affected by emotion, is not under voluntary control.

The labyrinthine righting reflexes also originate from the utricles, and serve to maintain the head in the vertical plane; these reactions initiate the righting reflexes of ordinary life (on rising from the ground the first movement is of the head) and are responsible for the neck and trunk components of the tilting reactions. Their hypoactivity causes failure to elevate the head, and instability due to absence of the tilting reactions; their overactivity on the other hand results in 'compulsive' righting or rolling.

The tonic neck reflexes, subdivisible into asymmetrical and symmetrical, are proprioceptive reflexes originating in the muscles and joints of the neck.

The asymmetrical tonic neck reflex is evoked by active or passive turning of the head, and this results in increased extensor tone in the limbs on the side to which the face is turned, with flexion of the opposite limbs. This reaction is demonstrable, though in a transient form, in the normal infant, until about the fourth month, and is actually present in some powerful movements of adult life. However, in many cases of cerebral palsy the posture induced by rotation of the head is obligatory and prevents the hands being brought together in the midline.

The symmetrical tonic neck reflex depends on extension or flexion of the neck, extension resulting in extension of the arms and flexion of the hips, while flexion results in the opposite, namely flexion or crumpling of the arms and extension of the hips. These reflexly induced postures are a normal part of the motor pattern of the infant beginning to crawl, but they are quickly integrated into other movements. Even in cases of cerebral palsy they are not as commonly demonstrable as are the asymmetrical reflexes, but when powerful, the activity of the symmetrical tonic reflexes means that if the child is kneeling with the head raised, extension of the hips is impossible, thus he can only crawl by 'bunny hopping'; while if he flexes his head he cannot maintain the crawling position because his arms give way.

Impulses from the upper three cervical segments are normally integrated with the labyrinthine input in the vestibular nuclei in order to signal the position of the body in relation to the head in space. The patterns of these two groups of tonic reflexes, the labyrinthine and the neck, are approximately the same, but opposite in effect, and they serve in the normal to centre the eyes when the head is turned. The tonic neck reflexes are lower in the physiological scale and therefore tend to be preserved when, because of damage to higher centres, the labyrinthine righting reflexes are in abeyance.

Neck and body righting reflexes. The body-on-body reflexes and body-on-neck reflexes operate to keep the trunk in a straight line; thus when the supine body is pulled up by the shoulders this reflex causes flexion of the neck and aids the labyrinthine righting reflex in bringing the head into the vertical position. The body-on-body reflex maintains the trunk erect and ensures orderly derotation when a turn has been initiated by the head or the pelvis. Though usually regarded as being 'centred' in the brain stem (about medullary level) these important reactions are susceptible to lesions quite far away in the nervous system: thus the body-on-neck reflex is commonly defective in disorders of the basal ganglia (like the protective stepping reaction, another 'brain stem' reflex). This bears out the hypothesis that many of the postural reactions are susceptible to influences at many levels, and so the absence of such a reaction is of no 'localizing' value, in the classical sense. However, we are not concerned here with localization but with the failure of specific systems.

The Moro reflex. This important primitive reflex consists of two phases, abduction of the arms with widespread fingers and abduction of the thighs with slight flexion of the knees, followed by a second phase of adduction of arms or clasping. The abduction phase accompanies the first inspiration at birth. This response soon vanishes and if present beyond 4 months is always a sign of abnormality.

Its absence in the neonatal period may be due to cerebral damage, while its asymmetry may give a clue to a brachial plexus palsy or a hemiplegia. The most effective stimulus is sudden extension of the neck as when the infant is laid upon a couch, the head being unsupported. André-Thomas' manoeuvre was to thrust the baby's flexed thighs abruptly headwards, causing an extension of head on neck. The reflex is quickly 'taken over' by auditory and visual stimuli as a general alarm reaction. Often in the abnormal child it will seem to occur spontaneously and sometimes one response appears to trigger another, resulting in a windmill type of involuntary movement of the arms. The response is present in the supine and vertical positions but absent in the prone position, suggesting that it is in part at least of utricular origin. An overactive Moro reflex may result in extension thrusts which make sitting impossible. Quite often in the athetoid infant it is impossible to detect the exciting stimulus, and it seems that these children accumulate or 'bank' subliminal stimuli until their threshold is reached.

The author has deliberately placed these 'lower brain stem reflexes' after the more elaborate reactions mediated by the basal ganglia because they dominate the scene only in the most severely handicapped child and because, in the majority of instances, the child with cerebral palsy who has difficulty with sitting, standing, balancing and walking, is found more often to have disorders of the reactions of equipoise and locomotion than troublesome release-phenomena due to over-activity of brain stem reflexes. Excessive extensor tonus or 'extensor thrusts', or an over-active asymmetrical tonic neck reflex may, of course, prevent the child from sitting, but far commoner causes are disorders of head and trunk elevation or of the simple counterpoising reactions.

Disorders of tone

By 'tone' is meant that responsiveness to stretch that distinguishes a normal muscle from a denervated one; the former offers resistance, the latter does not. The basis of all tone is the influx of proprioceptive impulses from the muscle spindles (the tautness of which is regulated by the gamma system) and from the upper three cervical segments and the labyrinths. This sensory input is continuous and is integrated mainly in the vestibular nuclei and the cerebellum. Tone can be divided into two obviously different varieties; on the one hand intrinsic tone, or the state of reactivity of the reflex arc revealed by active resistance above a critical velocity (in the normal child the critical velocity is so high that only the tendon tap will elicit the stretch reflex) and on the other hand postural tone or the state of continuous and unfatiguable contraction of postural muscles that is needed to overcome gravity and maintain posture.

In that all movements begin and end in a posture, normal postural tone is essential if normal movements are to be carried out: all disorders of co-ordination are associated with disorders of tone. It is thus of crucial importance to distinguish between the truly hypotonic muscle (i.e. one in which the stretch reflex is impaired) and the floppiness that results from impairment of postural reflexes.

In the abnormal state tone can be diminished (hypotonic) or increased (hypertonic). Under normal circumstances the tension of the spindle is maintained at approximately constant level so that it can respond immediately to stretch. If the muscle spindles are slack they fail to respond to stretch unless it is extreme; this occurs in hypotonia. If the spindles are taut they respond unduly to stretch and bombard the spinal motor neurones with impulses which will lead to excessive reflex contraction of the main muscle fibres; this occurs in spasticity which is the commonest type of hypertonus seen in childhood.

The spindle system is controlled by elaborate facilitatory and inhibitory systems throughout the spinal cord and brain stem. The facilitatory system is governed largely by the cerebellum, hence a cerebellar lesion deprives the system of its drive and results in hypotonia. The facilitatory system in the brain stem is far more widely distributed than the inhibitory system which is limited to the lower medulla. If the brain is damaged it is usually the facilitatory system that dominates the scene, permanently increasing the tension in muscle spindles. Spasticity is thus a frequent accompaniment of brain damage. The increase in tone is usually most evident in those muscles which maintain the body's posture against gravity, hence it is seen mostly in calf and anterior thigh muscles and the biceps. Many of the postures seen in spastic diplegia can be analysed in terms of spasticity of antigravity muscles, though usually one will also find evidence of disturbances of the basic postural reactions of the trunk.

Paralysis and disorders of the pattern of voluntary movements
Weakness is common to all forms of cerebral palsy, even those characterized by involuntary movements, for in these, although the involuntary movements themselves may be powerful, voluntary movements as such are weak or even absent. This state of affairs is seen particularly in patients with athetosis in the early months, when the combination of inertia, absence of postural fixation, and paralysis of gaze movements may give the misleading appearance of mental retardation, a classical pitfall of the unwary.

The weakness of severe cerebral palsy is at first generalized, involving the neck and trunk as well as the limbs and is usually associated with a general physical frailty, so that if deprived of adequate stimulation these children are still babies at the age of 5 years. Their parents are frightened of handling them and yet it is handling that they need most.

The paresis comprises a number of features. The initiation of a movement is slow, as if the brain were incapable of deciding which pathway to use or of selecting the most appropriate of several patterns of movement, and so the movement may start in the wrong muscle group. The sequence of innervation of muscle groups is inappropriate, the agonist often contracting first in an obstinate contrary movement. Discrete movement is impossible, e.g. extension of the wrist is associated with extension of all the fingers, while attempts at flexion result in flexion of all the segments of the limb or involve both limbs simultaneously in a crude symmetrical movement; in the lower limb, flexion at the hip can only occur together with flexion at the knee. Even in mild cases 'mirror movements' are often seen in the unaffected hand when an effort is made to use the affected one in a case of hemiplegia. Thus the essential features of the paresis of cerebral palsy are slowness of initiation, simultaneous contraction giving a crude and ineffective pattern and lack of fractionation of movements, in other words lack of the ability to acquire skill. In the normal person the process of fractionation, learned by the endless repetition of infancy, ensures that only the essential parts of a basic pattern of movement are retained. By a process of continuous monitoring each fraction of a movement runs smoothly into the next; the more skilled the act the more economically it is performed, the more in fact it becomes automated. We are only aware of the parts of a movement when engaged in the very earliest stages of learning a new motor act, when the stages are monitored by vision or internal language, as anybody can verify by learning to tie a new knot. Automation and its sequel, economy of effort, go to make up skill and skill is what the clumsy person, and still more so the cerebral palsied child, cannot achieve. If he is to master a movement at all he must bring his mind to bear upon it continuously, but there is a limit to what can be done by a damaged motor system. Mental subnormality, unless profound, does not necessarily mean that a child cannot profit from treatment, for in many such cases a skilled therapist can train the child to make some use of his few reflex and semi-automatic patterns.

The subject of voluntary movements (and paresis) needs to be looked at anew. There are two kinds of voluntary movements: the ballistic, as in striking with a hammer, and the guided, as in putting a thing in a hole. In cerebral palsy both these kinds of movement are usually impaired, though occasionally the ballistic movement is possible when the guided one is not, and so a child may be able to achieve an accurate swipe at a lever or person when he cannot manage a more 'controlled' movement though the two are equally 'voluntary'.

Involuntary movements

The picture painted so far is mainly of the diplegic or quadriplegic child with impaired postural reactions, weakness of voluntary movement, a reduced choice of patterns and consequent inefficiency, and with troublesome hypertonus due to release of the brain stem facilitatory system which governs the muscle-spindle setting. Such a child is characterized by his relative immobility and, in rare instances, can come near to the desperate state of 'de-efferented man', a creature with input intact, mentation unassessable, and output nil. The child with athetosis shares with these children the defects of the postural reactions but has in place of the positive symptom of hypertonus the positive symptom of involuntary movements. At their worst these can be of extreme severity and though the child may show a profusion of such movements he also shows immobility. Lacking fixity of the trunk he has no power of locomotion except perhaps by wriggling or rolling and he cannot perform a voluntary movement because each act is destroyed in advance by contrary movement.

Together with early hypotonia and impairment of postural fixation of the trunk, involuntary movements form the principal feature of athetosis (used here in its broad sense to cover the dyskinetic cerebral palsies), though involuntary movements are also often present in less marked form in other types of cerebral palsy because of the diffuse nature of the lesion. Almost any kind of 'unwanted' movement, from tremor to rapid choreic or slow dystonic movements, can occur in cerebral palsy, but the violent writhing and irregular movements are confined to athetosis.

The irregular arrhythmic movements affect almost all muscles, including the respiratory, but are most evident in the face, tongue, neck and arms. In infancy they appear first in the toes and fingers. Although 'caused' by damage to the basal ganglia they cannot originate in these structures because damaged tissues cannot originate movements. They must originate in undamaged parts of the nervous system, presumably the cortex, hence they are absent in early infancy when the cortex has not begun to function. They are absent in repose or when attention is deeply held, diminished by fatigue and fever, less evident in the prone position and most evident in the supine and vertical positions. They are provoked by emotion, insecurity, startle or the desire to perform a voluntary act. Any mother of an athetoid child will tell that he can be motionless when in complete postural equilibrium with his attention engaged (e.g. when watching the television) but only those who have attempted to feed and dress an athetoid child can know how troublesome the movements can be. At their least evident these comprise slow rippling or rolling movements of the tongue, retraction and protrusion of the lips or moderately rhythmical flexion and extension of the digits. At their most marked they constitute violent 'throwing' movements of the limbs or even the body, preventing any voluntary activity. 'Jack-knifing', i.e. sudden collapse of trunk on hips when an attempt is made to bring the child to the standing position, can be very troublesome.

Frequently cases of athetosis show over-activity of the tonic neck and labyrinthine reflexes. Occasionally it is possible to demonstrate a conflict between the grasp and avoiding reactions; often the visual avoiding reaction (head and eyes being averted from the object desired) forms part of the pattern. Usually the tactile avoiding reaction in the feet is excessive, resulting in the peculiar 'athetoid dance' when the child is stood up and this may be the earliest positive sign. Often the repeated semi-rhythmic rotary movements of the arms seem to originate from spontaneously arising and perhaps self-perpetuating startle reactions. A very common feature is a coarse proximal ataxia involving the arms and giving rise to an obvious intention tremor; the movement intended alternates with its opposite. Indeed, looking at these children struggling to do things one begins to suspect that any voluntary act is normally 'shadowed' by its opposite as a controlling device, but in athetosis the two patterns occur 'out of phase'. It seems fairly certain that the spasms are related not to attention as such but to the arousal mechanism that precedes activity. No form of physiotherapy, unless it results in profound fatigue, has anything more than a transient effect on the movements. This is not to say that therapy can play no part, for it can be usefully directed to the defects of postural fixation that invariably accompany the condition.

The association of athetosis with disorders of the basal ganglia caused by jaundice or anoxia is accepted. It is because the damage is thus localized that intelligence is so often preserved; indeed, the condition was originally described as 'ataxia with imbecility in which intelligence is preserved, despite appearances being so adversive'. Athetosis is, in fact, a pure disorder of motility. The most severe athetosis may be accompanied by total lack of speech but nevertheless high intelligence because of the sparing of the cortex, whereas when intelligence is low there is usually an admixture of rigidity which tends to slow the movements down.

An important feature of athetosis is its change with age (measured in decades). The infant is commonly hypotonic and shows defective postural reactions. Gradually involuntary movements appear and increase in violence through the years, though they may later become damped down by the development of rigidity. The adult athetoid is nearly always rigid with grossly hypertrophied neck muscles and often contractures and deformities.

Failure of development of cortical reactions

Many of the phenomena of cerebral palsy are the result of disinhibition of fairly primitive reflexes or of failure of higher centres to gain control of, or assimilate, basic movement patterns. These are termed positive or release phenomena and include hypertonus, involuntary movements and overactivity of primitive brain stem reflexes. In contrast, in negative phenomena, e.g. paresis and inco-ordination, there is absence of function due to disorder of the neural pathways necessary for those functions and, in addition, failure to develop certain reactions which require cortical function. Though commonly alluded to as cortical reflexes these reactions cannot be 'located' in the cortex (the grasp reflex, for instance, is present in the fetus, the neonate and the anencephalic) any more than the tilting reaction can be 'located' in the labyrinth, but they are all profoundly sensitive to cortical deficiency and are thus important indicators thereof and furthermore, have prognostic significance. The cortical reflexes of interest are the grasp reflex, the tactile and visual avoiding reactions, and the placing and supporting reactions.

The stimulus for the grasp reflex is contact with the palm or stretching of the finger flexors; this reflex fades after a few months. The grasp reflex in the toes is shown by flexion or 'crumpling' on contact with a supporting surface and until it fades, usually at 7–8 months, standing is not possible; from this time on the foot is needed for anti-gravity support and balance. The stimulus for the tactile avoiding reaction is light contact with the back of the hand or forearm; this normally develops later than the grasp reflex but tends to fade quickly. The stimulus for the placing reaction is contact with the front of the forearm or shin when the infant is suspended and brought briskly forward so that the limb being tested strikes the edge of the table, when foot or hand is deftly placed on the surface. Deceleration is undoubtedly an adjuvant and vision should theoretically be excluded but, for convenience, usually is not. The tactile placing reaction is normally present at birth and hardly ever fades unless the child is crying or ill. The supporting reaction follows placing but is less reliable as a test.

The placing reaction is of diagnostic value as it is commonly absent in the mentally subnormal. It shows a fairly precise correlation with the degree of mental retardation rather than with the severity of concurrent spastic paresis since the reaction can be demonstrated in quite spastic limbs, given time for response. A variation is Foerster's position in which the thighs are flexed but the knees remain straight so that the legs are parallel with but above the table. In athetosis the placing reaction in the arms is often absent, the limbs being folded away (like an undercarriage) but the placing reaction in the legs is present and leads on to the characteristic 'athetoid dance'. Placing reactions play a useful part in treatment because they are among the easiest reactions to elicit, are facilitated by repetition, and will lead on to a positive supporting reaction, except in cases showing the grossest mental retardation.

The tactile avoiding and grasp reactions can be regarded as being in opposition to one another, so that when the tactile avoiding reaction replaces the grasp reflex the infant automatically throws down an object placed in his hand; this is a transient phenomenon in normal development and its persistence beyond 10 months suggests mental subnormality. Damage to the frontal lobes 'releases' the grasp reflex, whereas tactile and visual avoiding reactions are 'released' by parietal lobe lesions. If the tactile avoiding reaction in the upper limbs is continuously enhanced the arm is folded away in a characteristic manner with the hand supinated and elbow flexed. This posture may also be seen in children with athetosis. Enhancement of the tactile avoiding reaction in the legs in experimental animals results in a peculiar gait likened to a 'dance on hot bricks' which is very similar to the 'athetoid dance'.

This way of looking at cerebral palsy may seem rather theoretical but is necessary if its very complex neurology is to be approached with understanding. However, it must be recognized that what is seen in infant or child is fact and what is read about is at best interpretation and at worst wrong. Finally it is apposite to ask what helps and what hinders the child with brain damage. Neglect, immobility, babying, fear of handling, ignorance, a rigid outlook on the part of the therapist, a bogus omniscience on the part of the physician; these all hinder. Intellect and drive, activity, enthusiasm, resourcefulness in the face of difficulties and realism in assessing motor deficits; these help, together with acceptance that any improvement in performance may take years, not months. The physician is an ephemeron in the life of his patient.

J. FOLEY

Associated Disorders

Available pathological evidence suggests that in most cases cerebral palsy is caused by a variety of agents acting upon a nervous system that was fairly normal in design in early embryonic life. Since damage to the cerebral hemispheres is usually diffuse, disorders of a non-motor kind are common in cases of hemiplegia, diplegia and ataxia (in which the lesion is not always limited to the cerebellum) but less so in cases of athetosis, in which the lesion may be strictly confined to the basal ganglia.

Many cases of cerebral palsy show one or more of what may be termed the associated disorders, the most important being sensory impairment (including defects of vision and hearing), perceptual and praxic defects, speech disorders, epilepsy and mental retardation.

In a given case the associated defects may be more important in general management than the motor abnormality; thus a child with mild diplegia or hemiplegia may show perceptual defects which in later school life far outweigh the physical disability. Since the detection of disorders of sensation and perception depends on the ability of the child to respond by gesture or speech, these deficiencies may become manifest relatively late, and their detection may necessitate a fairly prolonged period of observation. This is one justification for special centres as opposed to the observation of such children in ordinary paediatric outpatient departments.

DISORDERS OF SENSATION

Sensory testing as such is extremely difficult in children under 2–3 years (and also in older retarded children) as they cannot give accurate yes/no responses. The exclusion of vision is always difficult as children invariably try to peep. Testing of position sense demands of the child a knowledge of the simple dimensions up and down (expected at age 2 years) and two-point discrimination similarly demands a concept of number.

Impairment of tactile sensation is rare in all types of cerebral palsy except hemiplegia, in which it is important in one-third of cases. Other modalities may be involved, but impairment of position sense is the most disabling. A hemiplegic hand with such sensory loss is unlikely ever to be used except as a prop.

In general, disorders of perception (the agnosias, tactile and visual) are more common than actual sensory loss. It is often necessary to approach sensory loss in the young child backwards, as it were, by demonstrating first that there is a tactile agnosia, then training the child in suitable tests before attempting to demonstrate whether or not there is actual sensory impairment.

VISUAL DEFECTS

Visual and ocular defects are commonly associated with cerebral palsy. In a personal series of over 1000 patients, severe disorders (including cataracts) were present in 4 per cent. Some other surveys have reported a much higher incidence of blind or partially sighted children (14 per cent in Dundee, Douglas, 1961; 15 per cent in Sheffield, Holt and Reynell, 1967). In general, severe visual defects are found in children with mental retardation and severe physical handicap, most often a spastic type of cerebral palsy.

Nearly one-half of cerebral palsied children have squints. Although more common in the mentally retarded, squint is found in over one-third of mentally normal cerebral palsied children. All types of squint are seen and the incidence is little affected by the type of cerebral palsy.

Oculo-motor and visual disorders are discussed in more detail in Chapter 21, but the detection of some visual defects forms part of the initial neurological examination of the cerebral palsied child.

Cortical blindness is relatively rare and seems always to be associated with severe retardation, presumably because the occipital and parietal lobes have been simultaneously damaged. Unfortunately the detection of cortical blindness early in infancy is difficult even by means of evoked potentials, for the demonstration that an electrical volley arrives at the visual cortex does not mean that the infant can see, in the sense of integrating the signal into something meaningful; the same applies to cortical auditory evoked responses and hearing.

An unusual and puzzling result of bilateral parieto-occipital lesions is 'piecemeal vision' in which, though there may be no defect of visual acuity, only a small part of the visual field can be attended to at a given moment and the whole scene cannot be constructed from the part. Difficulties in sorting object from background, in depth perception, and in counting objects visually are probably related phenomena. Children with these difficulties have accurate vision for distant objects but can be baffled by nearer objects like stairs and furniture.

Hemianopia occurs in at least one-third of cases of hemiplegia; usually it causes little inconvenience until the child tries to read. Apraxic disorders of ocular movement are discussed below.

HEARING LOSS

The true incidence of hearing loss in cerebral palsied children is difficult to establish because of problems in testing. Incidence in the more comprehensive surveys ranges from 42 per cent (of whom 17 per cent had severe loss) in a study of 427 children by Fisch (1957) to 28 per cent (6 per cent severe) in a study of 226 children by Holt and Reynell (1967). The much lower incidence of severe hearing loss in the more recent study is most likely due to the decline of kernicterus complicating haemolytic disease of the newborn. Significant hearing loss is most common in athetoid cerebral palsy, with hearing for middle and high tones most affected. Less often hearing loss is associated with diplegia, particularly when due to severe perinatal anoxia.

The detection of hearing loss is of the utmost importance if the child is to be properly managed and if the beginning of speech is to be encouraged. Electronic averaging techniques provide a warning of what must later be confirmed by repeated clinical audiometry. The distinction between hearing loss and mental retardation can be very difficult in an apathetic and paralysed child under the age of 2 years. Accurate assessment of the type and degree of hearing loss will take many sessions, which is another reason why these children are best cared for in special centres. Hearing loss is further considered in Chapter 22.

SPECIFIC PERCEPTUAL AND EXECUTIVE DISORDERS

In adult neurology there is little difficulty in accepting the statement that brain damage can result in a large variety of specific disorders of perception and performance, which can all be incorporated into the general terms agnosia and apraxia. Some of these (e.g. topographical agnosia and dressing apraxia) are of precise localizing value.

Not unexpectedly almost every specific disorder that has been described in adults can be found sooner or later in a population of children with cerebral palsy. The child's general performance may be pulled down by an undetected specific defect and result in an apparent global impairment. It is thus important that every backward cerebral palsied child should be carefully tested by an experienced psychologist, in case the backwardness is due to a specific defect that can be ameliorated to some extent by special education.

The definitions of apraxia and agnosia imply that these are disorders of concepts which have already been formed. This being so, the disorders cannot be diagnosed until the child has reached the mental ages at which the appropriate concepts should have been developed. There must therefore be 'gnosic' and 'praxic' ages for a large variety of perceptual and praxic activities. Before these ages are reached the child with brain damage will show disabilities that are amorphous and he can only gradually reveal if his intellectual performance is normal in most respects but specifically retarded in certain others. It is important therefore to know how and when the child develops concepts.

The most significant studies in this field were those of Piaget. He studied a small number of children intensively and continually and deduced from their responses to questioning the nature of the development of the child's thought. There have been many objections to his work: the method cannot be applied statistically, or used as a basis for 'tests'; the observations depend to a considerable extent on the child's speech and there are important linguistic differences between French and English (e.g. the use of reflexive verbs); Piaget implies that the child's concept of space depends on exploration, whereas it is now known that a physically immobile child may develop a normal concept of space presumably by visual and auditory means alone. A further difficulty is the fact that Piaget found it necessary to devise his own terminology and the labelling of his slightly overlapping periods has caused much confusion.

Piaget divided the child's intellectual development into three main periods:

(1)   the sensorimotor stage of 'reversible actions', from 0–18 months,
(2a) the preconceptual and later intuitive stages, from 18 months–7 years,
(2b) the stage of 'concrete' or voluntary operations, from 7–12 years, leading up to
(3)   the dawn of deductive thinking at around puberty.

In this section we need be concerned only with periods 1 and 2a. The order in which the child passes through these periods is constant; the exact timing is not and the movement from one period to the next depends on, and is an indicator of, mental age but not chronological age. It is literally true that to understand Piaget's ideas it is necessary to have a baby at one's elbow.

Agnosias are disorders of recognition. Where sensation is unimpaired and mental images are intact, inability to recognize an object by one of the senses is known as an agnosia. Hence the agnosias are classified according to sensory modality: tactile, visual, auditory.

Perception is the attachment of meaning to sensation by matching with an internal code or concept. The concept is the basic mental symbol representing a class of objects, symbols or properties.

Conceptualization is thus the reduction of one of many objects to a common factor and this simplifies mental processes. For example, the concept 'house' spares the mind the trouble of comparing the object (picture or word) with all houses that have been seen previously. The concept is thus the basis of 'form constancy', that process by which the code is kept in the mind's eye while matching is being carried out. Conceptual thought is more efficient than 'concrete' or preconceptual thought, being less tied to the object. 'Concreteness' is one of the hallmarks of mental subnormality and is shown in an inability to generalize, to paraphrase and to condense.

Apraxia was defined by Kinnier Wilson (1908) as 'an inability to perform certain subjectively purposive movements or movement complexes with con-servation of motility, sensation and co-ordination'. 'Subjectively purposive' implies that the individual is aware of the act he is trying to perform; he is not agnostic for the goal but he cannot produce the pattern of movement required to achieve it.

The terms agnosia and apraxia cannot be applied to a child in his amorphous sensori-motor stage but they are useful once he emerges into his preconceptual stage.

It is not always easy to decide whether a disability is one of perception or of performance; some seem to be mixtures of both. The commonest disorders in children with spastic cerebral palsy are: difficulty in copying shapes (probably praxic rather than perceptual); difficulty in reproducing sequences visually or auditorily (examples being an order of pictures, a list of animals); picture completion; the imitation of actions; matching shapes; distinguishing right and left; detecting spatial relations in pictures (in front of, behind, below); figure background discrimination.

The agnosias

When identifying an agnosia it is necessary to take into account the gnostic age of the child, prove that there is no sensory loss for the modality in question, and exclude a nominal aphasia as the cause of the deficit by using pointing or matching. Care must be taken that failure to name an object is not confused with failure to recognize it; an individual with a nominal dysphasia may fail to name what he evidently recognizes.

The normal gnostic ages have been carefully worked out by Monfraix and the Tardieus (1961a and b). For example the normal child at 2 years can recognize a marble, cube and pencil by touch, while a child of 6 can identify nine out of twelve geometrical shapes. Using the Tardieus' tests a 'gnostic quotient' can be worked out.

Tactile agnosia will prevent the identification of an object or shape by touch, though it is instantly recognized by vision. It should be remembered that an individual may be able to match correctly objects that he cannot recognize.

Visual agnosia may be for objects, pictures, symbols (including words), faces or places. Visual acuity must be very low indeed before it impairs recognition and because of the phenomenon of 'completion of the image' a field defect does not of itself impair recognition, though there are bound to be some cases in which the responsible lesion is so situated as to cause both a hemianopia and a visual agnosia. Visual agnosia for outline drawings is much more common than agnosia for objects. Inability to detect spatial relationships in pictures is particularly common.

Auditory agnosia may rarely involve common household sounds and the condition then amounts to an auditory imperception. More often it involves the recognition of rhythms or of words; thus receptive aphasia can be regarded as one form of auditory agnosia.

Corporeal agnosias are disorders of the body image. Thus there may be an agnosia for a limb or half of the body, or for relationships of parts of the body in space. The commonest expressions of this disorder are finger agnosia and the inability to tell right from left. Bilateral agnostic defects may occur with unilateral cerebral palsy such as hemiplegia.

The apraxias

When identifying an apraxia it is necessary to take into account the praxic age of the child, to show that the act is understood and to demonstrate that there is no paralysis or, more importantly, no disorder of postural control, that will prevent the movement from being carried out.

The essential feature of an apraxia is that it is a disorder of a voluntary act. Thus a patient with a true glossal apraxia will be able to lick his lips involuntarily though he cannot do so to order and this distinguishes the condition from that of a supra-bulbar paresis.

The apraxias can be broken down into two main groups: disorders of doing and disorders of arranging.

Disorders of doing. In this group are included the apraxias for actions involving the use of objects such as toothbrush, comb and scissors. A much larger group of disorders involves movements of the face, trunk and limbs, e.g. difficulty in closing the eyes, showing the teeth, kissing, moving the tongue, following with the eyes, pointing, waving, putting one hand on a knee or an ear, sitting down on a chair without missing it or kicking a ball. These are all dominant hemisphere functions, if laterality has been established.

An inability to perform one of these movements does not amount to an apraxia until the child is chronologically well past the relevant praxic age. Apraxia for face and limb movements can cause considerable difficulty if speech, occupational and physiotherapists are not aware of its possible existence.

Disorders of arrangement include dressing apraxia, constructional apraxia and disorders of sequencing.

There are two kinds of dressing apraxia; getting lost in the clothes and being unable to don the clothes in the right order. The former is more common but a child may be able to dress only if the clothes are laid out in precisely the order in which they are to be put on. Dressing apraxia is of considerable theoretical importance because it can be 'out-grown' in time, suggesting that the other kinds of constructional apraxia can also be overcome given patience and understanding.

The term constructional apraxia has tended to be superseded recently by the more restricted term 'visuomotor disorder'. The older term is wider and implies that there is no disorder of movement as such. The simplest tests are those involving stick designs or building steps with bricks, while the more complex and demanding are those involving Kohs blocks and the Goldstein series of patterns. The copying of block designs is probably the best test of constructional apraxia. The apraxic will know that his design is wrong and will struggle on to rectify it, with no hope of success; the agnostic will settle back contentedly, convinced that his wrong design is right.

Drawing is a kind of constructional praxis and provides a useful test. An extension of drawing is the use of symbols for writing and hence a 'visuomotor' defect may constitute an important part of a difficulty in writing. The term dyslexia regrettably distracts attention from the dysgraphia which is almost always the more important facet of the dyslexic child's problems.

Ability in sequential arrangement (i.e. arranging in time or space) is heavily dependent upon short-term memory and age, e.g. the normal child cannot copy a sequence of beads until the age of $4\frac{1}{2}$. Every child is apraxic until he has reached the praxic age and has been taught the skill but there are some children with brain damage who persist in being incapable of the simplest spatial tasks and yet who have normal verbal and logical abilities. These specific disabilities, encountered especially in children with diplegia, are all the more important because they involve difficulties with sorting, matching and assembly such as may be required in the humblest of industrial occupations; there are very few occupations in which only verbal ability is required.

This rather theoretical and rigid classification of disorders of perception and performance forms a basis from which one can operate, but in practice the disability is found most often to be a mixture of agnosia and apraxia.

Ocular apraxias

Apart from squints, other abnormalities of ocular movement are common in cerebral palsy. The nature of an eye movement depends on the task. Scanning a scene or picture is carried out by a rapid sequence of saccadic (leaping) movements with a few regressions for checking purposes, all at a constant high velocity. On the other hand, the eye movements needed for copying are slower, subject to frequent checks and more laborious. It is the latter in particular that are deranged in cases of quadriplegia. Leaping and following are different varieties of movement and can be differentially impaired at brain stem level. They are interesting examples of 'ballistic' as opposed to 'guided' movements: the ballistic movement is fired off as an entity and is not checked in its trajectory by any sort of feedback, while the guided movement is checked moment by moment by sensory inflow.

Disorders of voluntary eye movement (i.e. the supranuclear gaze palsies) merge into the rather ill-defined ocular apraxias such as inability to turn the eyes at will this way or that, to follow, to scan or to make the eyes leap to a target. Gaze palsy, especially of upward gaze and convergence, is common in early athetosis and may give to the limp child the appearance of blindness. After about a year this palsy vanishes. 'Locking-on' is a rare symptom of bilateral lesions in adults; the eyes, having achieved a target, seemingly cannot be removed from it. 'Locking-off' is much more common but has not yet been formally described. It may well be a manifestation of the visual avoiding reaction and it is seen particularly in athetoids when the eyes fly away from the object of interest and yet the child, with head and eyes averted, seems able to see precisely what he is not looking at. Jerkiness of slow follow movements is seen in many children with 'minimal brain damage' and also in phenytoin intoxication. Study of the numerous disorders of eye movements in cerebral palsy has been hampered by the technical difficulties of electro-oculography in the child, but this difficulty can now be overcome in non-specialized centres by the use of videotape with a telephoto lens and an extension tube of a few millimetres.

CEREBRAL DOMINANCE

A great deal has been made of the fact that left-handedness is much more common in children with cerebral palsy, dyslexia and speech disorders than in the general population. It has been implied that left-handedness (or right cerebral dominance) and confusion between right and left are the cause of many learning difficulties. A simpler explanation is probably the correct one, namely that the proportion of left-handers in the child population with neurological abnormalities is the result of brain damage occurring early in life. Damage to a potentially left hemisphere dominant person will tend to shift dominance to the opposite hemisphere and if damage is done at random to a potentially normal population with a left/right dominance ratio of 80/20, the resultant ratio will approach 50/50.

Failure to achieve clear cerebral dominance may, however, add to the child's difficulties by impeding the process of information-sorting that goes on between the two hemispheres. Recently the localization of specific functions in the two hemispheres has become rather more precise. The various disorders can be listed as shown in Table 14.7 and even when dominance has not been firmly established they nevertheless tend to cluster in the way shown.

TABLE 14.7. Disorders associated with lesions of dominant and non-dominant hemispheres.

Dominant hemisphere	Non-dominant hemisphere
Disorders of language, symbolization and logical thought	Defects in pattern recognition
Limb and facial apraxias	Topographical disorientation
Modality, specific agnosias	Constructional apraxia
Finger agnosia	Dressing apraxia
Right-left confusion	Impairment of musical and rhythm
Acalculia	memory

These specific deficits described may show up clearly enough in the older child but important questions, which have not yet been answered, are: when can they first be detected in the younger child and how can they be detected as specific phenomena emerging from the normal preconceptual phase of a child's development? It is here that simple tests remain the most useful for the clinician; those of language development (such as the Reynell Scales, p. 118) on the one hand and on the other the simplest tests of praxic ability, bricks for building steps and elementary posting boxes which, unlike form boards, have the advantage of demanding arrangement in three dimensions. Appendix 14.1 details some such simple tests which might suggest specific difficulties in perception or performance, indicating the need for the much more elaborate repertoire of the clinical psychologist and the occupational therapist specializing in the problems of the child with brain damage.

SPEECH DISORDERS

Speech disorders (often preceded by sucking, swallowing and chewing difficulties) are present in up to 50 per cent of cerebral palsied children, even after excluding those whose slow language development is in keeping with their estimated mental age. Speech problems are found in the majority of children with athetoid cerebral palsy, in one-half of children with ataxia and in about one-third of diplegics. Feeding and speech problems are considered in Chapter 24.

EPILEPSY

Epilepsy is reported in about one-half of cerebral palsied children, being most commonly associated with quadriplegia and hemiplegia (particularly in patients of low intelligence) and least commonly with ataxia and athetosis. Epilepsy is further considered in Chapter 17.

MENTAL RETARDATION

If severely quadriplegic children in long-stay hospitals are included, surveys indicate that about one-third of cerebral palsied children are mentally retarded, over one-half are borderline or dull and about one-quarter are of average or above average intelligence. It is possible that some of the retardation previously reported is more apparent than innate and due to sensori-motor deprivation. Since the pathological lesions are diffuse it is not surprising that the most severe motor defect tends to go with the greatest degree of mental subnormality. Although this is usually the case, there are exceptions which can be very difficult to detect if the child happens also to be speechless. The most important exceptions of all are cases of athetosis with damage limited to the basal ganglia (p. 280).

There can be no *physical* signs of mental deficiency, the evidence for which can only come from study of the behaviour of the child. However, there are many physical accompaniments, the correlations of which with mental deficiency are so high that they are of diagnostic and prognostic value. The following signs are suggestive of associated retardation: delay in the acquisition of postural reactions in the absence of any positive or 'release' phenomena; absence of the placing and supporting reactions; Foerster's variation of the placing reaction; dorsiflexion of the feet and external rotation of the legs in the supine position; continuous distractibility, probably due to a defect in the cortical mechanism that normally suppresses stimuli learned to be unimportant, thus the child must react to any and every stimulus in his environment or, conversely, immovable fixity of attention; endless preoccupation with one toy and motor stereotypies. Persistent mouthing of objects beyond 12 months and refusal to feed are probably expressions of hypothalamic or temporal lobe damage. Other phenomena occasionally seen are now known to result from precisely localized lesions, e.g. aggression is correlated with damage to the amygdaloid nuclei and some forms of self-mutilation both in man and in experimental animals are known to have a biochemical basis.

DETERIORATION IN CEREBRAL PALSY

By definition cerebral palsy is due to a non-progressive lesion and so deterioration should not occur; occasionally, however, it does. Deterioration can be real, and irreversible, or apparent, and in some instances reversible. Real deterioration is the result of wrong diagnosis: a slowly progressive condition has been mistaken for cerebral palsy. Examples are the leucodystrophies, craniopharyngioma, tuberous sclerosis, ataxia-telangiectasia, and progressive anoxic gliosis due to fits. Apparent or reversible deterioration is more common, and due to numerous factors. The early assessment may have been inaccurate, the severity of the condition being misjudged in the first 2 years, when the child's neurological machinery has not been subjected to the full testing load of postural and psychological demands. Undetected minor epilepsy, or more often chronic intoxication with anticonvulsants, may cause serious deterioration which can be rectified once recognized. Pain due to an undetected dislocation of hip is an occasional cause. Emotional stress in a family coping with a handicapped child, and the child's gradual awareness of his lot in comparison to that of others, may result in declining performance. Inadequate, wrong or too doctrinaire treatments are common causes, as may be the wheel-chair outlook encouraged for convenience. However, the commonest cause of apparent deterioration is the overloading of the child's defective motor and mental equipment that occurs when he encounters the demands of real schooling for the first time; this is the second epoch in which he needs intensive therapy, the first being his first 2 years.

J. FOLEY

Orthopaedic Aspects

There are few indications for operative surgery in the cerebral palsied child under the age of 5 years. Nevertheless, as long-term management is the hallmark of treatment in this condition, it is right that the orthopaedic surgeon should be brought into the picture at an early age with a view to planning possible intervention in the future. After many years in which surgery in cerebral palsy was viewed with suspicion bordering on alarm, the issues are now clearer and there is general acceptance of the view that, given specific indications, a carefully planned surgical procedure can effect a major step forward in the management of some of these children.

The outstanding indication for surgery is the presence of fixed deformity in a joint since once this is established, prolonged efforts by the physiotherapist can only effect a moderate improvement. The deformity may arise from spasm or organic contracture in the muscles and tendons controlling the joint, from contracture of the joint capsule or from a combination of these. Each will need consideration in a surgical procedure.

By comparison tendon transfers, to effect improved muscle action on a joint, are of limited value in cerebral palsy. Even under ideal conditions, any transfer of a muscle-tendon unit results in some loss of power. When this is combined in cerebral palsy with the associated loss of central co-ordination of movement, the results tend to be very disappointing. The indications for this type of surgery are very few.

In nearly all cases, assessment for possible future surgery must include a firm indication that the child has the inherent capacity to take advantage of the increased potential that the surgery will produce. In other words, there can be no indication whatever for corrective surgical procedures to relieve deformity of the knee or ankle in a child who, for central reasons, is clearly quite unable ever to achieve any independent locomotion. The only exception to this rule is seen in the problem of gross adduction deformity of the hips when, because of extreme crossing of the legs, perineal toiletting is very difficult. In this case, adductor tenotomies can bring about a dramatic relief in the burden for the parents even if for other reasons the child is never going to be capable even of standing.

All surgery in this condition should be of the simplest nature and the child mobilized as soon as possible. Admission to hospital should be for a minimum period and is usually only necessary for about 3 days.

Upper limb

The characteristic cerebral palsy position of the upper limb (the so-called 'bird's-wing' deformity) is not unacceptable from a functional point of view.

There are, therefore, very few indications for surgery in this limb and certainly none in the very young child. The one operation which can produce a dramatic improvement in the functional use of the hand and fingers, as well as improving the cosmetic appearance, is arthrodesis of the wrist. However, this must be reserved until bone growth at the lower forearm epiphyses is almost complete, i.e. 14–16 years.

Lower limb

To achieve normal standing balance it is essential to have the soles of both feet firmly on the ground. The child whose knees are in fixed flexion and whose ankles are in equinus has no proper base and here surgery has the maximum amount to offer. It is usually best if the equinus deformity is tackled first.

The ankle. During the period up to 5 years, equinus deformity is treated by attention to passive stretching exercises, stimulation of dorsiflexor muscle action and possibly one or more periods in plaster of Paris casts, maintaining the ankle in the maximum correction possible. However, if no significant progress is being made, if the heel remains high and is accompanied by a tight heel cord, the operation of elongation of the tendo-achillis should be seriously considered from the age of 5 years onwards.

A slightly curved incision is made longitudinally on the medial side of the tight tendo-achillis. A long Z-shaped incision is made in the tendon, allowing the divided surfaces to slide on each other, so that lengthening can be achieved without separation of the ends. Some care is required in measuring the exact amount of lengthening as over-correction deprives the child of any spring in the gait, an essential element in 'take-off' for walking. The best final position is with slight tension developing in the tendon with the ankle exactly at 90°. At the same time any contracture of the posterior joint capsule can be divided. After suture of the tendon, the wound is closed and below-knee walking plaster applied. The child returns home the next or the following day and is encouraged to stand on the plaster straight away under the continuing surveillance of the same physiotherapist as before. The cast can be removed after 4–6 weeks.

Two local factors influence the prognosis after this surgery. Fixed deformity only arises because of unequal muscle action on either side of the joint. If the dorsiflexors of the ankle are found to be weak, then the tendency for recurrence of the deformity is increased. On the other hand, good dorsiflexor action and correction of the equinus deformity carry the best outlook for the future. Another factor in the very young is the effect of growth in the leg. Normal relations in the limb depend on exactly equal growth of the constituent parts. However, if organic changes within the muscle-tendon unit cause it to grow at a slower rate than the bones of the leg, some recurrence of equinus deformity may occur in spite of the continuing efforts of the therapist. A second lengthening of the tendon may then be required after an interval of a few years and before growth is completed.

The correction of an equinus deformity may produce unexpected bonuses in improved position of the knees and hips, and a child who previously seemed unlikely ever to stand independently, let alone walk, may now become able to do both and move significantly nearer to independent existence.

The knee. Many cerebral palsied children show a flexed position of the knees on standing. The first requirement is to establish the cause. It may be found that the knees can be passively corrected into full extension when the child is lying down, but on standing the knees flop into a flexed knee position. This is due to weakness of quadriceps action and palpation at the back of the knee will confirm that the flexor tendons are slack. No operative surgery will help in this situation which is best dealt with by fitting polythene casts to support the knees when weight-bearing.

On the other hand, examination may show limitation of passive extension of the joint due to spasm/contracture of the hamstring tendons, to contracture of the posterior capsule or both. If the tendons are responsible, they will be seen and felt to stand out as tight cords under the skin at the back of the joint.

Marked improvement will follow a modified Egger's operation. Two short incisions are made posterolaterally and posteromedially to display the biceps tendon on the lateral side, and the semitendinosus, gracilis, sartorius and semi-membranosus tendons on the medial side. These are divided just proximal to their insertions below the knee and then attached to the soft tissues on the back of the femoral condyles above the joint. If all the tendons are divided there is some risk of later development of genu recurvatum or 'back knee'. To safeguard against this, it is customary to leave one of the tendons (frequently the semi-membranosus) intact on the medial side. After closure of the wounds a plaster of Paris cylinder is applied extending from the groin to the ankle with the maximum extension possible. If some limitation of extension remains, the cause is posterior capsule tightness but this can usually be overcome by serial changes of plaster over the coming weeks, gaining a little more extension each time.

As in the case of ankle surgery, the child is retained in hospital for the minimum time possible, is then returned to the physiotherapist who has been managing long-term care, and standing and walking is encouraged from the outset. The casts are retained for 4 weeks and then bi-valved. The child is gradually mobilized, the therapist using his discretion about the length of time the bi-valved casts should be totally or partially retained for walking and for wear at night.

The hip. Congenital dysplasia of the hip can occur in a cerebral palsied child with the same frequency as in a normal child. However, the presence of an adduction deformity and scissor position of the legs frequently brings with it an increased risk of outward subluxation of the femoral head. This is not uncommon in children in the under 5 age group.

Once again, the need is to keep operative procedures as simple as possible. Surgery is not indicated unless there is definite expectation that the child will walk. Many children require nothing more complicated than a subcutaneous tenotomy of the tight adductors on the medial side of the groin. The legs can then be held out in the abducted position by broomstick plasters, in which plaster cylinders are applied to each leg and the hips are held in maximum abduction by the fixture of a transverse bar (or broomstick) between the two casts. The casts are retained for 3 weeks, followed by abduction exercises and possibly the use of an abduction pillow between the legs at night.

Once correction has been obtained additional surgery is seldom necessary, although a further subcutaneous tenotomy may be performed a few years later if required. More complicated procedures, such as psoas release, obturator neurectomy or shelf operations to stabilize the hip, are only occasionally indicated.

At all times, the objectives of orthopaedic management in cerebral palsy should be to achieve a dramatic step forward in the programme of treatment, with the minimum of disturbance to the child and without any interruption of care from the physiotherapist and others that the child knows well.

K.M. BRYANT

The Physical Management of Cerebral Palsy

The object of all physiotherapists treating physically handicapped children is to help them to live as normal a life as their handicap allows.

In his therapy sessions, the child will gradually develop new abilities of posture, locomotion and manipulation which must be meaningfully utilized and consolidated in all aspects of his daily life if maximum independence and optimum function are to be achieved. It is therefore apparent that efficient day-long management is quite as important for this as specific techniques of physiotherapy.

Each area of activity is complicated by some or all of the child's physical deficits and the deficits themselves can be aggravated by some activities and methods of handling. This question of total management is complex and full consideration of it is beyond the scope of this short discussion. Therefore only the main points will be raised and a few suggestions made. A list of publications giving more detailed information will be found at the end of this chapter.

EVERY-DAY ACTIVITIES

Dressing
Problems with dressing and undressing a cerebral palsied child can arise long before he is old enough to dress himself. If spastic, he may stiffen up when being handled. If he is athetoid, his incessant movements will hamper dressing. In either case, he will probably be at his most difficult when lying on his back and should therefore be dressed prone across the knees. An older child who can roll but cannot sit manages better in side-lying.

The clothes themselves are important, especially when the child is trying to dress himself. All garments should be slightly larger than necessary, with loosely fitting sleeves and wide necks. They should fasten at the front; preferably with velcro, studs or zips with large rings for easy grasp. If buttons are unavoidable, then the buttons should be fairly large and go easily through the buttonholes. Trousers or skirts with elasticated waists are easier to put on and to take down when in a hurry for the lavatory. Socks without turned heels and mitts rather than gloves also simplify the task.

Long before a child is ready to dress himself, he should be talked through dressing and undressing, so that he learns the names of his garments and which parts of his body they cover, as well as how to put them on and remove them.

Undressing is learned first and he will probably begin spontaneously by pulling off mittens, socks and shoes. Clothes with sleeves present more of a problem and he should learn to remove them by stages, beginning with the final manoeuvre of taking his arm out of the last sleeve and working backwards. If he shows signs of dressing apraxia (p. 288), i.e. persistent and unremitting difficulty in recognizing the function of garments or in donning them properly despite adequate use of arms and hands, then dressing and undressing a large doll may help to resolve this.

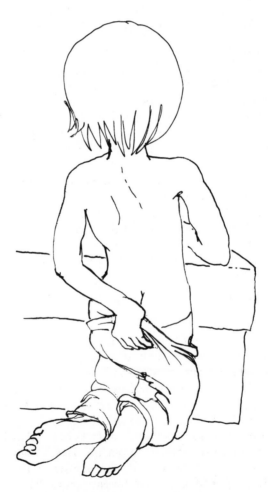

FIG. 14.1. Putting on trousers kneeling.

Positions for dressing depend on the child's level of physical competence and some common difficulties are: poor sitting balance, so that one arm is always needed for support; difficulty in using the hands independently, and poor grasp.

Putting on trousers, skirts or pants is particularly difficult, because few children have achieved sufficiently good standing balance to leave both hands free. They should be taught how to dress their lower half one-handed while kneeling with support (Fig. 14.1) or lying on the floor (Fig. 14.2a and b).

Like all self-help skills, learning to dress should be tackled at the appropriate time of day, thus becoming part of the day's routine.

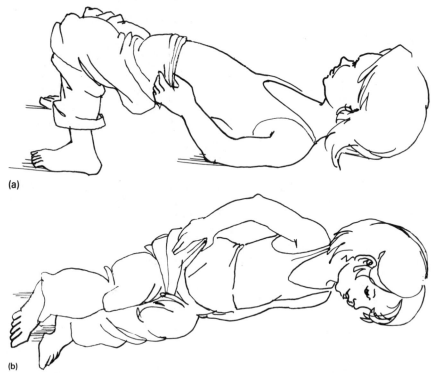

(a)

(b)

Fig. 14.2a and b. Putting on trousers lying on the floor on back and side.

Washing

Some of the points made when discussing dressing are also relevant to the washing and bathing of a handicapped child.

If he shows strong extensor thrust, it is easier to wash a very young child in a prone position, instead of bathing him. If there is only slight to moderate tendency to extension, than a small bath or large sink which permits only a semi-reclining position should contain this. Such a child should have his hips fully flexed as an additional precaution before he is placed in his bath.

A wide variety of bath seats are marketed to meet the needs of children who are too flexed to sit with their legs extended, who have no sitting balance or who have athetoid movements of the legs (Fig. 14.3a and b). Suppliers are listed below.

If athetoid movements are severe, then the bath should be padded with sheets of foam rubber.

Sponges are preferred to towelling face-cloths for children who are hypersensitive to touch, while loofahs stimulate the sluggish. A child who is ready to wash his own face but who cannot grip his face cloth, should have a wash glove instead. Face washing should be encouraged since hands to face is also an important ability for self-feeding.

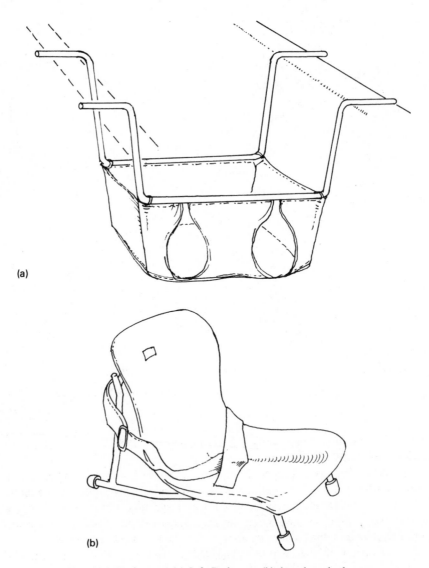

(a)

(b)

FIG. 14.3. Bath seats; (a) Safa-Bath seat; (b) Amesbury bath seat.

Many children are averse to tooth-brushing, but will often accept this if musical or electric toothbrushes are used. Electric toothbrushes are also useful for desensitization in children who have problems of hypersensitivity in the oral area.

Potting

Rules for toilet training which are valid for normal children are also applicable to handicapped children, although the handicapped child will probably be older when training begins and will take longer about it. Frequent and regular potting is necessary, and the child must be told why he is being potted and praised when he is successful. Because of his physical problems, however, he will need extra support and a potty offering good stability and some pelvic support should be chosen (Fig. 14.4a and b).

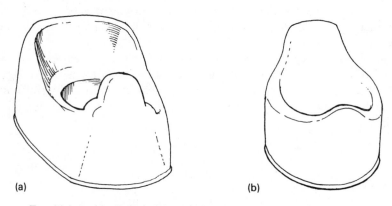

(a)   (b)

Fig. 14.4a and b. Potties giving good stability and some pelvic support.

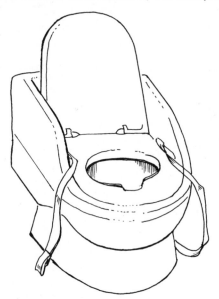

Fig. 14.5. Baby Relax Toilette.

If a stable potty alone is not enough, then the pot can be placed in a cardboard carton, in a corner of the room or against the wall between two stools. A good potty chair for severely handicapped children is available from the Spastics Society and the Baby Relax Toilette (Fig. 14.5) is useful for a child with partial sitting balance.

As with all self-help skills, assistance should be withdrawn as soon as possible.

Feeding

There are many reasons why a cerebral palsied child may be difficult to feed and later on, may have difficulty feeding himself. Problems can arise primarily from disorganization of the organs and muscles directly involved, such as tongue thrust, bite reflex, strong gag reflex, hypersensitivity of oral areas, poor lip closure and drooling. Secondary disruptive disabilities are tonic reflex activity, incomplete head control, poor sitting balance, weak grasp, incomplete hand/eye co-ordination, inability to get the hand up to the mouth and athetoid movements of the arms and head.

Children like to see what they are getting to eat and if their food is placed in front of them they will not lose their balance looking for it. The exception to this is the child with tongue thrust and/or a bite reflex. If he is fed from the side, so that he does not see the spoon until the last moment, this will minimize anticipation.

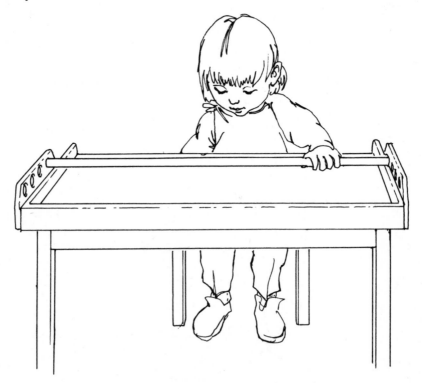

Fig. 14.6. Table with bar devised at Cheyne Spastic Centre.

Spoons should be shallow to permit easy removal of food by the lips and small and rounded to avoid stimulation of a gag reflex. If he has a bite reflex then the spoon should be of bone or polythene and not of metal.

Position is of major importance. The head must be kept upright and not allowed to extend, to aid swallowing and to avoid extensor thrust. A chair and table of the right size and height are also essential for good self-feeding. These are discussed below. Keeping the free hand forward on the table aids sitting balance and a bar fixed across the table providing a stable hand hold is helpful to athetoid children (Fig. 14.6).

POSTURE AND MOBILITY

Positions
Until he can change his position for himself, the cerebral palsied child is dependent on others to change it for him. A good position is one that obeys the following rules:

it should counter any deformity the child's particular deficits put him at risk of developing;

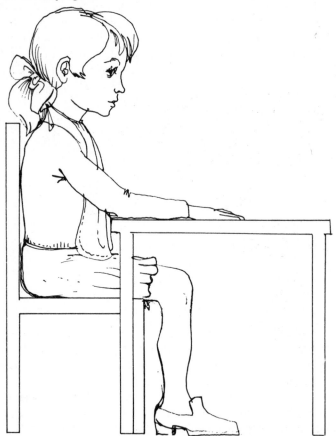

FIG. 14.7. Correct chair and table height for self-feeding.

it should be the optimum position for his current activity;

it should have in it an element of therapy, e.g. standing to play at a table when consolidating standing balance for later walking;

no position is a good position if the child is left in it until he is stiff and uncomfortable, frequent changes of position are important;

static positions should alternate with movement. Therefore, the non-ambulant child should have frequent periods on the floor.

When planning the child's home and nursery programme, his therapist should choose several positions for him and indicate their use for specific activities, e.g. prone over a wedge to play for a child who cannot sit safely and lacks complete head control.

Furniture

Tables and chairs tailored to the requirements of individual children are essential for comfort and functional ability, as well as playing a significant part in the prevention of deformity.

The best chair for most children is the one which maintains a right angle at hip, knee and ankle (Fig. 14.7). A child with extensor thrust should, however, be given a chair with a sloping seat which will increase his degree of hip flexion. If sitting balance is insecure, then the chair should have arms. Corner seats make it possible for children with imperfect sitting balance to sit on the floor (Fig. 14.8) and if pommels are added, they are also able to maintain good

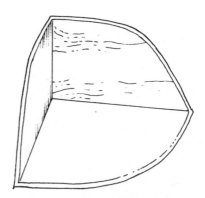

FIG. 14.8. Corner seat.

abduction of the thighs. This is an excellent way of avoiding the invidious W-sitting position which reinforces internal rotation deformities of the hips and increases the possibility of sub-luxation (Fig. 14.9).

The 'bean-bag' chair offers a choice of several comfortable positions to the extended child who cannot sit (Fig. 14.10). All are semi-reclining positions, however, and do not offer much chance to see or to use the hands. For hand function, a prone wedge should be substituted.

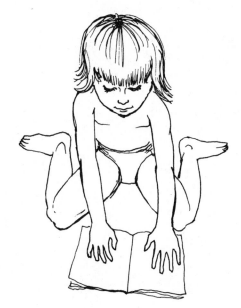

FIG. 14.9. W-sitting.

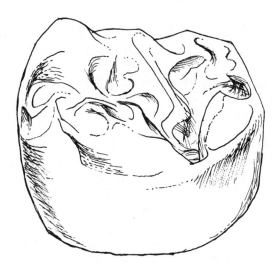

FIG. 14.10. Bean bag (sag bag) chair.

A severely athetoid child with extensor thrust should have a specially made chair of canvas-deck-chair shape; firm, but well padded and with adequate side supports (Fig. 14.11).

Holt *et al.* (1972) stressed the importance of ensuring that wheelchairs are adapted to suit the individual child and showed the need for special clinics to review periodically the suitability of aids provided.

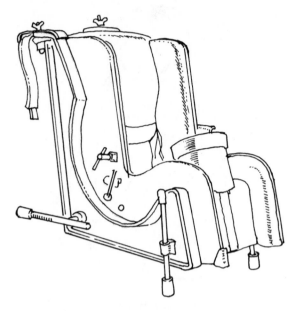

Fig. 14.11. Chair for athetoid child.

A table or play tray of the wrong height can effectively prevent full use of the hands. If sitting balance is good and arm movements not too inco-ordinated, the table should be waist height and allow for the knees to be comfortably tucked underneath. An unsteady child will find it easier to use his hands if the table is high enough for him to rest his elbows on it, thus shortening the lever of movement, without having to lean too far forward and disrupt his sitting balance.

Lifting and carrying
If a child has some acceptable way of getting around, then he should only be carried when he is tired or if time is pressing. How he is lifted and carried depends on the type and pattern of his disability.

A child who is stiff in extension will be stiffest when lying on his back and before he is picked up, he should either be drawn up into sitting, or rolled on to his side. Parting his legs and carrying him astride the hip with his arms forward and across one's shoulders reduces the chance of his stiffening up while being carried and also allows him some view of his surroundings.

Conversely, a small child whose tone is predominantly flexor, is better carried in extension, either on his side and facing forwards (Fig. 14.12) or prone with support under chest and thighs.

If a floppy child is carried facing forward with his back to the carrier and with his hips flexed, this will encourage him to maintain an upright posture.

Athetoid children are easier to lift if they are first turned into prone. If taken up from a chair then the arms should be drawn well forward across the

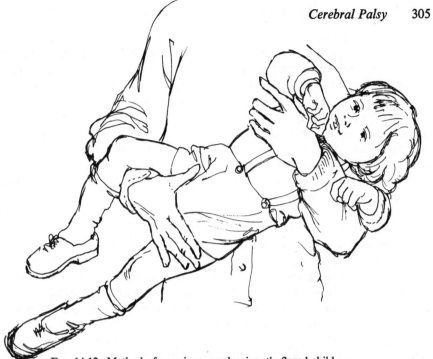

Fig. 14.12. Method of carrying a predominantly flexed child.

chest before lifting. These children are more safely and comfortably carried if their hips are well flexed and their shoulders protracted (Fig. 14.13).

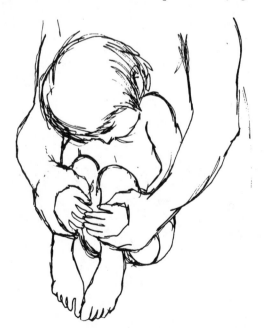

Fig. 14.13. Method of carrying an athetoid child.

Pre-walking mobility

Almost all diplegics develop the activity known as 'sealing'. This is a progression in prone in which the extended trunk and legs are dragged along the ground by rolling the forearms forward one over the other, under the chest. Some learn to move quite quickly like this, but the strong muscle work in arms which are working in an abnormal pattern of movement reinforces the abnormal pattern of extension/adduction of the lower limbs. If possible, children should be induced to use rolling as an alternative. It is the most desirable initial method of moving about because of the relaxing element of trunk rotation involved.

Crawling is acceptable if it is in a good reciprocal pattern and without undue internal rotation of the legs at the hips.

Bunny-hopping must be discouraged whenever spasticity is present because, being a strongly flexor activity, it increases incipient flexor deformity at hips, knees and ankles, which can in turn reduce the prospect of walking.

As soon as sitting balance is secure, it is better to get the child upright and astride a toy horse or engine on wheels or a suitably sized tricycle. Pushing himself about with his feet strengthens his legs and learning to pedal develops good reciprocal leg action. The dimensions of these toys is very important. Seats of foot propelled mounts should be at a height which enables the child to get his feet comfortably flat on the floor and not too wide for the amount of abduction he can manage without recourse to internal rotation at the hips.

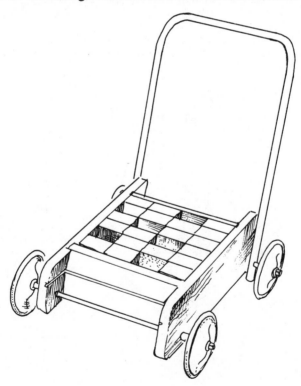

Fig. 14.14a.

Some children are reluctant movers, but will often attempt movement at the instigation of another child while declining to do so for their therapist. If children of similar abilities are taken together in small groups of three or four, the energetic encourage the indolent. Such classes also provide valuable additions to individual therapy.

Activities should be simple and basically functional along the lines laid down by Professor Peto (see below) and his technique of rhythmic intention should also be employed.

Walking aids
Fig. 14.14a–d shows a selection of walking aids suitable for small children; all are manufactured commercially (list of suppliers of all equipment below).

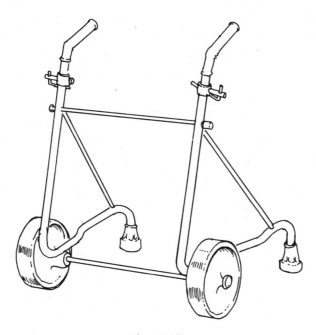

FIG. 14.14b.

The type chosen will depend on the degree of assistance required, either for balance or weight-taking and on the degree of disability in the arms. The aim will be to find the aid which will enable the child to walk in the most normal pattern he can achieve. Wheeled aids often seem to run away with the child. Finnie (1974) suggested an ordinary straight backed chair for use in the home.

SOME APPROACHES TO PHYSICAL TREATMENT OF CEREBRAL PALSY

There are several very different schools of thought about the physical treatment of cerebral palsy; each is largely based on its own interpretation of the salient neurological phenomena, but while concepts and methods may differ, there is

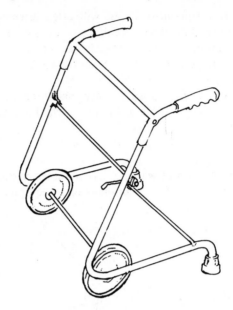

Fig. 14.14c.

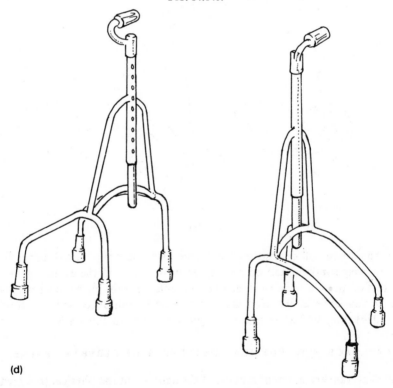

(d)

Fig. 14.14. Walking aids: (a) weighted walker; (b) rollator; (c) rollator with Cheyne bar; (d) quadripods.

one unifying belief. All authorities are consistent in declaring that regular treatment from the earliest possible age is the best way of ensuring that the cerebral palsied child will achieve his maximum potential.

The Bobath method

Dr. Karel and Mrs. Bertha Bobath, neurologist and physiotherapist respectively, have made exhaustive studies of most types of abnormal neurological behaviour (Bobath and Bobath, 1975) and they hold the view that the arrest or retardation of normal motor development resulting from cerebral palsy is manifested in two particular ways. Firstly there is prolonged retention of the primitive total patterns of earliest childhood and, where moderate to severe spasticity is present, the release of tonic reflexes can place considerable limitation on the quality and range of active movement.

Secondly, the normal postural reflex mechanism, which forms the background of normal active movement, is delayed and/or imperfectly developed; poor head control, lack of trunk rotation and the absence of balance and other adaptive reactions are evidence of this.

Together, the Bobaths have developed the neurodevelopmental system of treatment which is probably the most highly regarded and widely practised. The aims of treatment may be summarized as follows: to inhibit abnormal reflex activity and facilitate movement (the one leading to the other) and to facilitate the normal postural reactions which are prerequisites for balance and normal movement.

The methods of treatment stem directly from these aims and have been described with admirable clarity by the originators and their associates (Bobath and Bobath, 1964; Bobath, 1967; Manning, 1972), therefore only a few relevant points will be made here.

Initially only static reflex inhibiting postures were used, but while these were effective for normalizing tone, they also inhibited active movement. Now, treatment is by reflex inhibiting patterns which are not static and, by making use of key points of control, inhibiting the release of abnormal, disabling reflexes, at the same time allowing movement.

Abnormal postural reflex activity originates mainly from head and neck, shoulder girdle and spine and by controlling these key points, active movement is simultaneously facilitated in the limbs.

One of the objectives of the neurodevelopmental method is to guide the child through the normal sequences of motor development; namely, rolling over, sitting, coming up onto hands and knees for crawling, standing and finally walking. Rolling from supine to prone can be facilitated quite simply if the child's head is flexed and rotated, when the trunk will follow. Extension and rotation of the head similarly facilitates rolling from prone to supine. If there is much spasticity, however, the desirable element of trunk rotation will be excluded. In such cases, using the shoulders as key points of control in the same pattern of movement allows a greater degree of rotation while controlling spasticity in the working muscles and allowing the child the added advantage of free movement of the head and neck.

It is necessary to develop righting and equilibrium reactions concurrently with inhibition and facilitation. Sometimes, postural reflexes develop automatically when abnormal patterns of movement have been broken, but more often, they too must be facilitated. A child must also be given the chance to feel a posture by being passively supported. Next, he must learn to hold it for longer and longer periods while support is progressively withdrawn. Finally, he must learn to maintain his position against outside forces, either as his supporting surface is disturbed or in the face of direct pressure.

The Vojta method

Dr. Vaclav Vojta is a paediatric neurologist who works in Cologne, West Germany, with very young children described as being at risk of developing a movement disorder. Both his interpretation of the problem and his methods of treatment are less complex than those of Dr. and Mrs. Bobath.

Vojta believes that there is present in the normal child an innate ability to respond to posture and he calls this Postural Reactability. He defines this phenomenon as an automatic active response in which the whole neuro-muscular complex is changed (Jones, 1975).

In order to test a child's postural reactability, he has devised a system of seven reflexes, arranged in specific developmental sequence and should a child show five or more abnormal responses out of seven, he is considered to be in need of treatment.

By stimulating trigger points, Vojta produces the two reflex patterns of rolling and creeping. He has called creeping the total marshalling of all co-ordinate movement.

The continued repetition of these patterns, by reflex stimulation, eventually translates an initially automatic response into an active movement.

Although relatively straightforward, the treatment is quite intensive, the patterns being repeated for 10–15 minutes four times daily. If the child is an out-patient, the parents are taught to carry out treatment at home under the close supervision of a therapist.

The Temple Fay method

Dr. Temple Fay, a neuro-surgeon, worked in Philadelphia, USA during the 1940s and 1950s. Like Vojta, Fay used patterning as a method of treatment and his patterns bear some similarity to those of Vojta, but the manner in which they were elicited was different and so was his interpretation of the neurological problem (Fay, 1946).

Fay believed in evolutionary levels of functional development and visualized motor development as progressing through four distinct stages: reptilian infantile squirming, amphibian movements, mammalian reciprocal motion on 'all fours' and advanced motor skill of walking.

When a lesion in the cortex precludes this normal sequence of motor development, then the primitive reflex movements of infancy, centred at lower levels and released by lack of cortical control, could be utilized to promote basic active patterns of movement. Once mastered, these movement patterns provided a foundation from which to tackle the more advanced functions of reciprocal crawling and walking.

Thus Fay and Vojta are at one, but whereas Vojta first procures his movements by reflex stimulation, Fay relied on passive positioning to trigger movement. He laid particular stress on two patterns, both carried out with the patient prone; the homo-lateral or alligator pattern and the contra-lateral, crossed or amphibian pattern.

The Temple Fay system of patterning is of current interest because of its connection with the next system to be described.

The Doman Delacato method

This is the method of treatment developed in Philadelphia during the past two decades by Glen Doman, a physical therapist and Carl H. Delacato, an educational psychologist (Doman, 1974).

The systems of treatment so far discussed have all been techniques of physio-therapy, mainly concerned with gross motor development and intended primarily for use by trained physiotherapists. Doman and Delacato aim to promote all aspects of development, using the child's parents, family and friends as his therapists. They have defined six areas of competence; mobility, language, manual, visual, auditory and tactile. They use the patterns of Dr. Temple Fay to improve mobility, and many of their techniques in the other spheres are standard techniques in general use.

The essence of their system is its remarkable intensity. Average programmes encompass a 7-hour day, but this can be up to twice as long for a very severely handicapped child. A 30-minute programme is devised, made up of 1, 2 or 3-minute periods devoted to such things as reading, visual, auditory and tactile stimulation, language, bath-room training and crawling. This half-hour prog-ramme is repeated non-stop throughout the day, punctuated only by meal times and six patterning sessions of 5 minutes each. Three or five people are required for each period of patterning.

The Peto method

This method of training and treating cerebral palsied children, called Conductive Education by its originator, was devised by Professor Peto of Prague, where his work is now being carried on at the Peto Institute by his successor, Dr. Maria Hari.

Like that of Doman and Delacato, the Peto method is a way of life. That is its only resemblance to any other system of treatment.

Being well aware of all the many receptive and executive difficulties which can occur in one child, Professor Peto became concerned about the number of specialists to whom the child must adjust, as well as the differences in emphasis and outlook that can arise in a multi-disciplinary team and cause possible confusion. Consequently, Peto decided that all the therapy and education a child required should be given in a resident setting by the same person. The Peto Institute is thus both an in-patient treatment centre and a training school for these all-round therapists whom he called conductors.

The Peto system has been well described by Cotton (1970; 1975). The chief elements are as follows:

As already stated, one therapist is responsible for all spheres of development; gross motor, sensori-motor, self-help skills and education.

Children with similar levels of physical ability receive treatment in groups and not in individual sessions.

Each task to be tackled, be it getting up from a chair or washing the face, is broken up into its component sequences of movement and each basic movement is practised separately until all are mastered, when they are run together to form the desired function.

The technique of Rhythmic Intention is used at all times. First of all, the conductor will state the task, e.g. 'We are going to stretch our arms'. Then the children will repeat this together and as they actually carry out the movement, they will reinforce it with another vocal formula: 'We are stretching our arms', or by counting as they move. Thus, the children simultaneously develop speech and give each movement or activity additional auditory stimulus.

Simple class-room furniture such as ladder-back chairs, slatted topped beds-cum-tables and wooden staves, all designed for easy grasping, are the main items of equipment used for motor development.

None of these methods has yet been subjected to independent clinical trials and evidence of efficacy is mostly empirical. There are of course several factors hindering the structured evaluation of any system of physical treatment, viz. the relatively small numbers of children likely to be available for any particular trial; the wide range and variety of motor handicap presenting, which makes matching for comparison very difficult; the diversity of associated sensory disorders which further complicates comparisons; the ethical problem of leaving a control group without treatment; wide variations in personality, motivation and intelligence of patients and differing parental attitudes.

The eclectic approach
More specific systems of treatment have been devised for cerebral palsy than for any other condition amenable to physical treatment, yet many physiotherapists have opted for an open approach for the following reasons.

As already stated, there is no independent clinical proof for preferring one method to any other.

Those variables which prejudice structured clinical trials also discourage too rigid a therapeutic approach. The endless permutations of handicap which can occur mean that each child presents his own picture of difficulty which can best be countered by his own individual programme of treatment. This is not a concept borrowed from the philosophy of Doman and Delacato. Their programmes are specific for each child only as regards the total amount of treatment prescribed and the time allotted to each selected area of stimulation. The actual techniques applied appear to vary little from child to child.

Concentrating exclusively on one system of treatment will leave unmet the needs of any child whom it does not happen to suit.

Keeping an open mind allows for the introduction of other techniques used in general neurological practice, particularly some of the techniques of proprioceptive neuro-muscular facilitation (PNF) developed by Kabat and Knott (Knott and Voss, 1956). Levitt (1966) has described the most useful of these techniques.

Some of the specific systems, particularly that of Doman and Delacato, call for more effort than most parents (especially those with other children) are able to contribute. The drawing up of individual treatment and home management programmes enables realistic goals to be set for each family.

Scrutton and Gilbertson (1975) have reservations about the eclectic approach, but Levitt (1969; 1977) has argued convincingly in its favour. The essence of the eclectic approach is that it sets out to treat the physical deficits of cerebral palsy by the most suitable technique(s) whatever their source, instead of applying a standard format of therapy to the collective diagnosis. Signs and deficits are analysed and arranged in order of gravity, so that priorities and aims of treatment can be established. The matching of deficit and treatment is not done in isolation but as part of the whole, so that improvement in one area is not achieved at the cost of deterioration in another. A simple example of this might be concentration on the attainment of secure sitting, or the exploitation of the sitting position once achieved to such an extent that the child develops flexion contractures at hips and knees.

As already stressed, detailed assessment as described in Chapter 10 precedes treatment. This is particularly relevant to young children for whom gross motor development must take priority, even if there is developmental delay in other areas. In the normal sequence of development, it is the mastering of certain basic motor skills that precedes and makes possible fine motor and intellectual achievements.

Broad aims of treatment are to facilitate optimum motor development and function and to prevent the development of deformities and contractures which would hinder and distort that function.

It is hoped that the following examples of treatment schemes will show how these aims can be met by drawing on ideas from all sources. To allow for as many examples as possible and for the sake of clarity, only clear diagnostic presentations are used, only the salient points of the assessments picked out and treatment suggestions have been kept to a minimum.

Diplegia. Age 3 years 2 months (real age allowing for prematurity 2 years 10 months).

Significant signs and deficits

Tone. Moderate increase in both legs, particularly in the abnormal pattern of extension/adduction/internal rotation. Slight increase in arms, detected in internal rotators of shoulders and flexors of elbows.

Tonic reflex activity. Release of tonic neck reflexes responsible for difficulty in holding the prone kneeling position, legs soon extend (STNR), tendency to collapse into flexion on left side if head is turned to right when prone kneeling (ATNR).

Postural reactions. Persistence of ATNR. Absence of sideways and forward parachute responses. Absence of equilibrium reactions.

Most disabling inabilities. Head control incomplete, cannot sit unaided, no reciprocal kick, can only move by sealing.

Suggested techniques

For head control. Pull to sit and lower, therapist holding child's arms and maintaining child's legs in abduction/extension/external rotation.

For sitting balance. Stimulation of equilibrium reactions in sitting on a large therapy ball or roll (Fig. 14.15a and b) in front of a mirror. Passive positioning on mat in front of a mirror, preferably in stride sitting or tailor sitting if easier to start with; only minimal finger-tip correction.

To minimize TNR influence (two therapists required). Position child passively in prone kneeling, then rock gently forward and back.

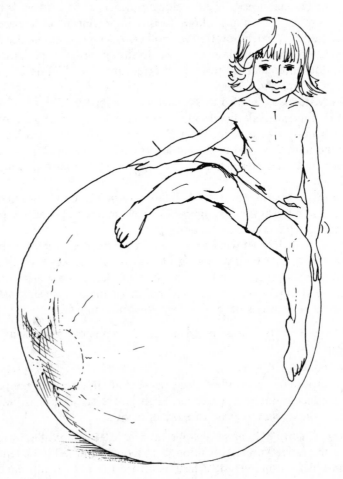

FIG. 14.15a.

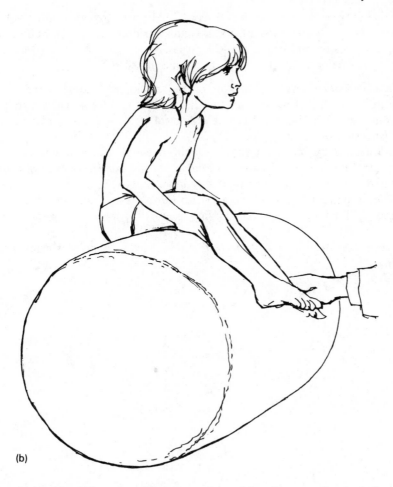

(b)

FIG. 14.15. Stimulation of equilibrium reactions sitting (a) on a therapy ball, and (b) on a roll.

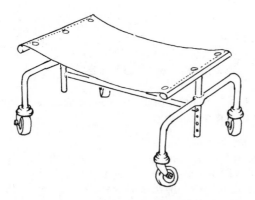

FIG. 14.16. Cheyne crawler.

To encourage reciprocal action of legs. Child supine on mat with head kept central and arms inhibited in abduction/extension/external rotation. Initiate reciprocal flexion and extension of legs passively, child will take over. Use a nursery rhyme or song, i.e. encourage a conditioned reflex.

For locomotion. Present method of movement by sealing is reinforcing abnormal patterns of movement. Substitute rolling and gradually introduce a crawling aid (Fig. 14.16). When teaching rolling, stress trunk rotation as a further means of stabilizing tone.

This child's age and pattern of disability require the neurodevelopmental approach. In addition, if passive stretching of tight adductors or hamstrings is required, this should be done indirectly in such a young child by the wearing of Cheyne pattern leg gaiters (Fig. 14.17) during rest periods and later, while practising standing; by correct carrying (p. 304); by stride sitting in a suitable chair.

The efficacy or otherwise of all treatment is tested by handling during therapy sessions.

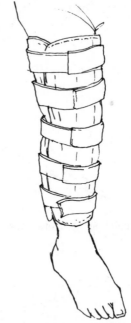

FIG. 14.17. Cheyne gaiters.

Dystonic infant. Age 9 months. Signs of neurological abnormality present for several months and not diminishing.

Significant signs and deficits
Generalized increase of tone in legs. When held vertical, legs scissor. Cannot sit. Persistence of ATNR. No sideways or forwards parachute reactions. (N.B. despite the great difference in their chronological ages, this child and the previous one are very close in gross motor age.)

Suggested technique
Vojta's crawl pattern would be suitable for this child.

Left-sided hemiplegia. Age 2 years.

Significant signs and deficits
Tone and posture. No appreciable increase of muscle tone in the left leg; when held supported in standing, both legs adopt a posture of slight flexion and internal rotation with eversion of the feet. Moderate increase of tone in left arm which is mostly held in the typical hemiplegic posture of internal rotation at the shoulder, flexion at the elbow and forearm pronated. Hand is mostly fisted, with the thumb adducted across the palm.

Postural reactions. Absence of left sideways parachute reaction. Forward parachute incomplete on left. Equilibrium reaction in sitting, but limited response to left.

Physical abilities. Sitting balance secure in all positions, gets out of sitting and comes up to sit from lying prone or supine. Rolls from prone to supine over right or left, prefers over right.

Main inabilities. No mode of progression. Not attempting to pull up to stand. Ignores left arm and hand.

Suggested techniques
For moving around. Facilitation of continuous rolling. Place favourite toys just outside his reach, increase distance.

For standing. Practice in front of a mirror with manual support at knees from therapist. Legs placed in abduction/external rotation to correct abnormal posture. Elicit positive supporting reactions.

To encourage awareness of left arm and bilateral use of hands. Training of sideways save to left and support reaction in left arm. Offer toys requiring two hands such as large balls, drum and sticks, hammer and pegs. Painting of pictures in the palms and games like 'round and round the garden'. Passive shaking of left arm to induce relaxation of fist. Throwing and catching balls (child in stride sitting). Passive placing of hands in wheelbarrow position if he will tolerate this. Many young hemiplegic children dislike being prone.

Dystonic athetosis. Age 4 years 10 months.

Physical deficits and inabilities. Total. No head control. No voluntary movement. Shoulders retracted.

Tone. Varies with position; hypertonic in supine in position of total extension, floppy when turned into prone.

Extraneous movements. Frequent bursts of severe athetoid movements both proximal and distal, sometimes triggered and always aggravated by loud noises and sudden movements around him, less frequent in prone.

Suggested techniques
Treatment initially directed towards gaining relaxation, some head control, getting arms forward.

For relaxation and head control. Prone on a large therapy ball, arms well forward and internally rotated at the shoulders, elbows extended. Encouragement to voluntary extension of head (adapted from Bobath).

Also for head control, additional. Semi-flexed reclining in a bean bag chair, arms held forward and adducted. Head turning to order. Progress to kneeling stride over therapist's thigh with chest support (Fig. 14.18).

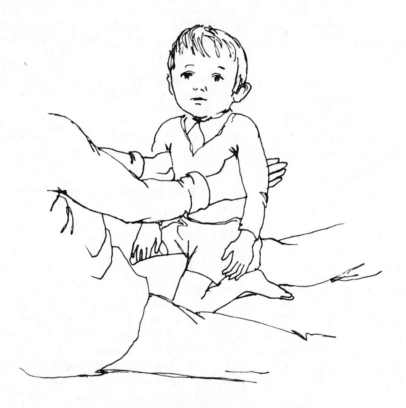

FIG. 14.18. Kneeling stride over therapist's thigh.

To get arms forward to mid line: position in supine on soft mat with head supported in flexion (avoiding stimulation over occiput), femora abducted, hips and knees well flexed. Practise the PNF pattern of extension/adduction/internal rotation, arms separately first and then together against light directional resistance. In PNF, extension brings the arms down to the trunk.

A special chair (Fig. 14.11) was made for this child at the Dundee Limb Fitting Centre to a design suggested by Nash.

Cerebellar ataxia. Age 2 years.

Physical deficits and inabilities

Tone. Generally hypotonic with abnormal range of movement at all joints. Reaching and grasping clumsy and inco-ordinated. Constant, overt exaggeration of normally undetectable postural responses to changes of position and to maintain position, particularly in standing. Stands with support only.

Gait. Wide-based, reeling, high stepping. Walks only with support, otherwise cruises round furniture.

Suggested techniques

Those techniques of postural stabilization and of directional movement against resistance (Knott and Voss, 1956) which would be relevant in cases of adult ataxia would be equally suitable for this child, but a 2-year-old cannot be expected to understand and tolerate such a stylized routine.

Suggested modifications are: walking with a rollator (Fig. 14.14b) against strong resistance provided indirectly by the therapist pressing down on the handles; climbing stairs against resistance applied at the ankles; engaging the child's attention with favourite toys while standing at a table of suitable (chest) height, while stabilizing the pelvis from behind and in same position, encouraging transference of weight.

Suppliers of Equipment

'Safa' bath seat
Supplies Officer, Spastics Society, 12 Park Crescent, London W1N 4EQ

Amesbury bath seat
Amesbury Surgical Appliances, 28 Pontygwindy Industrial Estate, Caerphilly, Mid-Glamorgan CF8 2WH

'Watford' potty chair
Spastics Society

Folding Canvas Corner Seat
Temple Engineering Co., P.O. Box No. 1, High Street, Cowes, Isle of Wight

Bean bag (Sag bag) chair
Sylvia Rice, 120 St. Stephens Avenue, London W1Z 8JD

Rollator with Cheyne bar
J. & A. Carter Ltd., Westbury, Wiltshire

First size rollators
Day's Medical Aids, Litchard Industrial Estate, Bridgend, Mid-Glamorgan

Toddl-aids (for walking)
Ellis, Son and Paramore Ltd., Spring Street Works, Sheffield, S3 8PB

Cheyne crawler
J. & A. Carter Ltd.

Cheyne pattern gaiters
M. Masters and Sons Ltd., 177/184 Grange Road, London, SE1 3AE

Therapy balls and foam wedges
Spastics Society

M.I. NASH

Sensori-motor Stimulation

Knowledge of the sequences and stages of development in normal children is a prerequisite for assessing what are the difficulties of the handicapped child which interfere with his ability to develop and learn from his sensory motor experiences. Referring to the first 18 months of life, Piaget wrote 'we call it the sensory-motor period because the infant lacks the symbolic function; that is, he does not have representations by which he can evoke persons or objects in their absence. In spite of this lack, mental development during the first 18 months of life is particularly important, for it is during this time that the child constructs all the cognitive substructures that will serve as a point of departure for his later perceptive and intellectual development' (Piaget and Inhelder, 1969). Thus it would seem that sensori-motor development is the cornerstone of the child's intellectual development.

In the normal child 'there is a continuous progression from spontaneous movement and reflexes to acquired habits and from the latter to intelligence' (Piaget and Inhelder, 1969). In contrast the handicapped child is often passive and unable to react spontaneously with his environment because of his physical deficits. The practice of sensori-motor stimulation is based on the premise that the sequence of development is of vital importance; 'what matters is the order in which the developments occur not the age at which they are attained. It [i.e. *Piaget's approach*] is thus applicable to all children no matter how slowly or how quickly they develop' (Woodward, 1970).

After assessment of present developmental achievements, a programme can be planned, designed to build upon the handicapped child's current abilities in a developmentally appropriate sequence and at an appropriate rate.

Sensori-motor and perceptual developmental in the normal child
The first year of life is the time when the infant begins to form concepts about himself and the world around him which will be the basis for later behaviour. This is the 'input-sensation' stage of development.

The infant's first responses and activities are motor ones and therefore his earliest learning experience is motor learning. His point of reference is his own body. With his body he experiements by tasting, looking and touching, thus making contact with his environment.

Rooting, sucking, swallowing and crying are present from birth so it is not surprising that the neonate's first point of attention is his mouth. The next focus of attention is his eyes. His mother's face is of great importance to the young infant. Recent experiments (Carpenter, 1975) have demonstrated at age 1 week a difference in eye responses to the face and voice of his mother from those given when he sees and hears another adult. Normally there is a very close mother-infant relationship both physically and emotionally and his mother becomes the bridge and the stimulus between the infant and his environment.

The newborn 'has no sense of self-identity, no sense which distinguishes between the world of things and the world of persons' (Gesell, 1950). Gradually he learns to differentiate between animate and inanimate objects in his environment. As the infant matures he discovers his physical self by movement and touch and later becomes aware of his personal self.

During the early months the infant's world is made up of pictures which he learns to recognize but which have no substance, permanence or spatial position. However, even now he is beginning to make the necessary links between sensory input, interpretation, perception and output that make development meaningful. The pictures gain stability and permanence by the infant making contact with the objects he sees through movement and manipulation. Interpretation follows and the information gained is stored.

The first stage in this process is hand-eye contact; 'the eye learns under the tutelage of the active hand' (Gesell *et al.*, 1941). By 3 months the hands are predominantly open and come together in the mid line. With his hands now within his range of focus the infant will study them intently. This stage of hand regard is an important preparation for later accurate controlled hand movement. First the infant moves the hand and watches as it moves, then as the eyes become more efficient 'the eye begins to lead, the hand follows along to confirm the result. . . . As the perceptual information and the motor information become more closely correlated . . . the eye can monitor the hand.' Finally, 'the eye can explore and the hand can duplicate; the hand can explore and the eye can visualise' (Kephart, 1971).

The physical development of head and trunk control broadens the infant's horizons as by 4 months this allows him to sit propped. He shows considerable interest in his surroundings, watching the movement of people and refusing to be left alone. He tries to relate objects to his own body by reaching out towards them, frequently over-shooting. By 6 months, when he has mastered reach and grasp everything is brought to the mouth to be tested as the infant's mouth is still his most effective method of exploration. At about this age he makes another step in the development of skilled movement, imitating actions such as tongue protrusion, waving and coughing.

As his hands are now useful tools the infant stops looking at them and instead uses them to explore his body and environment. The positions the infant uses in this body play are a preparation for later independent sitting; he will grasp his feet, bring them to his mouth and suck his toes. A major extension of this body play is play with his mother, touching her face and feeling and pulling her hair.

When objects within reach can be grasped, the infant turns them around and watches them as he did his own hands. When he drops a toy he will adjust his position to see where it has gone. When the infant first begins to test objects by using his hands he pats them with the flat palm but as his tactile awareness improves, he is able to palpate with the tips of his fingers. He uses this new-found tactile appreciation to good effect when he tests and feels the texture of food, putting his hands in the dish and squeezing food between his fingers with evident enjoyment. The increase in tactile awareness leads to a considerable increase in manipulation. The infant pushes and pulls objects and bangs them together. The index finger is used to poke through holes. Later the insides of objects have a particular fascination and the child spends much time poking objects into holes, putting them in and out of containers, putting on and taking off lids. This object play is self-orientated and in the second year the child keeps all his toys to himself as possessions are very important to him.

As mobility increases the child experiments with that mobility (e.g. repeatedly pulling to stand and then letting go) and uses it to further explore his environment. Once he can crawl and then walk he gets into everything (cupboards, drawers, handbags) and nothing within reach is safe from his exploring hands.

Sensori-motor awareness and perception form the basis for further skills. Motor learning results in a body of motor information, concerned with what movements are possible, how they are made and what are the results. Tactual and kinaesthetic data are used to monitor the course of the movement and to provide knowledge of its results. These data are closely allied to, and possibly inseparable from, movements since they occur only in the presence of movement and since movement always produces one or both. The body of motor information therefore is largely tactual and kinaesthetic in nature. It is a body of action information by and about movement. On the other hand visual and auditory information have initially no movement implications; they provide static information which needs no response for its fulfilment (Kephart, 1971).

The deprivation of motor experience, sensation and stimulation suffered by the cerebral palsied child

The cerebral palsied or otherwise physically handicapped child will not have normal experience of voluntary movement. His opportunities of exploring in his own way and in his own time will be restricted by physical inability. For some, experience of locomotion is totally that of being carried from place to place.

The handicapped child may also have difficulty in manipulation and his ability to learn may be impeded by lack of range and control of movement. Experiences of distance, spatial relationships, speed changes, height and depth, shape, size, weight, texture and temperature may be extremely limited. The opportunity to achieve a visual–motor–tactile match may be further restricted by persistent primitive reflexes such as the Moro and asymmetrical tonic neck reflexes.

The normal child repeats a movement for the sheer enjoyment of performing it, and through repetition it becomes a skilled movement. He finds many ways of doing the same thing; will run, hop, skip and jump when going on an errand. He is constantly on the move. In the normal infant and young child, motor learning follows certain steps. First comes the differentiation of single movement out of a global mass and the child learns how to move a part voluntarily and for a purpose. Next the child will isolate this movement from the movement of the rest of his body. Finally these single movements will be knit together into co-ordinated patterns with each separate motion synchronized with the whole (Kephart, 1971; Chaney and Kephart, 1968). The cerebral palsied child may be unable to learn in this way through movement.

By moving about the normal child becomes aware of his body's position in space and the area his body occupies. He learns to judge distance in relation to his body and from the experience of moving, falling and righting himself. The handicapped child's knowledge of spatial relationships may be impeded by lack of experience, poor awareness of body position, slow development of tactile and visual skills as well as the inaccurate body concept built up by abnormal movement patterns.

The handicapped child's curiosity may be stunted because of failures in the past or under-developed because he is unable, or unwilling through fear, to make use of his environment. Fear of movement and of new situations is often apparent in the physically handicapped child whose motor and sensory responses are unreliable. His awareness of his own body may be vague and inaccurate. He may feel insecure and unsure of what, where or who he is. He lacks the inner drive of the normal child towards independence. Indeed everything is stacked against the handicapped child's possibility of developing independence, being physically and emotionally dependent on his parents for a protracted time. Many mothers seem to have a need to protect and cosset their handicapped children to excessive degrees.

The mother–child relationship is often tense because of the mother's anxieties and because, from the earliest months, the infant's responses may have been abnormal. Sensori-motor stimulation is by its nature a two-way interaction. The mother responds naturally to a normal infant thus starting the chain of action–reaction. The cerebral palsied infant may not respond and gradually the mother (i.e. the stimulus) stops trying to obtain a response, although this infant needs more stimulation.

The play of the normal child is spontaneous and a reward in itself, whereas the handicapped child tends to be passive. He needs encouragement and 'pushing', as he attempts a task step-by-step, if he is to complete it. Finnie (1974) comments on the different responses from normal that the cerebral palsied child makes in play situations: 'his handicap prevents him from learning through play in a natural way, so unless he has help and encouragement he will not be able to learn as he plays or to reach his potential'. She continues, 'give him as wide a range of experience as you can, including the stimulation of feeling, seeing and listening and encourage him at all times to explore himself'.

If one observes and notes down all the activities undertaken by a normal 2 to 3-year-old in the space of 10 minutes and compares these observations with the activities of a cerebral palsied child of the same age, then one realizes to some extent what limited movement ability means in terms of deprivation.

Sensori-motor stimulation programmes
The object of a sensori-motor stimulation programme for a cerebral palsied child is to awaken his drive and stimulate his interest so that he will learn through interaction with his environment. Initially this involves the constant feeding in of sensory experiences and information to the child. Sensori-motor stimulation, either at home or in a treatment session, is aimed at helping the handicapped child to make more and better use of anything in his environment, such as people (the most important stimuli), objects (what they are for, how to use them) and toys (for imaginative and constructive play).

With practice the mother can become the best therapist. At first she will be the one initiating most activities but as the child begins to respond she can then use that response to build on. She is taught to make use of any activity in which the child shows interest. Parents need to learn how to observe their child and his responses and to know and understand the rationale of the therapy programme: why it is being done, what it is hoped to achieve and how to assess the child's progress. It is vital to pitch the programme at the child's developmental level; if it is too advanced he will not respond.

'As the handicapped child matures more slowly and with difficulties he needs to be given earlier and more specific stimuli than normal children. He needs more repetitive play to reinforce learning (one must avoid the child's play becoming stereotyped). He needs to be presented with more provoking situations to stimulate his reactions' (Seifert, 1973).

The value of early sensori-motor stimulation can be seen in the change in parents' attitudes. Often they become more relaxed and confident in handling their child and in playing with him. They begin to suggest and try out new ways of obtaining a response from the child. The child himself becomes more alert and responsive.

Some examples are given below of sensori-motor stimulation programmes for cerebral palsied children attending the Cheyne Centre, London.

A. was *a severely mentally retarded boy with athetoid quadriplegia*, aged 1 year 9 months. He did not show any interest in people or things and did not seem to recognize either parent. His only responses were crying when uncomfortable and primitive pleasure sounds; sometimes he showed hand regard for short periods. When laid prone his arms splayed backwards. Sitting was not possible as his attention was frequently interrupted by extensor head movements whenever he tried to do anything.

At therapy sessions a parent was always present. In addition parents were asked to note when A. was at his most responsive at home (e.g. after feeding, after morning or afternoon sleep) and use that time for the following programme.

Training visual fixation and following: mother was instructed to look at the child, smile and coo when feeding him; he was shown the spoon of food or the cup, when he fixated on these he was rewarded with food or drink. A brightly coloured noise-making toy was presented in the mid-line at a short distance away (no more than 1 m). When A. fixated on the toy it was gradually moved in widening arcs, starting with movements from mid line to side and then up and down. As following movements became established the noise-making toy was replaced by a silent one. Mother also used her own voice and face to obtain following eye movements. When the desired eye movements were achieved A. was rewarded with a smile, cuddle or cooing.

Tactile awareness: a tactile mattress was made (Fig. 14.19), the idea taken from the feeling cushion (Lear, 1974). This was covered with materials of different texture. Baby toys, which were easy to grasp and mouth and which gave a response even from a slight physical movement, were attached to the mattress by short tapes. After the daily bath A. was rubbed with a rough towel to increase

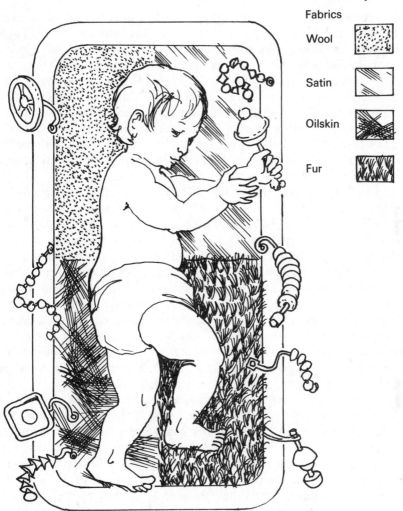

Fabrics

Wool

Satin

Oilskin

Fur

FIG. 14.19. Tactile mattress for sensori-motor stimulation.

sensory awareness and then placed on the mattress naked, except for protective pants. He was placed in different positions so that body, hands and feet came into contact with different textures. He was encouraged to hold on to toys and carry them to his mouth.

Body play: A.'s hands were brought to his mouth so that he could suck his thumb. He was encouraged to grasp and hold on to his mother's finger.

After 3 months of almost daily intensive occupational and physiotherapy, reinforced at home, A. was able to sit unaided for a short period, feeding had improved and he was generally more alert, playing for short periods with toys and being more responsive to people.

B. was *a severely physically handicapped child with athetoid quadriplegia,* aged 2 years 2 months. He was hypertonic with strong Moro response and completely 'spasmed' out of his baby buggy. He had little control of his eyes or head. However, his eyes seemed bright and he was responsive to his parents, particularly his mother, suggesting reasonable mental potential. Initially it was necessary to find positions for play in which B. did not spasm. The most useful were side-lying, supported sitting in a high-backed chair with a tray under the armpits for support of arms and a hammock for lying in. A similar routine to the one described above was employed for training visual awareness and following. At home, mobiles that moved in one plane (side to side or up and down) were hung over B.'s hammock to encourage him to watch. Clockwork toys were also used for this. B.'s family were instructed to speak to him always at his eye level so that he could fixate on the speaker.

Bringing hands together in the mid-line was practised with B. in side-lying. Even though his hands were tightly fisted, toys were strung together and draped over his hands to encourage him to look at them and to bring his hands to his mouth. As he had particular difficulty in getting his hands together in the mid-line, a circular plastic ring was sometimes used to keep his hands loosely together, so that he could hold on to an object placed between them. At home B. was helped to feel his face, hair, feet and other body parts, while language was used to describe the parts of the body and the direction of movement.

After 2 months eye control improved and concentration began on eye–hand co-ordination. Mother was instructed always to present toys and activities in the mid-line. Objects that made a noise when moved and which varied in sound and texture were dangled within arm's reach. Toys which could be knocked or pushed with a gross arm movement (e.g. skittles, wobbly toys which will not stay fallen) were also used. Mother experimented with types of objects that B. could pick up most easily (e.g. Match-Box cars), which were then used as the basis for imaginative play with a running commentary by mother. Games such as finding objects hidden under foam, in warm soapy water or hidden in a bowl of sand were useful to eliminate the grasp reflex. B. was encouraged to hold on to a bar, fixed on his tray at arm's length, and this steadied his body and facilitated voluntary grasp and feeding. As B. had no method of self-locomotion he was carried to explore parts of the house and garden with constant language to explain all that he saw and where possible he was allowed to handle household materials.

In treatment sessions B. was taught to select by eye pointing or arm movement one of two objects placed at distance from each other. The parents were then encouraged not to anticipate B.'s every need but to let the child indicate by eye movement, body movement or attempts at speech. Once he had made some effort he was rewarded with the desired object or activity. A Yes/No response was sought whenever possible.

In 5 months eye control had improved so much that it was becoming possible to make an assessment of comprehension by eye pointing.

C. was *a hyperactive boy with hemiplegia and poor eyesight* (following head injury), aged 4 years 5 months. He attended the Cheyne Centre preschool nursery from age 3 years. The programme described was to prepare him for school entrance. Aims of treatment were to improve concentration, to improve C.'s awareness of direction and space, particularly in relation to constructional tasks as a preparation for writing, and to practise visual and motor sequencing in preparation for reading.

C. had specific difficulty in copying any constructional task as his field of vision was limited. Initially directions were carried out in relation to C.'s own body. Concepts of up/down, top/bottom, left/right were reinforced with appropriate body movements.

Constructional tasks started with match-sticks on a black background as C.'s visual handicap was such that he could only attend to a small area of the visual field at one time. Emphasis was placed on copying simple patterns using spatial words to reinforce the task. Next, longer coloured sticks were used; copying patterns with these involved remembering some of the visual sequence as C. was unable to see all the pattern with one glance. He was encouraged to feel the pattern while looking at it. Sets of small cars were also used for sequencing as the child enjoyed these. Sequences were copied by C. using an identical set of cars.

Simple prewriting exercises using a felt tip pen followed. C. was encouraged to look carefully as he used the pen, but the materials were so structured as to be within his visual capability.

C. attended for 3 months' therapy. Now he attends a school for partially sighted children, is reading and beginning to write.

Group treatment

The nursery group at the Cheyne Centre consists of up to twelve cerebral palsied children of normal or mildly retarded intelligence, whose mental ages range from $2\frac{1}{2}$–5 years. These children attend daily and their weekly programme (Table 14.8) consists of individual and group treatment. Priorities in treatment are worked out at regular meetings of staff working in the nursery, i.e. house-mother and occupational, speech and physiotherapists. Everyday activities such as toiletting, dressing, feeding, and mobility and preschool activities are incorporated into the programme.

Two groups sessions weekly are conducted by the occupational therapist and last 1 hour. In one session the children sit round a table and in the other they are 'free-sitting' on the floor or on a circle of chairs. When sitting on chairs in a circle, those unable to sit alone are helped to maintain sitting balance by holding the bars of a ladder-backed chair, which may be weighted down with sandbags. The child sits facing the back of this chair which thus provides a secure and stable grab rail. Even severely physically handicapped children can learn to gain some control of sitting if they stabilize themselves in this way.

The aims of the free-sitting group are symmetry in sitting, maintenance of sitting balance when using hands freely, body awareness, tactile and olfactory awareness.

An example is given of a typical group session. Initially, to evoke a vocal response on command each child answers his own name with 'I am here' or other vocal response for those without speech.

TABLE 14.8. Example of a nursery programme

	Monday	Tuesday	Wednesday	Thursday	Friday
9.30 to 10.30	Preschool work (OT) or individual physio/ speech therapy for some children.	Free play —————— each morning ——————			
10.30 to 11.30	Table group (OT) concentrating on hand function	Free play or individual treatment	Free sitting group (OT as described in text)	Gross motor group, physiotherapy, concentrating on pulling to standing, walking, crawling etc.	Swimming, including undressing/dressing practice or painting/ water play.
11.30 to 12.00	—————— toiletting and preparation for lunch ——————				
12.00 to 13.00	— — — — — Lunch time — — — — —				
13.00 to 14.00	—————— Rest time ——————				
14.00 to 15.00	Standing and walking group (PT & OT) *Some* children attend	Language group (Speech therapy)	Singing or band	Language group (Speech therapy)	Standing and walking group. (PT & OT)
15.00 to 15.45	—————— Tea and getting ready to go home ——————				

The children are reminded how to sit with feet flat on the floor, buttocks back, feet and knees together. Many of the techniques used are taken from Peto's conductive education system (Cotton, 1975) and instructions are reinforced with rhythmical intention aimed to stimulate body and spatial awareness (p. 311). Concepts of up, down, beside, on top of and so on are emphasized with body movements. Gross arm movements are practised with action songs and other rhymes are used to improve trunk control and balance in sitting. Attention is drawn to different parts of the body with more action songs.

Each child is handed a coloured ring when he names the colour correctly or selects a colour named (colour discrimination). The rings are used to practise the movements involved in dressing ('I put my arms into my ring'; 'I put my ring on top of my head'). To stimulate bilateral visuo-motor activity a rope is passed from child to child and each is requested to thread his ring on to it.

The last 10 minutes is used for either feeling, tasting and smelling or for playing tactile games. Household supplies such as flour, cornflakes, sugar, coffee, spaghetti and currants are placed on saucers. Each child is encouraged to feel, taste and smell the foodstuffs whilst appropriate language is used to describe taste, colour, smell, texture and use of items. In one tactile game a bag of small bricks, covered with different textures, is passed around. Younger children are asked to 'find me one that feels just like this' and older children are asked to pick out a certain number of bricks depending on the level of development of their concept of numbers. Descriptive words are used for reinforcement. An animal's face with cut-outs lined with matching textures is used as a focal point; each child takes a turn to fit his bricks into the cut-outs of appropriate texture. The group session finishes with a song.

J. MULHALL EGAN

References

Aetiology and Prevention

ARMSTRONG D. and NORMAN M.G. (1974) Periventricular leucomalacia in neonates. Complications and sequelae. *Archives of Disease in Childhood*, **49**, 367.

BANKER B.Q. and LARROCHE J.-C. (1962) Periventricular leukomalacia of infancy. A form of neonatal anoxic encephalopathy. *Archives of Neurology*, **7**, 386.

BAX M. (1964) Terminology and classification of cerebral palsy. *Developmental Medicine and Child Neurology*, **6**, 295.

BICKERSTAFF E.R. (1964) Aetiology of acute hemiplegia in childhood. *British Medical Journal*, **2**, 82.

BRAND M.M. and BIGNAMI A. (1969) The effects of chronic hypoxia on the neonatal and infantile brain. A neuropathological study of five premature infants with the respiratory distress syndrome treated by prolonged artificial ventilation. *Brain*, **92**, 233.

BRANDT S. (1962) Causes and pathogenic mechanisms of acute hemiplegia in childbood. In *Acute Hemiplegia in Childhood*. eds. Bax M. and Mitchell R. *Little Club Clinics in Developmental Medicine, No. 6*. London: Heinemann.

CHILDS B. and EVANS P.R. (1954) Birth weights of children with cerebral palsy. *Lancet*, **i**, 642.

CHRISTENSEN E. and MELCHIOR J. (1967) *Cerebral Palsy. A clinical and neuropathological study. Clinics in Developmental Medicine, No. 25*. London: Heinemann.

CHURCHILL J.A. and COLFELT R.H. (1963) Etiologic factors in athetotic cerebral palsy. *Archives of Neurology*, **9**, 400.

CHURCHILL J.A., MASLAND R.S., NAYLOR A.A. and ASHWORTH M.R. (1974) The etiology of cerebral palsy in pre-term infants. *Developmental Medicine and Child Neurology*, **16**, 143.

DAVIES P.A. and TIZARD J.P.M. (1975) Very low birthweight and subsequent neurological defect (with special reference to spastic diplegia). *Developmental Medicine and Child Neurology*, **17**, 3.

DESMONTS G. and COUVREUR J. (1974) Congenital toxoplasmosis. A prospective study of 378 pregnancies. *New England Journal of Medicine*, **290**, 1110.

DRILLIEN C.M. (1972) Aetiology and outcome in low-birthweight infants. *Developmental Medicine and Child Neurology*, **14**, 563.

DRILLIEN C.M., INGRAM T.T.S. and RUSSELL E.M. (1962) Comparative aetiological studies of congenital diplegia in Scotland. *Archives of Disease in Childhood*, **37**, 282.

DRILLIEN C.M., INGRAM T.T.S. and RUSSELL E.M. (1964) Further studies of the causes of diplegia in childhood. *Developmental Medicine and Child Neurology*, **6**, 241.

EVANS P.R. (1948) Antecedents of infantile cerebral palsy. *Archives of Disease in Childhood*, **23**, 213.

FITZHARDINGE P.M., PAPE K., ARSTIKAITIS, M., BOYLE M., ASHBY S., ROWLEY A., NETLEY C. and SWYER, P.R. (1976) Mechanical ventilation of infants of less than 1501 gm birth weight: Health, growth, and neurological sequelae. *Journal of Pediatrics*, **88**, 531.

GAMACHE F.W. and MYERS R.E. (1975) Effects of hypotension on rhesus monkeys. *Archives of Neurology*, **32**, 374.

GARTNER L.M., SNYDER R.N., CHABON R.S. and BERNSTEIN J. (1970) Kernicterus: High incidence in premature infants with low serum bilirubin concentrations. *Pediatrics*, **45**, 906.

GERRARD J. (1952) Kernicterus. *Brain*, **75**, 526.

GRIFFITHS M. (1967) Cerebral palsy in multiple pregnancy. *Developmental Medicine and Child Neurology*, **9**, 713.

GRIFFITHS M.I. and BARRETT N.M. (1967) Cerebral palsy in Birmingham. *Developmental Medicine and Child Neurology*, **9**, 33.

GRUNNET M.L., CURLESS R.G., BRAY P.F. and JUNG A.L. (1974) Brain changes in newborns from an intensive care unit. *Developmental Medicine and Child Neurology*, **16**, 320.

GUSTAVSON K-H., HAGBERG B. and SANNER G. (1969) Identical syndromes of cerebral palsy in the same family. *Acta Paediatrica Scandinavica*, **58**, 330.

HAGBERG B., HAGBERG G. and OLOW I. (1975a) The changing panorama of cerebral palsy in Sweden 1954–1970. I. Analysis of the general changes. *Acta Paediatrica Scandinavica*, **64**, 187.

HAGBERG B., HAGBERG G. and OLOW I. (1975b) The changing panorama of cerebral palsy in Sweden 1954–1970. II. Analysis of the various syndromes. *Acta Paediatrica Scandinavica*, **64**, 193.

HAGBERG G., HAGBERG B. and OLOW I. (1976) The changing panorama of cerebral palsy in Sweden 1954–1970. III. The importance of fetal deprivation of supply. *Acta Paediatrica Scandinavica*, **65**, 403.

HEMSATH F.A. (1934) Birth injury of the occipital bone with a report of thirty-two cases. *American Journal of Obstetrics and Gynecology*, **27**, 194.

ILLINGWORTH R.S. and WOODS G.E. (1960) The incidence of twins in cerebral palsy and mental retardation. *Archives of Disease in Childhood*, **35**, 333.

INGRAM T.T.S. (1964) *Paediatric Aspects of Cerebral Palsy*. Edinburgh: Livingstone.

ISLER W. (1971) *Acute Hemiplegias and Hemisyndromes in Childhood. Clinics in Developmental Medicine Nos. 41/42*. London: Heinemann.

JACOBI G., v. LOEWENICH V., EMRICH R., RITZ A. and JANSSEN W. (1974) Results of post mortem cerebral contrast studies in prematures and newborns. *Journal of Perinatal Medicine*, **2**, 135.

KOROBKIN R. (1975) The relationship between head circumference and the development of communicating hydrocephalus in infants following intraventricular haemorrhage. *Pediatrics*, **56**, 74.

LILIENFELD A.M., PASAMANICK B. and ROGERS M. (1955) Relationship between pregnancy experience and the development of certain neuropsychiatric disorders in childhood. *American Journal of Public Health*, **44**, 637.

LITTLE W.J. (1862) On the influence of abnormal parturition, difficult labours, premature birth and asphyxia neonatorum, on the mental and physical condition of the child, especially in relation to deformities. *Obstetrical Transactions*, **3**, 293.

MACHIN G.A. (1975) A perinatal mortality survey in South-east London, 1970–73: The pathological findings in 726 necropsies. *Journal of Clinical Pathology*, **28**, 428.

MARRIAGE K.J. and DAVIES P.A. (1977) Neurological sequelae in children surviving mechanical ventilation in the neonatal period. *Archives of Disease in Childhood*, **52**, 176.

MYERS R.E. (1975) Four patterns of perinatal brain damage and their conditions of occurrence in primates. *Advances in Neurology*, **10**, 223.

SCHNEIDER H., SCHACHINGER H. and DICHT R. (1975) Telencephalic leucoencephalopathy in premature infants dying after prolonged artificial respiration. Report on 6 cases. *Neuropädiatrie*, **6**, 347.

SCOTT H. (1976) Outcome of very severe birth asphyxia. *Archives of Disease in Childhood*, **51**, 712.

SIMMONS M.A., ADCOCK E.W., BARD H. and BATTAGLIA F.C. (1974) Hypernatremia and intracranial haemorrhage in neonates. *New England Journal of Medicine*, **291**, 6.

SMITH J.F., REYNOLDS E.O.R. and TAGHIZADEH A. (1974) Brain maturation and damage in infants dying from chronic pulmonary insufficiency in the post-neonatal period. *Archives of Disease in Childhood*, **49**, 359.

STEINER H. and NELIGAN G. (1975) Perinatal cardiac arrest. Quality of the survivors. *Archives of Disease in Childhood*, **50**, 696.

SYMONDS E.M. (1976) The evaluation of fetal well-being in pregnancy and labour. In *Recent Advances in Paediatrics*, *5*, ed. Hull D. Edinburgh: Churchill Livingstone,

TERPLAN K.L. (1967) Histopathologic brain changes in 1152 cases of the perinatal and early infancy period. *Biology of the Neonate*, **11**, 348.

WIGGLESWORTH J.S., KEITH I.H., GIRLING D.J. and SLADE S.A. (1976) Hyaline membrane disease, alkali and intraventricular haemorrhage. *Archives of Disease in Childhood*, **51**, 755.

WYNN M. and WYNN A. (1976) *Prevention of Handicap of Perinatal Origin. An introduction to French policy and legislation*. London: Foundation for Education and Research in Child Bearing.

Classification
INGRAM T.T.S. (1964) Definition and classification of cerebral palsy. In *Paediatric Aspects of Cerebral Palsy*. Edinburgh: Livingstone.

HAGBERG B., SCANNER G. and STEEN M. (1972) The dysequilibrium syndrome in cerebral palsy. *Acta Paediatrica Scandinavica, Supplement* **226**.

Physical Aspects
ANDRÉ-THOMAS S. and SAINT-ANNE DARGASSIES (1952) *Études Neurologiques sur le Nouveau-Né et le Jeune Nourisson*, p. 434. Paris: Masson et Cie.

ANDRÉ-THOMAS S., CHESNI Y. and SAINT-ANNE DARGASSIES (1960) *The Neurological Examination of the Infant. Little Club Clinics No. 1*, p. 50. London: Heinemann.

GAMPER E. (1925/6) Bau und Leistungen eines menschlichen Mittelhirnwesens (Arhinencephalie mit Encephalocele) zugleich ein Beitrag zur Teratologie und Fasersystematik. *Zentralblatt für die geoamte Neurologie und Psychiatrie*, **102**, 154; **104**, 49.

HAGBERG B., HAGBERG G. and OLOW I. (1975) The changing panorama of cerebral palsy in Sweden 1954–1970. *Acta Paediatrica Scandinavica*, **64**, 187.

LITTLE CLUB (1959) Memorandum. Terminology and classification of cerebral palsy. *Cerebral Palsy Bulletin*, **2**, 27.

LUNDBERG A. and PHILLIPS G.C. (1973) T. Graham Brown's film on locomotion in the decerebrate cat. *Journal of Physiology (London)*, **231**, 90.

MARTIN J. PURDON (1967) *The Basal Ganglia and Posture*, pp. xii, 152. London: Pitmans.

Associated Disorders

DOUGLAS A.A. (1961) Ophthalmological aspects. In *Cerebral Palsy in Childhood and Adolescence*, ed. Henderson J.L. Edinburgh: Livingstone.

FISCH L. (1957) Hearing impairment and cerebral palsy. *Speech*, **21**, 43.

HOLT K.S. and REYNELL J.K. (1967) *Assessment of Cerebral Palsy* Vol. II. London: Lloyd-Luke.

MONFRAIX C., TARDIEU G. and TARDIEU C. (1961a) Disturbances of manual perception in children with cerebral palsy. *Cerebral Palsy Bulletin*, **3**, 544.

MONFRAIX C. and TARDIEU G. (1961b) Development of manual perception in children with cerebral palsy. *Cerebral Palsy Bulletin*, **3**, 553.

WILSON S.A.K. (1908) A contribution to the study of apraxia with a review of the literature. *Brain*, **31**, 164.

Physical Management

BOBATH B. (1967) The very early treatment of cerebral palsy, *Developmental Medicine and Child Neurology*, **9**, 373.

BOBATH K. and BOBATH B. (1964) The facilitation of normal postural reactions and movements in the treatment of cerebral palsy. *Physiotherapy*, **50**, 246.

COTTON E. (1970) Integration of treatment and education in cerebral palsy. *Physiotherapy*, **56**, 143.

COTTON E. (1975) *Conductive Education and Cerebral Palsy*. London: Spastics Society

DOMAN G. (1974) *What to do About your Brain-injured Child*. London: Cape.

FAY T. (1946) Observations on the rehabilitation of movements in cerebral palsied children. *West Virginia Medical Journal*, **42**, 77.

FINNIE N.R. (1974) *Handling the Young Cerebral Palsied Child at Home*, 2nd Ed. London: Heinemann.

HOLT K.S., DARCUS H. and BRAND H.L. (1972) Children's wheelchair clinic. *British Medical Journal*, **4**, 651.

JONES R.B. (1975) The Vojta method of treating cerebral palsy. *Physiotherapy*, **61**, 112.

KNOTT M. and VOSS D.E. (1956) *Pro-prioceptive Neuromuscular Facilitation*. New York: Hoeber and Harper.

LEVITT S. (1966) P.N.F. techniques in cerebral palsy. *Physiotherapy* **52**, 46.

LEVITT, S. (1969) Physiotherapy. In *Cerebral Palsy and the Young Child*. ed. Blencowe S.M. Edinburgh: Churchill Livingstone.

LEVITT S. (1977) *Treatment of Cerebral Palsy and Motor Delay*. Oxford: Blackwell Scientific Publications.

MANNING J. (1972) Facilitation of movement: the Bobath approach *Physiotherapy*, **58**, 403.

SCRUTTON D. and GILBERTSON M. (1975) *Physiotherapy in Paediatric Practice*. London: Butterworth.

Sensori-Motor Stimulation

CARPENTER G. (1975) Mother's face and the newborn. In *Child Alive*, ed. Lewin R. London: Temple Smith.

CHANEY C.M. and KEPHART N.C. (1968) *Motoric Aids to Perceptual Training*. Columbus, Ohio: Charles E. Merrill.

COTTON E. (1975) *Conductive Education and Cerebral Palsy*. London: Spastics Society.

FINNIE N. (1974) *Handling the Young Cerebral Palsied Child at Home*, 2nd Ed. London: Heinemann.

GESELL A. (1950) *The First Five Years of Life*. London: Methuen.

GESELL A., ILG F.L. and BULLIS G.E. (1941) *Vision: Its Development in Infant and Young Child*. New York: Hoeber.

KEPHART N.C. (1971) *The Slow Learner in the Classroom*, 2nd Ed. Columbus, Ohio: Charles E. Merrill.

*LEAR R.(1974) *Do It Yourself*. London: Noah's Ark Publication.

PIAGET J. and INHELDER B. (1969) *The Psychology of the Child.* London: Routledge and Kegan Paul.

SEIFERT A. (1973) Sensory motor stimulation for the young handicapped child. *Occupational Therapy*, **36**, 559.

WOODWARD W.M. (1970) Cognitive processes, Piaget's approach. In *The Psychological Assessment of Mental and Physical Handicap*, ed. Mittler P. London: Methuen.

Further Reading

Physical Aspects

BROWN J.K., INGRAM T.T.S., SHANKS R.A., SHAW J.F. and STARK G. (1973) Disorders of the central nervous system in *Textbook of Paediatrics*, eds. Forfar J.O. and Arneil G.A Edinburgh: Churchill Livingstone.

DENNY-BROWN D. (1962) *The Basal Ganglia and their Relation to Disorders of Movement*, p. 144. London: Oxford University Press.

GORDON N.S. (1976) *Pediatric Neurology for the Clinician. Clinics in Developmental Medicine Nos. 59/60.* London: Heinemann.

MONNIER M. (1970) *Functions of the Nervous System*, Vol. 2, pp. xviii, 658 Amsterdam: Elsevier Publishing Company.

PEIPER A. (1963) *Cerebral Function in Infancy & Childhood.* (Translated Nagles B. and Nagles H.) ed. Wortis J. New York: New York Consultant's Bureau.

Associated Disorders

ABERCROMBIE M.L.J., GARDINER P.A., HANSEN E., JONKHEERE J., LINDON R.L., SOLOMON G. and TYSON M. (1964). *Perceptual and Motor Skills, Monograph Supplement* **3**, V18, 561.

BEARD R. (1969) *An Outline of Piaget's Developmental Psychology.* London: Routledge and Kegan Paul.

BRAIN W.R. (1955) Aphasia, apraxia and agnosia. In *Kinnier Wilson's Neurology*, ed. Bruce A.N. 2nd Ed., Vol. 3, London: Butterworth.

GARDINER P., MAC KEITH R.C. and SMITH V. (1969) *Aspects of Developmental and Paediatric Ophthalmology. Clinics in Developmental Medicine, No. 32.* London: Heinemann.

SMITH V.H., ed. (1963) *Visual Disorders and Cerebral Palsy. Clinics in Developmental Medicine, No. 9.* London: Heinemann.

WILLIAMS M. (1970) *Brain Damage and the Mind.* Harmondsworth, Middlesex: Penguin Books.

Orthopaedic Aspects

SAMILSON R.L. ed. (1975) *Orthopaedic Aspects of Cerebral Palsy. Clinics in Developmental Medicine Nos. 52/53.* London: Heinemann.

Physical Management

ELLIS E. (1967) *The Physical Management of Developmental Disorders. Clinics in Developmental Medicine, No. 26.* London: Heinemann.

HOLT K.S. ed. (1975) *Movement and Child Development. Clinics in Developmental Medicine, No. 55.* London: Heinemann.

Sensori-motor Stimulation

BARTRAM G.E. (1973) *Not Yet Five*, 2nd Ed. London: E.S.A.

BRERETON B. LE G. and SATTLER J. (1975) Cerebral Palsy: Basic Abilities: A plan for training the pre-school child. 2nd. Ed. Sydney: Spastic Centre for New South Wales.

†HARKNESS C. and SANDYS H. (1972), *Teaching a Handicapped Child to Feed.* London: Friends of the Centre for Spastic Children.

*HAYES B. (1975) *Encouraging Language Development.* London: Noah's Ark Publication.

*JAFFE D. (1975) *Design and Make Magnetic Board Toys.* London: Noah's Ark Publication,

*KNOWLES S.E. and MOGFORD K. (1975) *Toys for Children with Hearing, Speech and Language Difficulties*. London: Noah's Ark Publication.

MONFRAIX C., TARDIEU G. and TARDIEU C. (1961) Disturbances of manual perception in children with cerebral palsy, *Cerebral Palsy Bulletin*, **3**, 544.

MONTESSORI M. (1972) *Dr Montessori's Own Handbook*. New York: Schoken Books.

†MOORE G. (1973) *Teaching a Handicapped Child to Dress*. London: Friends of the Centre for Spastic Children.

*NEWSON E. (1973) *Why Toys?* London: Noah's Ark Publication.

*RICHARDSON A. and WISBEACH A. (1976) *I Can Use My Hands*. London: Noah's Ark Publication.

*TOY LIBRARIES ASSOCIATION (1974) *ABC of Toys*. London: Noah's Ark Publication.

* Available from Toy Libraries Association, Sunley House, Gunthorpe Street, London E1 7RW.

† Available from 63 Cheyne Walk, London SW3 5NA.

Appendix 14.1

A Screening Scheme
for the Initial Assessment of Perceptual-motor Function

In the preschool child assessment of perceptual motor function is complex. Standardized assessments are available from 4 years of age upwards but these can take more than an hour to administer, which is far beyond the time available to one child in a clinic or screening visit. Early identification of perceptual motor dysfunction is desirable so that, where possible, treatment can be started before school entrance. These factors have highlighted the need for a brief 'pre-assessment' (Table A14.1) which could indicate whether or not a more comprehensive assessment by a psychologist and/or occupational therapist is required.

The equipment is compact and readily available except for the formboards, which can usually be made up in workshops or occupation centres for the disabled or by local joiners. A scale diagram is given for both the 3-shape and 12-shape boards (Figs. A14.1 & A14.2).

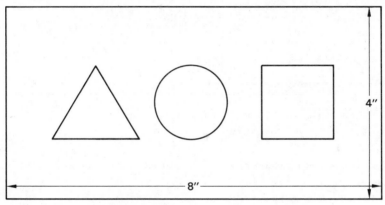

Instructions for making formboards
1. Cut two rectangles of $\frac{1}{4}''$ plywood to measurements given.
2. Cut shapes from one piece of plywood.
3. Join two rectangles of plywood with glue and panel pins.
4. Smooth edges of shapes so they fit into holes with ease.

Fig. A14.1. Scale diagram of three-shape formboard.

PRAXIS AND BILATERAL INTEGRATION

Equipment: none.

Child (C) and examiner (E) sit facing each other. E asks C to perform the task, or demonstrates the activity for him to copy.

E looks for hesitation, slowness or inability to perform the activity inconsistent with any motor disability C may have; disregard of one side of the body, and tendency to avoid crossing the mid-line.

VISUAL AND SPATIAL DISCRIMINATION

Equipment: Picture books (e.g. Ladybird); pairs of simple pictures, e.g. houses, babies, dogs; 3 and 12-shape formboards; ring pile up toy; $12 \times 1''$ cubes; piece of card (A4 size) to act as screen.

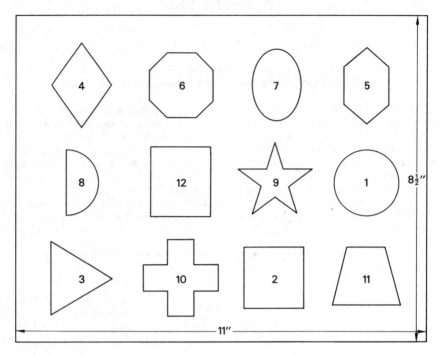

Fig. A14.2. Scale diagram of twelve-shape formboard.

Fine visual discrimination
E encourages C to look at pictures in the book, talks about the details and asks C to show them.

Recognition of form
C seated at table, E facing him.
(1) Three to four pictures are placed in front of C who is asked to give E the one which is like the picture held up by E for him to see.
(2) Three-shape formboard is placed in front of C with shapes opposite the appropriate holes. C is asked to put shapes into the holes where they belong.
(3) Empty twelve-shape formboard is placed in front of C. Shapes are presented to C in order of increasing difficulty for him to fit into appropriate holes (as given in Fig. A14.2).

   In these tests E looks for overdependence on trial and error inappropriate for age, forcing of shapes into incorrect holes, failure to turn shapes in the hand and fitting shapes on one side of the board only.

Recognition of size
C seated at table, E facing him.
   For 3 year level E selects three rings from pile up toy; largest, smallest and middle one. These and the pole of the toy are placed in front of C, who is asked to place the biggest one, middle-sized one and smallest one on the pole in that order. At 4 and 5 years, four and six rings are graded respectively.
   E observes if C depends on a trial and error approach inappropriate for age.

Constructional skills with cubes
C seated at table, E facing him.
   According to C's age, E either demonstrates the construction or builds a model behind the screen.

TABLE A14.1 Developmental norms which may be used as indicators of a preschool child's perceptual motor abilities.

Age in years	Praxis and bilateral integration	Visual and spatial discrimination	Tactile and proprioceptive discrimination	Eye–motor control
2	Shows hair, nose, eyes, mouth, hand, foot. Imitates raising arms above head, clapping hands, revolving hands round each other.	Recognizes fine details in pictures. Completes three-shape formboard.		With pencil imitates vertical line and sometimes V.
2½		Recognizes minute details in pictures. Matches simple pictures. Aligns cubes to form train.	Indicates which object placed in hand; of cube, marble, pencil, cotton reel, match box.	Imitates horizontal line, circle and sometimes V and T.
3	Shows eyebrows, cheeks, chin, arms and legs.	Matches three to four shapes of twelve-shape formboard. Grades three rings in order of size.	Identifies which finger touched by showing on own hand.	Copies circle, V, H, T. Imitates cross.
3½	Imitates closing fist and wiggling thumb, right and left hands.	Builds bridge of three cubes from model.		
4	Imitates spreading fingers and bringing thumb into opposition, right and left hands. Shows common joints.	Matches eight shapes. Grades four rings in order of size. Builds three steps with six cubes after demonstration	Recognizes five to seven of twelve shapes placed in hand. Indicates where touched, one or two stimuli.	Copies cross, V, H, T, O.
5	Counts fingers of one hand with index finger of other. Raises right and left hand on request.	Matches ten shapes. Grades six rings in order of size. Builds three steps with six cubes from model.	Recognizes seven to eight of twelve shapes placed in hand.	Copies square, triangle, V, H, T, O, X, L, A, C, U, Y.

E observes C's approach to the task, the speed and accuracy of construction, whether or not he recognizes errors and the effectiveness of his corrective measures.

TACTILE AND PROPRIOCEPTIVE DISCRIMINATION
Equipment: 2 sets of objects (cube, marble, pencil, cotton reel, matchbox); 12-shape formboard; card screen.

Stereognosis
C sits at table with one hand and then the other placed palm upwards on the table, E sits beside him holding the screen to obscure C's view of his own hand.

According to age level either one set of objects or the empty formboard is placed in front of C, who is asked to point to which of the objects or shapes has been placed in his hidden hand. Both hands are tested.

Identification of tactile stimuli
(1) Finger agnosia. C sits at table with hand behind screen. E sits beside C and touches fingers of his hand in random order. After each finger has been touched the screen is removed and C asked to point to the finger touched. Both hands are tested.
(2) Identification of double tactile stimuli. E stands behind C and touches him in two places simultaneously on available skin (e.g. hands, forearms, sides of face), on right or left or both sides of the body. C is asked to point to where he has been touched.

The types of error made are noted; does C ignore any touch on one side of the body or when touched on both sides does he only show one place?

EYE–MOTOR CONTROL

Equipment: 2 pencils; paper; sample cards of shapes and letters.

C seated at table, E facing him. Paper is placed in front of C with pencil in the middle, pointing away from him. C is asked to imitate (after demonstration) or copy (from diagram) shapes and letters appropriate to age level.

E notes which hand is used to hold pencil, type of grasp and if the pencil is controlled effectively to produce a recognizable facsimile.

GENERAL OBSERVATIONS

The following questions should be borne in mind throughout the screening. If responses are inappropriate for C's age these points may be further indicators of perceptual-motor dysfunction.

Is attention span appropriate for age? Is C easily distracted?

Is handedness well defined or inconsistent?

Is hand function unduly clumsy for age?

How does C react to tasks? Does he withdraw, refuse to attempt the task or try to divert E's attention from it?

Does C recognize when he has made a mistake and what is his emotional reaction to failure?

How does C position his head to look at objects? Is it obvious that eye and hand are not in co-ordination?

Does C move around the room freely, avoiding obstacles, seating himself in a chair or finding a toy under the table?

Children with perceptual-motor dysfunction are likely to present a scatter of problems under each of the headings above. Single problems could be insignificant but a pattern of responses below the child's mental age level merits further investigation.

References

AYRES A.J. (1973) *Southern California Sensory Integration Tests Manual*. Los Angeles: Western Psychological Services.
GESELL A., ed. (1950) *The First Five Years of Life*. London: Methuen.

MONFRAIX C., TARDIEU G. and TARDIEU C. (1961) Disturbance of manual perception in children with cerebral palsy. *Cerebral Palsy Bulletin*, **3**, 544.

SHERIDAN M.D. (1968) *The Developmental Progress of Infants and Young Children*, 2nd Ed. London: Her Majesty's Stationery Office.

E. M. FAIRGRIEVE

CHAPTER 15

Minor Abnormal Neurological Signs in the First Two Years of Life

Brain damage or dysfunction is not necessarily manifest in overt mental retardation or neurological defect. Less obvious developmental delay and signs of minor neurological impairment are seen frequently in follow-up clinics for infants considered to be at high risk on account of known adverse factors operating in the pre-, peri- or immediate postnatal periods and also, though less often, in infants and young children attending other clinics for routine development screening.

The prognostic significance of minor abnormal neurological signs requires further long-term study but the frequency with which such signs are associated with problems of maternal caretaking and of early development and behaviour is not in doubt. Demonstration of these signs assists in the management of concurrent problems and, since present evidence suggests that children showing these signs may be at increased risk of educational and behavioural problems in the early school years (Chapter 16), there is a case for continued supervision of such children after the immediate problems have resolved. In addition, recognition of the transient or continuing minimal nature of the abnormal signs in the majority of infants exhibiting these will avoid the assumption that the infant is developing cerebral palsy and the unnecessary distress that is caused to parents by misdiagnosis.

Most infants who are found to have minor abnormal neurological signs present either in the early months of life with the irritable baby syndrome or later with developmental delay and/or other problems of behaviour such as sleeplessness, overactivity and marked temper.

Irritable Baby Syndrome

Apart from systemic disease (e.g. infection or congenital malformation), irritability, constant crying and feeding difficulties may be due to maternal inexperience and mismanagement. Too small teat hole is the commonest single cause of slow feeding, poor weight gain and crying due to hunger and to colic from air-swallowing. However, such symptoms are also commonly associated with minor neurological abnormality and all irritable infants should be examined with this in mind.

The combination of minor abnormal neurological signs and severe problems of behaviour and management in the early months of life in the absence of systemic disease or obvious maternal mishandling constitutes the irritable baby syndrome. It is an early manifestation of the dystonic syndrome (p. 343) in which problems of behaviour and management predominate.

There is frequently a history of some adverse factor in the perinatal period, most commonly low birth-weight or evidence of hypoxic or traumatic birth injury. The infant may have exhibited transient abnormal neurological signs in the newborn nursery (Chapter 3), in which case there is usually a quiescent period with definite minor abnormal signs reappearing at 4–8 weeks. Alternatively the abnormal signs may be noted for the first time at that age. The appearance or reappearance of these signs is associated with increasing difficulties of management.

The mother describes the baby as constantly crying, sleepless ('the slightest sound wakes him'), jumpy and easily startled by noise or change of posture. If asked to show exactly what the baby does when disturbed the mother will often demonstrate a typical startle response. A variety of feeding difficulties are described; slow sucking or frequent cessation of sucking, excessive wind, frequent small vomits, not settling to sleep after feeds. Difficulties of handling include dislike of the bath, the baby described as arching his back or throwing himself backwards in extension and 'going stiff' when mother attempts to place him in the water, and similar problems in the caretaking activities of undressing, dressing and nappy changing. The mother who has had other normal infants may comment that this one 'feels different', is 'stiff' or 'tense' and does not 'cuddle' in the same way as her other babies.

Home based remedies for the problems may well have been tried; changing feeds to other milks, adding cereals in the belief that crying denotes hunger, giving gripe-water and other anti-colic preparations and abandoning the daily bath. When medical advice is sought the anti-cholinergic preparation dicyclomine hydrochloride (Merbentyl®) is often prescribed and it is not uncommon to find irritable babies who are receiving this drug before each feed, with little relief of symptoms. Merbentyl® is specific for the condition known as evening colic, in which a spectrum of symptoms occurs, ranging from mild irritability and failure to settle after the early evening feed to intermittent attacks of screaming with drawing up of the legs, repeated for several hours, the screaming continuing even when the infant is picked up. The attacks usually occur in the evenings between 18.00 and 20.00 hours, the baby being perfectly good at other times during the day. If irritability and crying is restricted to certain periods of the day and if the symptoms respond dramatically to Merbentyl® the diagnosis of evening colic can be made with some confidence. The irritable baby syndrome does not respond to this drug and its use should not be continued beyond a few days' trial period.

Observation reveals a hyper-alert, overactive infant, who, when laid supine, rolls vigorously from side-to-side with jerky unco-ordinated movements of limbs appropriate to a younger age. Typically this is most obvious when the infant is first unwrapped from his shawl. Spontaneous ATNR posture, prolonged or fixed (p. 136) is seen frequently. This response is also easily elicited passively. When the infant is being laid down and again when being lifted up a brisk Moro reaction may be elicited. In prone the infant may exhibit vigorous crawling movements to the extent that with slight pressure on the soles of the feet he 'crawls' up the couch.

When held in vertical suspension the infant typically assumes the dystonic posture (p. 147). Primitive walking is easily elicited and exaggerated and may be prolonged for age. Tendon reflexes are usually brisk and clonus may be demonstrated, especially jaw clonus which may be spontaneous.

In moderate or severe cases of the irritable baby syndrome the mother is very likely to show signs of stress. The irritable, constantly crying infant who feeds poorly, goes into stiff, extended (and to the mother 'rejecting') postures when handled or when attempts are made to lift and comfort him and never sleeps for long by day or by night is a source of considerable anxiety to parents, quite apart from the physical exhaustion that comes from broken nights and wearisome days.

The demonstration of the abnormal neurological signs described gives the doctor confidence in reassurance to mother that the baby's behaviour is in no way her 'fault', that his tendency to go into extension when handled is an automatic reflex response and does not mean that she is being rejected and that other caretakers would have the same problems as she is having.

Feeding is facilitated if the infant is positioned in semi-upright sitting with the head slightly flexed forwards. He may sleep more contentedly and be less easily startled if placed prone or firmly swaddled. When the mother shows signs of excessive strain we do not hesitate to sedate the infant with chloral (e.g. triclofos sodium, 250–500 mg, two to four times daily before feeds).

In most cases behaviour improves spontaneously by 12–16 weeks and the abnormal neurological signs resolve. In some the irritability resolves, but dystonic signs, developmental delay and other problems of behaviour persist. In others, persistence of irritability is due to maternal anxiety and it may be necessary to break what has become a vicious circle by arranging a period of separation of mother and infant, at least for a part of the day, by evoking the aid of granny or by admission to a day nursery for a few weeks. This will give mother a rest and confirm that with calm handling the infant does or does not behave calmly. In a small proportion of cases the irritable baby syndrome is the first indication of a developing cerebral palsy.

The constantly crying infant, whatever the cause, is at particular risk of baby battering (Chapter 20). The mother of any infant exhibiting this sort of behaviour should be closely and sympathetically questioned about the effect on herself and her husband. It can be put to the mother that the temptation to batter a crying infant into silence is an understandable and not uncommon reaction of normal parents under excessive strain. Immediate steps should be taken to relieve strain, if necessary by hospital admission, if there appears to be any danger to the infant. Even in the absence of immediate dangers of this sort it is reasonable to suppose that a normal loving mother–infant interaction may be damaged by the traumatic effects of living with an excessively irritable baby during the first few months of his life (Shaw, 1977).

Minor Abnormal Neurological Signs Presenting Later

Unless neurological status is being systematically monitored in follow-up studies it is unlikely that minor abnormal neurological presentations will come to light in the absence of associated problems.

That infants with abnormal signs are more likely to have developmental problems than those without was demonstrated in a study of infants of very low birth-weight (Drillien, 1972). Fifty-four per cent of low birth-weight infants with these minor signs showed significant developmental delay at 1 year compared with 17 per cent of similar weight infants who appeared to be neurologically intact.

Further experience has been gained from a study of 100 infants and young children who, over a 2-year period, were referred to an assessment unit from a development screening programme on account of slow development and/or problems of behaviour. All these referrals followed development screening at either 5, 9 or 15 months. The total of 100 does not include those who on further examination were considered to be mentally retarded, or to be developing cerebral palsy or a neuromuscular disorder.

TABLE 15.1. Abnormal neurological presentation in young children referred to an assessment unit on account of developmental delay or disturbed behaviour.

	Abnormal neurological signs (ANS)								
Reason for referral	Nil		Dystonic		Hypotonic		All ANS		Total.
	No.	%	No.	%	No.	%	No.	%	No.	%
Developmental delay, global	16	64	5	20	4	16	9	36	25	100
Developmental delay, especially motor	8	15	19	35	28	50	47	85	55	100
Behaviour	3	15	17	85	—	—	17	85	20	100
Total	27		41		32		73		100	

The principal reasons for referral, whether or not abnormal neurological signs were detected and the predominant abnormal neurological presentations found are detailed in Table 15.1. Minor abnormal neurological signs were found in nearly three-quarters of these young children with developmental and behavioural problems, but whereas only 36 per cent exhibited these signs when the problem was one of global delay, the incidence rose to 85 per cent when gross motor delay was particularly prominent and when there were severe problems of behaviour and management in the first year of life.

Two abnormal presentations predominated, the dystonic syndrome and hypotonia, with some overlap between the two.

The dystonic syndrome
In this series the dystonic syndrome was exhibited by 20 per cent of infants with global delay, 35 per cent of those with relative excess of motor delay and 85 per cent of those with behaviour disturbance.

Variable increase in extensor tone on changes of posture is always present in the dystonic syndrome. Other common findings on examination are exaggeration and prolongation of primitive reflexes, brisk phasic reflexes, asymmetries and motor delay. Dystonic posturing of legs and arms is well seen with the infant held in vertical suspension when legs are held extended and adducted with plantar flexion of feet and arms extended, abducted and internally rotated or flexed across the chest (Fig. 15.1); in both arm postures the hands are usually

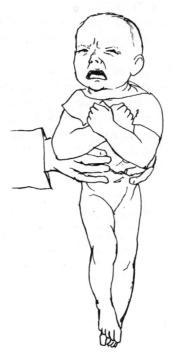

FIG. 15.1. Dystonic posture in vertical suspension in an irritable baby aged 10 weeks.

tightly fisted and frequently the thumbs are held across the palms. When the infant is lowered to the floor extension of first toes is often seen and when the infant's feet touch the floor there is a strong extensor thrust. He may also begin to walk forward on toes because of a retained walking reflex and at older ages, when walking is voluntary, may still be up on his toes. At 9–10 months it may be difficult to decide whether walking is reflex or voluntary on this manoeuvre. Primitive reflexes such as the Moro, ATNR and progression reflexes are easily elicited and retained well beyond the usual age. Tendon jerks are often brisk, crossed adductor response may be present and ankle and jaw clonus may be demonstrable.

When the infant is laid down on the couch and again when he is lifted up, he tends to go into sudden extension. Sitting balance is delayed and the infant may need to be strapped in for sitting rather than propped, to prevent slipping down. Mother may report that the baby does not like to sit and when this is

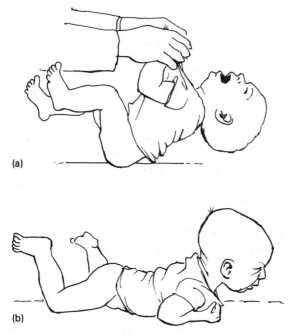

Fig. 15.2a and b. Contrast in head posture in supine pull to sit and prone in an irritable baby aged 10 weeks.

attempted 'he doesn't seem to bend in the middle'. On pull up from supine the infant may show excessive head lag for age which is in contrast to apparent maturity of head control when prone (Fig. 15.2a and b). In prone he may raise his head and upper chest off the couch to the extent that he rolls over, several months before this would be expected. Mother may report that the baby has a 'strong back' and likes to stand, which he does on tip-toes 'like a ballet dancer'. The infant's apparent maturity in standing is also in contrast to head lag on pull up and in this manoeuvre he may come right up to stand onto his toes.

Increases in tone may be obvious with limitation of abduction at hips, difficulty in dorsiflexing the feet beyond 90° and a definite pronator catch found at wrists. Abnormalities may be noted in grasping and reaching. Strong hand preference may be reported. At rest the hands may still be fisted and reach be slow and ataxic or show a characteristic dorsiflexion at wrist and spreading of fingers.

What has been described would be considered a severe degree of the dystonic syndrome. More often the presentation is less obvious and the abnormal neurological signs detected vary in number and severity. Dystonic posturing is usually more obvious in legs than arms, although the signs can be equally prominent in both upper and lower limbs. In a minority abnormalities of posture, tone and reflexes are restricted to the arms.

One-third of dystonic infants in the sample described exhibited asymmetries, most often after 6 months when the other abnormal signs were beginning to resolve. Asymmetries were more commonly seen in the upper limbs and demonstrated by abnormal postures remaining on one side and disappearing on the other, unequal fisting of hands and unequal response in sideways and forward parachute manoeuvres. In the legs asymmetries of posture, tone and reflexes may be seen. In one-fifth of the sample the dystonic signs disappeared to be replaced by hypotonia, usually generalized and at 9–10 months or later.

Hypotonia
In the 2 year series quoted hypotonia was found in 16 per cent of infants with global delay and in 50 per cent of those with more obvious motor delay; in contrast no infant with a predominant behavioural problem presented thus. In a few the infant was reported to have been hypotonic from birth but in most hypotonia was noted at 5 months or older. Asymmetry was unusual; most often hypotonia was generalized. Hyperextensibility at wrist and knee, easy overabduction at hips and easy dorsiflexion of the feet on to the tibiae were common. In one-third tendon jerks were brisk, in the rest unexceptional or somewhat reduced.

Outcome of Minor Abnormal Neurological Signs in Infancy

The abnormal presentations described could presage the development of a diplegia, hemiplegia or cerebellar ataxia. However, abnormal signs in the first year highly suggestive of a developing cerebral palsy may completely resolve or leave a residuum of minor abnormality (such as clumsiness) that could not be considered as even a mild cerebral palsy. In the low birth-weight study mentioned above, one-quarter of infants of weight 1500 g or less exhibited signs highly suggestive of cerebral palsy in the first year; two-thirds of suspect infants did not develop cerebral palsy. This underlines the importance of reserve in what is said to parents particularly of infants who are younger than 6–9 months.

When the infant exhibits signs of brain damage in the immediate postnatal period and those signs persist or become accentuated in the first 6 months of life the risk of permanent damage is very high. If abnormal signs are first detected at 2–4 months and are still present at 9 months and show no sign of resolving there is a considerable risk of later abnormality, but more often the abnormal signs are disappearing by this age, in which case the prognosis is relatively good.

With severe dystonia there is likely to be motor delay which is obvious to parents who are also likely to have noticed that the baby feels stiff to handle. Usually they accept the explanation that the stiffness of muscles, which they have observed, is holding the baby back and that this stiffness may well resolve. Unless the paediatrician is fully convinced in his own mind that the baby has cerebral palsy the terms 'spastic' and 'brain damage' should be avoided until after 9–10 months.

In the majority of infants showing the dystonic syndrome abnormal neurological signs have disappeared by 12–15 months apart from those who progress to hypotonia. These and the infants presenting initially with hypotonia may still show generalized decrease in tone often with slight intention tremor in hands until 2 years or later.

Of those children in the sample described who have been followed up for periods of 9–18 months, one-half who were found to have minor abnormal neurological signs were considered developmentally and behaviourally accept-able at their last examination, one-quarter still showed developmental delay and one-quarter had considerable problems of behaviour. In contrast, of those children who presented with developmental delay (usually global) and no abnormal neurological signs, all were still significantly delayed at their last examination; in most, developmental status was unchanged. Thus it appears that early developmental lags accompanied by definite though minor abnormal neurological signs carry a better prognosis for later functioning. One may expect developmental spurts as abnormal signs resolve.

The long-term significance of early neurological dysfunction is uncertain. There is some evidence (p. 123) that such children are at high risk of educational difficulties and may well constitute an important component of the syndrome loosely termed 'minimal cerebral dysfunction' (Chapter 16).

References

DRILLIEN C.M. (1972) Abnormal neurologic signs in the first year of life in low-birthweight infants: possible prognostic significance. *Developmental Medicine and Child Neurology*, **14,** 575.

SHAW C. (1977) A comparison of the patterns of mother-baby interaction for a group of crying, irritable babies and a group of more amenable babies. *Child care, health and development* **3,** 1.

CHAPTER 16

The Clumsy Child

In the past 25 years the long-term neurological disabilities affecting young children have received increasing attention. Included in this category are severe mental and physical handicaps and additional syndromes with few or any abnormal physical signs. In this sense these syndromes may be minimal but they can cause major problems as far as the child and his family are concerned.

Minimal Cerebral Dysfunction

This term was formulated in revolt against the concept of minimal brain damage, as very often evidence of acquired damage in these conditions is non-existent (Bax and Mac Keith, 1963). What is often referred to as minimal brain dysfunction constitutes a heterogeneous group of behaviour syndromes, learning disorders, and motor disabilities. Ingram (1963) included under chronic brain syndromes: minimal cerebral palsy, clumsy children, the hyperkinetic syndrome, specific retardation of speech development, dyslexia, and a variety of symptoms such as distractability, impulsiveness, irritability and emotional immaturity.

There is no doubt that the term served a useful purpose in the past by drawing attention to a large number of children who are often in urgent need of help. Even if there are arguments in favour of continuing to use it, in an administrative sense, to include a variety of disabilities which do not fit into categories such as mental defect, cerebral palsy and epilepsy, there are dangers in this because it may be thought that a diagnosis has been made, when in fact only a label has been attached to the child. What is required is a detailed analysis of the child's difficulties. Is there a significant delay in language development, are there defects of perception or of motor organization, is the child unacceptably overactive or emotionally immature or, as is almost always the case, is the child suffering from a number of these disorders? It can be accepted that these children are almost always multiply handicapped, as even the most specific learning disorder is likely to be associated with a secondary emotional reaction of some kind. A number of different primary disorders quite often occur in the same child; this is not surprising as they have common aetiologies. Only by a careful analysis of the child's difficulties can sensible plans be made to give the help which is needed.

If it is accepted that 'minimal brain dysfunction' signifies that a child has minor degrees of disability affecting a variety of functions, it is apparent that some are more easily recognized than others. Disorders of language, minor degrees of cerebral palsy and the more obviously emotionally disturbed children should be classified accordingly and are considered elsewhere. However, many children who have in the past been included in the category of 'minimal cerebral dysfunction' are in fact suffering from an impairment of perceptual motor function. Their difficulties can be of a fairly subtle kind and manifest themselves only in certain situations, for example, when writing in the classroom or playing games as a member of a team. When they do, failure is likely and this may lead to emotional and behavioural disorders.

Perceptual Motor Disabilities

Many neurological diseases can result in clumsiness, e.g. cerebellar lesions, chorea and peripheral neuropathies, but if circumscribed and progressive conditions are excluded those remaining can be considered under the heading of developmental perceptual motor disabilities.

Incidence
It has been estimated that 5–6 per cent. of children in primary schools are clumsy to a degree that will significantly interfere with their progress (Brenner *et al.*, 1967; Gubbay, 1975). This means that there are likely to be one or two children in each class who are in need of special help.

Aetiology
Genetic factors have been implicated but most of the evidence is anecdotal. There are families in which more than one child is excessively clumsy without there being anything in the past history to suggest acquired causes. It is possible that these children are predisposed to suffer from perceptual motor disabilities just as others, given the opportunity, may develop exceptional skills.

More boys than girls have difficulties of learning. This may be related to the effect of the Y chromosome, if its presence slows the development of the male. The slower maturation will have a direct effect, and will also expose the male brain for a longer period to the results of noxious agents. The more immature the brain, the more it is likely to suffer damage. Also there is a longer time for males to suffer from imperfections of their genome (Ounsted and Taylor, 1972).

Clumsy children suffer from the same kinds of pre-, peri- and postnatal complications that occur in children who subsequently develop cerebral palsy. A study in Manchester did not suggest any one particular cause except possibly for evidence implicating hypoxia during pregnancy. Francis-Williams (1976) has shown that children who exhibited neurological dysfunction in the newborn period were significantly more liable to learning difficulties at the age of 8–9½ years than a control group with a normal birth history (p. 123).

The clinical problem
Delay in motor development is common, the child being late to sit, stand and walk. Inco-ordination may affect large movements, the finer movements, eye–hand co-ordination, or all aspects of motor function. Instead of an increasing grace of movement the child's gait remains awkward with frequent tripping

and falling. Skipping, jumping and hopping take a long time to develop. Fine movements can be hard to perfect so that the child cannot help with dressing at the expected ages, particularly with the doing up of buttons and laces. Manipulation of toys is difficult. It is not surprising that articulation is often affected as it involves muscular co-ordination of a complex degree.

Clumsy children come under additional pressure on school entry when their performance will be under critical review and subject to comparison with their peers. It has to be admitted that fidgety and restless behaviour in the classroom must be a source of annoyance to the teacher but sometimes this is not the child's fault. If eye–hand co-ordination is the particular disability, tasks such as catching balls will be difficult and the poor performance at games can have serious social consequences. Writing will be especially affected and lack of neatness and even illegibility can be a constant source of friction between child and teacher. Very often the difficulties will be recognized but this is not always so. The child who cannot talk properly is obvious to all but the one whose movements are awkward can easily be regarded as a nuisance and accused of not trying. It is not uncommon to hear that a child has been told to repeat a task again and again until it is successfully accomplished, and that it is only a matter of trying harder, when in fact the task is quite beyond his ability. Is it to be wondered that emotional complications are almost inevitable in these circumstances?

When emotional problems arise, usually as a result of failure, the child is likely to stop trying. Apathy and depression may be the dominant mood of such children, but overactivity and lack of attention and concentration are commoner. The latter can occur as a primary disability but can also result from inappropriate teaching and boredom.

Analysis of the disability
It is not only important to discover if a child is clumsy in the performance of large or small movements or both, but also the reasons for this. In some children the disability is due to severe perceptual disorders so that concepts of shape and size are poorly formed and orientation may be impaired. Such disabilities will make the acquisition of early reading skills more difficult, and, in the case of defects of orientation, writing will be particularly affected with letters arranged back to front and in the wrong order to a greater degree than can be passed as normal.

The development of perception depends on information conveyed by the sensory input channels, particularly vision and hearing and any impairment, e.g. a squint or severe refractive error, may have a deleterious effect. The child's intellectual level will have a significant effect on the ease with which percepts are formed; as will memory and imagery, attention, and concept formation. As far as the last factor is concerned the severely physically handicapped child is at a particular disadvantage as exploration of the environment is considerably restricted. This can result in an apparent perceptual disability which in reality is due to lack of experience.

Other children do well on tests of perception but apparently fail in motor organization. That is to say they cannot easily build up the patterns and memory of movements that underlie the acquisition of any motor skill. If any of us wish to perfect a motor task we have not done before we will have to practise at it and only when it becomes 'automatic' will we cease to be clumsy.

In establishing an efficient organization of motor function, intersensory integration is essential as is the concept of the body image. For instance, a carpenter's tool or tennis racquet will only be used efficiently when it becomes as much a part of the body image as the hand controlling it. An intention tremor or athetosis will affect both motor organization and perception to some degree; there is no division between these functions, only a proportionate involvement which has implications for management (Wedell, 1968).

Assessment

Piaget found that children under the age of 4 years lacked mental representation of objects and relationship of their parts and they were unaware of properties such as the number of sides, verticals or parallels (Beard, 1969). Such features of normal development must be taken into account in the assessment of young children.

If it is suspected that a child is clumsy for his age, a careful history of pre-, peri- and postnatal events must be obtained. Parents and teachers must be questioned about their evidence for suggesting that the child's movements lack co-ordination. It must be remembered that children may be referred because of symptoms such as headache, abdominal pain or nocturnal enuresis which on further enquiry are found to be symptoms of increasing stress in the school situation due to a learning disorder of this kind.

Unless the disability is marked, a routine neurological examination may be unrewarding. Careful observation of the child in the clinic as he plays with toys or is asked to carry out everyday tasks may indicate very clearly that he is abnormally clumsy; then a more detailed analysis of the disability will be needed. Tests that can be used include the Frostig Developmental Test of Visual Perception (Frostig, 1964), the Test of Motor Impairment (Stott *et al.*, 1972), the extended Griffiths Mental Development Scale (Griffiths, 1970) and the Weschler Intelligence Scale for Children (Weschler, 1949; 1963). Some have developed standardized scales of their own (Peters *et al.*, 1975). Such tests will reveal the strong as well as the weak points of the child's performance and on this information a remedial programme can be developed for the particular child.

In addition, there are a number of special investigations that must be done. It is as important to check the vision of a child with a perceptual motor disability as it is to examine the hearing of a child with delayed language development. Apart from helping to analyse the child's perceptual and motor disabilities psychometric tests will establish the over-all intellectual level, as the co-ordination of movements must be judged in relation to the mental rather than the chronological age. If complicating emotional and behavioural disorders are a prominent feature these will need to be assessed. Their treatment may be more difficult than that of the underlying disorder of learning and sometimes psychiatric advice is needed.

When there is a severe degree of disability, help in the assessment of these children will be required from a number of different disciplines including the teaching profession. This can be given most efficiently in Assessment Centres where those with varying expertise are working as members of a team, as it is all too easy to cause confusion in the management of the child.

Early identification

The more severely affected child is likely to be recognized by parents and is often identified in the good nursery school. Recognition of the disability at an early age may prevent many of the emotional and behavioural complications. However, many children are not identified early, particularly the less severely affected. As the tests suggested for a detailed assessment of this disability are very time-consuming, there is a strong argument for including some items of perceptual function and motor organization in the developmental screening of preschool children and in the school entry medical examination. Then without necessarily attaching labels, the teacher can be alerted to the need to watch a particular child's progress and to give extra help if necessary. Bax and Whitmore (1973) included in the entrant examination a short battery of neuro-developmental tests, viz. for squint, hearing, speech comprehensibility, facial symmetry, motor impersistence, tongue tremor, hand patting, finger-nose pointing, imitation of gesture, diodochokinesia, pencil grip, drawing of a circle, square and triangle, gait, heel–toe walking and hopping.

Management of the clumsy child

Much of the work in nursery and infant classes is obviously just what is needed in terms of perceptual training. Teachers and psychologists are likely to work out their own methods suited to particular children. If the main problem is a lack of motor organization, constant practice, suitably motivated, is presumably the answer. However, instructions to carry out certain tasks may not be understood by a child with a severe perceptual disability. It may be necessary to break down the task into simple parts and demonstrate these in detail. For example, when teaching the child to tie shoe-laces each manoeuvre must be taken in turn and practised until it has been perfected. It is relatively common to find that children with perceptual motor disabilities score 10 to 20 points higher on the verbal items of the Wechsler Intelligence Scale for Children than they do on performance items, so full use should be made of the child's verbal ability.

The physiotherapist and the occupational therapist have an important part to play in helping children with perceptual motor difficulties. Following assessment of the particular child's difficulties a programme of exercises is devised which the child, with the help of parents, can practise at home, and also practical ways are worked out for the child to overcome the disability in everyday life (Gordon and Grimley, 1974). Exercises will include those for larger movements such as balancing, positioning the limbs and traversing an obstacle course, and those for fine co-ordination like cutting out pictures, drawing shapes and the use of peg boards.

While stressing the importance of trying to overcome these difficulties, it is also important, especially for the older child, to find ways of circumventing them.

For example, if writing remains illegible in spite of a great deal of practice, it may be better to learn to type. It is also vital that all the child's efforts are not devoted to battling to acquire skills which his peers seem to accomplish much more easily than he does. He must be placed in a position where success is possible. To be of any use, assessment must high-light strengths as well as weaknesses. Advice must be given to child, parents and teachers (Dare and Gordon, 1970). For example, the child must be told that constant practice can improve his performance but that some activities will need to be circumvented. Parents must be convinced of their child's disability, that it is no one's fault and that they can assist in treatment. The teacher must be encouraged to discuss the concept of the clumsy child and to help in planning a remedial programme based on test results.

Conclusions

Perceptual motor disabilities resulting in clumsiness are common in young children. They are often associated with other disabilities, e.g. delayed speech development and poor concentration. If unrecognized, emotional and behavioural disorders will almost certainly arise. These children seem to constitute most of those previously included in the term minimal cerebral dysfunction.

The majority are likely to progress satisfactorily in the primary school if given adequate understanding and extra help in the classroom. A screening test on school entry will alert the teacher to these children's needs. Those more severely affected must be assessed in greater detail and some will require special educational provision. There is often no dividing line between minimal cerebral palsy and disabilities of the type described in this chapter, but the particular label attached to the child may well influence people's attitudes and care must be taken not to add to the child's disabilities.

The child is entitled to help if this is required. He must be rewarded for the extra effort that is often necessary and not blamed for not trying. Assistance must be given in finding ways around the disabilities and success in some fields must be assured.

References

BAX M., and MAC KEITH, R. (1963) *Minimal Cerebral Dysfunction. Little Club Clinics in Developmental Medicine No. 10.* London: Heinemann.

BAX M. and WHITMORE K. (1973) Neurodevelopmental screening in the school entrant medical examination. *Lancet*, **ii**, 368.

BEARD R.M. (1969) *An Outline of Piaget's Developmental Psychology.* London: Routledge and Kegan Paul.

BRENNER M.W., GILLMAN S., ZANGWILL O.L. and FARREL M. (1967) Visuo-motor disability in school children. *British Medical Journal*, **4**, 259.

DARE M.T. and GORDON N. (1970) Clumsy children: a disorder of perception and motor organisation, *Developmental Medicine and Child Neurology*, **12**, 178.

FRANCIS-WILLIAMS J. (1976) Early identification of children likely to have specific learning difficulties: Report of a follow up. *Developmental Medicine and Child Neurology*. **18**, 71.

FROSTIG M. (1964) *The Marianne Frostig Developmental Test of Visual Perception*, 3rd Ed. Palo Alto, California: Consulting Psychologists Press.

GORDON N. and GRIMLEY A. (1974) Clumsiness and perceptuo-motor disorders in children. *Physiotherapy*, **60**, 311.

GRIFFITHS R. (1970) *The Abilities of Young Children*. London: University of London Press.

GUBBAY S.S. (1975) *The Clumsy Child*. London: W.B. Saunders.

INGRAM T. (1963) Chronic brain damage syndromes in childhood other than cerebral palsy, epilepsy and mental defect. In *Minimal Cerebral Dysfunction*, eds. Bax M. and Mac Keith R. *Little Club Clinics in Developmental Medicine No. 10*, London: Heinemann.

OUNSTED C. and TAYLOR D.C. (1972) *Gender Differences: Their Ontogeny and Significance*. Edinburgh: Churchill Livingstone.

PETERS J.E., ROMINE J.S. and DYKMAN R.A. (1975) A special neurological examination of children with learning disabilities. *Developmental Medicine and Child Neurology*, **17**, 63.

STOTT D.H., MOYES F.A. and HENDERSON S.E. (1972) *Test of Motor Impairment*. Guelph, Ontario: Brook Educational Publishing.

WEDELL K. (1968) Perceptual-motor difficulties. *Special Education*, **57**, 25.

WECHSLER D. (1949) *Wechsler Intelligence Scale for Children*. New York: Psychological Corporation.

WECHSLER D. (1963) *Wechsler Pre-school and Primary Scale of Intelligence*. New York: Psychological Corporation.

CHAPTER 17

Epilepsy

Epilepsy may be defined as a recurrent paroxysmal disturbance of central nervous system function, associated with a self-limiting excessive neuronal discharge. It is a symptom complex of multiple aetiology, characterized by repetitive stereotyped disturbances of movement, consciousness, sensation and behaviour depending on which part of the brain is involved.

Aetiology

The term secondary (symptomatic) epilepsy indicates that a cause has been found. Primary (idiopathic) epilepsy indicates that the cause is unknown although in some of these patients autopsy reveals anatomical changes, whilst in others brain structure is normal and seizures must have been due to disturbed neuronal metabolism.

Aetiological factors are outlined in Table 17.1.

TABLE 17.1. Aetiological factors of the epilepsies

PRIMARY OR 'IDIOPATHIC' EPILEPSY
  Genetic factors

SECONDARY OR 'SYMPTOMATIC' EPILEPSY
  Prenatal
  Drugs
  Radiation
  Infections particularly rubella, cytomegalovirus and toxoplasmosis
  Placental insufficiency
  Chromosomal abnormalities

  Perinatal
  Anoxia
  Trauma

  Postnatal
  Metabolic: hypoglycaemia, hypocalcaemia
  Toxic: lead encephalopathy, atropine poisoning
  Infections: meningitis, encephalitis, cerebral abscess
  Trauma: sub-dural haematoma, non-accidental injury
  Vascular: thromboembolic complications, cortical thrombophlebitis, vascular anomalies, hypertensive encephalopathy
  Tumours: glioma, meningioma
  Degenerative: lipid storage disorders, 'slow virus' infections (e.g. subacute sclerosing panencephalitis)
  Hypersensitivity: ? Infantile spasms

Genetic factors
Seizures are reported in 12 per cent of parents and siblings of children who have had at least one convulsive episode and an EEG pattern of the spike-wave type. This same EEG pattern is also found among 45 per cent of their close relatives, prevalence being highest in the age group 5–16 years. This suggests that the spike-wave EEG abnormality is an expression of an autosomal dominant gene, but that other factors are required to produce seizures (Metrakos and Metrakos, 1972).

Biochemical factors
The neurochemical and neurophysiological processes involved in a seizure are the same ones utilized in normal cerebral function. The neurone is electrically excitable due to movement of ions across the cell membrane. This excitability is transmitted down the cell's axon and via transmitter substances to other neurones. Inhibitory mechanisms prevent synchronous firing. In epilepsy either an excess of normal excitation or a deficiency of normal inhibitory function permits the abnormal synchronous firing that constitutes a seizure. The disturbance may originate in any area of the cortex or in the deeper centres.

Neuropathological factors
There is no single specific pathology for epilepsy. Seizures may occur with almost any pathological process affecting the brain or without any obvious anatomical, physiological or metabolic disorder. Cerebral pathology may be related to factors in the pre-, peri- or postnatal periods (Table 17.1).

Classification

Seizures can be classified on the basis of the principal clinical manifestations, on their localization by means of electroencephalography, and by the aetiological factor responsible for the seizure state.

Generalized seizures
Major seizures (grand mal) consist of loss of consciousness and posture and a sequence of motor (tonic and clonic) and secondary autonomic events. The tonic phase lasts 10–20 seconds followed by clonic or jerking movements usually lasting 30–60 seconds although they can last longer. Autonomic features include tachycardia, increased blood pressure, mydriasis, flushing, glandular hypersecretion (especially bronchial) and apnoea. The clonic phase is followed by complete muscular relaxation lasting 5–10 minutes during which incontinence may occur. Generalized tonic-clonic seizures are uncommon in the first year of life because the infant's central nervous system is immature and unable to respond in this way (Lombroso, 1974). The ictal EEG pattern commonly takes the form of generalized spike and wave complexes of $1\frac{1}{2}$–3 per second.

Minor seizures (absences, petit mal). The classical petit mal absence is characterized by impairment or loss of consciousness and of memory (but without loss of posture), having abrupt onset and ending and brief duration of 5–15 seconds, occasionally up to 1 minute. Minor motor phenomena consisting of the eyes rolling upwards and flickering of eyelids may be observed. Attacks may occur many times daily and interfere significantly with concentration and learning. These attacks are rarely seen before the age of 3 years and the majority cease in adolescence.

The ictal EEG contains the well-known generalized 3 per second rhythmic spike and wave discharge (Fig. 17.1) which can often be precipitated by making the child hyperventilate for 2 or 3 minutes.

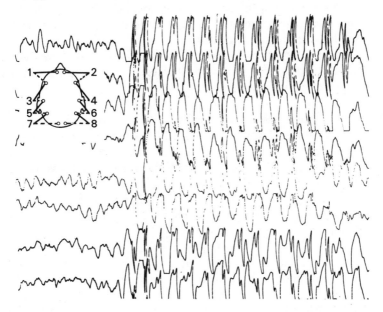

FIG. 17.1. EEG showing generalized 3 per second spike and wave complexes accompanying a petit mal attack.

Atypical absences, with more prominent motor manifestations (e.g. lip-smacking, picking at clothes) and less abrupt onset and ending, are usually associated with diffuse cerebral pathology, refractory nature to medication and poor prognosis. The EEG pattern (petit mal variant) shows bursts of diffuse symmetrical and irregular sharp and slow wave complexes at about 1–2 per second. Minor seizures that are clinically similar but lack these EEG changes may arise from a cortical focus in a temporal lobe.

Akinetic seizures (drop attacks, atonic seizures) consist of a sudden intense hypotonia of all postural muscles resulting in the child falling to the ground. There is usually immediate recovery, the attack lasting seconds only. However, there is considerable risk of coincidental injury.

Unilateral seizures
Seizures completely affecting one half of the body occur almost exclusively in

children especially under the age of 5 years. They appear to result from neuronal discharge in the entire contralateral cerebral hemisphere and its subcortical connections. The clinical manifestations and ictal EEG pattern are identical to those of generalized seizures apart from their unilateral nature.

Partial seizures (focal attacks)

A focal attack often starts with the so-called aura. This is some sensation experienced by the child and is related to the area of cerebral cortex in which the seizure arises. In the young child, who cannot describe his experience, the parent may observe a sudden change in behaviour; the child is upset and runs to his mother. The older child may be reluctant to describe his aura as he feels it to be peculiar, strange and frightening.

Symptomatology depends on the area of cortex involved. Consciousness is not lost unless the discharge spreads to the deeper sub-cortical structures and the seizure becomes generalized.

Frontal cortex (motor): clonic movements are limited to one body region, e.g. thumb and index finger, lips and eyes. In adversive seizures the eyes and head turn away from the side of the discharging focus. These seizures may be followed by post-ictal unilateral weakness (Todd's paralysis) lasting for several hours up to a day or two.

Parietal cortex (sensory): localized paraesthesiae are experienced or less commonly dysaesthesiae.

Occipital cortex (visual): brief impairment of vision or crude hallucinatory experiences (e.g. flashing lights, bright colours) occur.

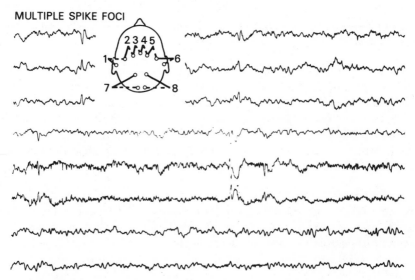

MULTIPLE SPIKE FOCI

FIG. 17.2. EEG showing independent spike foci in the left and right mid-temporal regions.

Temporal lobe (psychomotor): symptoms are extremely varied and include unpleasant epigastric sensations accompanied by fear; hallucinatory experiences affecting smell, taste, hearing, vision and movement (vertigo); dreamy states with feeling of unreality; affective disorders with episodes of anxiety, fear or depression and primary automatisms. The child may suddenly stand still, stare or turn pale. Chewing and lip-smacking, purposeless fumbling, patting of the hands and picking at clothes may be seen. The child may move aimlessly around the room and occasionally utter stereotyped or nonsensical phrases. Temporal lobe seizures are difficult to recognize in younger children because they are unable or find it difficult to describe their aura and the EEG focus tends to 'migrate' or change its location with maturation of the brain. The EEG features consist of spikes or sharp waves localized to a temporal lobe (Fig. 17.2).

Myoclonic seizures
Myoclonus means brief muscular jerks which, when recorded electromyographically, are shown to last between 10–200 milliseconds with an average of 50 milliseconds. Epileptic myoclonus is classified as generalized, unilateral or partial. Generalized myoclonus consists of bilateral massive jerks or of diffuse multi-focal 'fragmentary' myoclonus. Myoclonus is usually symptomatic of serious cerebral pathology, e.g. cerebral degenerative disorders, toxic encephalopathies and infantile spasms. The ictal EEG consists of generalized discharges of variable wave form, usually multiple spikes or sharp waves followed by one or more slow waves.

Investigation and Diagnosis

A full history is taken from the parent and from the child if he is old enough. A complete physical and neurological examination is made including scrutiny of the skin for stigmata of neurocutaneous syndromes (tuberose sclerosis and neurofibromatosis) and ophthalmoscopy for signs of raised intracranial pressure and for chorioretinitis and abnormal retinal pigmentation which may signify intrauterine toxoplasmosis, cytomegalovirus or congenital rubella.

Diagnostic procedures
The following may be indicated to identify aetiological factors and to determine the type of seizure and focus, if any.

Blood tests. Although uncommon, except in the newborn, hypocalcaemia and hypoglycaemia should be excluded. Amino acid chromatography will exclude inborn errors of metabolism such as phenylketonuria. In younger children specific serological tests may exclude intrauterine infections.

Radiological examinations. In infancy skull x-ray may show evidence of raised intracranial pressure or skull asymmetries suggesting early brain damage. In older children bony erosions and abnormal calcifications may be seen.

Contrast studies, such as air encephalography and cerebral angiography, are major procedures and require hospitalization. They may be indicated when a progressive neurological disorder is suspected and there are focal abnormalities on examination and EEG.

Lumbar puncture. This procedure is not indicated in the usual forms of epilepsy but is mandatory if infection is suspected and usually contraindicated if there is evidence of raised intracranial pressure.

Electroencephalography. Paediatric encephalography presents special problems. A satisfactory record may be difficult to obtain and its interpretation is often complicated because of the changes that occur with increasing age. Maturation of the EEG bears some relationship to cerebral morphogenesis; the younger the child the slower the dominant rhythm (Fig. 17.3). The EEG is just one of the

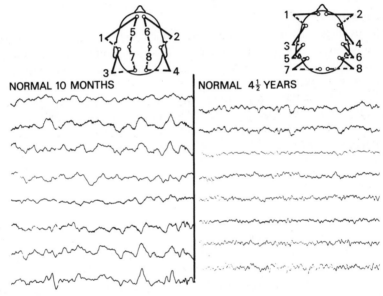

NORMAL 10 MONTHS   NORMAL 4½ YEARS

FIG. 17.3. EEG at 10 months of age with dominant rhythm 2–4 Hz; and at 4½ years of age with dominant rhythm 6–8 Hz.

investigations which will contribute to the patient's management. As it is uncommon to obtain an ictal recording, it is necessary to depend on the interseizure patterns for diagnostic assistance as these may show abnormal discharges which are *formes frustes* of seizure discharges. This finding can be of great assistance in identifying attacks as epileptic and in indicating the type of seizure, particularly in the younger child who is unable to describe his symptoms and when there have been no reliable witnesses of the attacks. As single records are often normal or show only non-specific abnormalities, serial records are more informative and if necessary can be combined with activating techniques, e.g. sleep, drugs.

Isotope brain scanning using radioactive trace techniques. This is a safe procedure and of proven value as a screening test in patients with suspected focal abnormalities such as subdural effusion, neoplasm, abscess and vascular anomaly.

Computerized transverse axial tomography. This new non-invasive technique has proved very successful in demonstrating intracranial lesions. When it becomes more readily available it should greatly reduce demand for air encephalography and cerebral angiography.

Differential diagnosis

In some circumstances breath-holding, night terrors and masturbation may simulate epileptic seizures. These conditions are discussed in Chapter 25. Infantile spasms may be confused with startle reactions or colic.

Syncopal attacks may occur rarely in young children. Malingering or hysteria is not seen at this age.

Benign paroxysmal vertigo is characterized by brief attacks of vertigo, nausea and marked unsteadiness. There is no loss of consciousness but the child may fall. Attacks last from a few seconds to several minutes and may recur at intervals of several days to several months. The attacks may occur in epidemics and affect more than one family member. The condition is sometimes confused with temporal lobe epilepsy. Caloric tests often reveal uni- or bilateral canal paresis.

Migraine is due to spasm of cerebral vessels. Children may present with odd symptoms such as dizziness, hemianopia, tingling and numbness in one hand spreading to arm and face. Nausea and vomiting are common as are facial pallor and headache. Attacks last for half an hour or longer. Rarely a transient hemiparesis may occur and speech be affected.

In all these conditions EEG's are normal.

Treatment

The primary cause of epilepsy can rarely be removed. Often the cause is a genetic tendency or a non-progressive pathological process which results in a proneness to occasional excessive and disorderly discharges of neurones. The aim of treatment is to suppress this excessive discharge completely and permanently, mainly by means of anticonvulsant drugs. Psychological and social factors must also be considered in management.

Anticonvulsant drugs should secure maximum control of seizures with minimum of unwanted side-effects. Incomplete control of seizures may be better than a patient handicapped by overdosage. The results of treatment must never be worse than the effects of seizures.

A single seizure with fever (p. 365) or a series of seizures occurring with central nervous system infection or head injury do not usually necessitate regular anticonvulsant therapy. However, should recurrent seizures develop this will be required.

Drug therapy should be simple (usually avoiding more than two drugs), given regularly and in adequate dosage. Serum drug levels should be monitored regularly.

The drugs recommended for controlling the various clinical types of seizures are given in Table 17.2, in order of preference for first and subsequent trials

TABLE 17.2

Clinical seizure type	Drug*	Dose	No. of doses in 24 hours	Therapeutic drug levels
Major Focal (including temporal lobe)	Phenytoin	Oral 5 mg/kg/day increasing as required	2	30–65 µmol/L
	Carbamezepine	Oral 15–20 mg/kg/day	2–3	15–30 µmol/L
	Sodium valproate	Oral 20–40 mg/kg/day	3–4	350–700 µmol/L
	Clonazepam	Oral 0.05–0.1 mg/kg/day	2	65–150 µmol/L
Absences and petit mal	Ethosuccimide	Oral 15–25 mg/kg/day	3	28–540 µmol/L
	Sodium valproate	Oral see above		
	Clonazepam	Oral see above		
	Ketogenic diet	Oral.		
Myoclonic epilepsy	Nitrazepam	Oral 2–15 mg/day	2–3	
	Clonazepam	Oral see above		
	Sodium valproate	Oral see above		
	Carbamezepine	Oral see above		
	Ketogenic diet	Oral.		
Infantile spasms	ACTH	I.M. 20 i.u./day	1	
	Synacthen	I.M. 0.5 mg/alt. days		
	Nitrazepam	Oral see above		
	Clonazepam	Oral see above		
Febrile convulsions	Phenobarbitone	Oral 3–5 mg/kg/day	2	80–160 µmol/L
	Primidone	Oral 10–15 mg/kg/day	2–3	
	Sodium valproate	Oral see above		

Major status	Diazepam	I.V. 0.2 mg/kg/dose	Can repeat in 30 mins. or by continuous I.V. drip.
	Clonazepam	I.V. 0.5–1.0 mg/stat	
	Paraldehyde	I.M. 0.1–0.3 ml/kg/dose	Can repeat in 30 mins.
	Thiopentone sodium	I.V. under supervision of anaesthetist	
Minor or 'petit mal' status	Diazepam	I.V. 0.2 mg/kg/dose	Can repeat in 30 mins. or by continuous I.V. drip
	Clonazepam	I.V. 0.5–1.0 mg/stat	
	ACTH	I.M. see above	
	Synacthen	I.M. see above	
Myoclonic status	ACTH	I.M. see above	
	Synacthen	I.M. see above	
	Diazepam	I.V. see above	
	Clonazepam	I.V. see above	

* Drugs listed in order of preference.

of medication. Medication is commenced in a low dose and increased to the point of complete therapeutic effect or until undesirable side-effects appear. If only a partial therapeutic effect is obtained despite the appearance of toxic symptoms, the first drug should be reduced until toxic symptoms disappear while a second drug is introduced and increased appropriately. Judging by the patient's response, he can be retained on these two drugs if satisfactory but if this combination proves ineffective the first drug is gradually withdrawn and a third drug introduced. Trials of different medications may be required in the more refractory cases but a combination of more than two anticonvulsants is best avoided. It is helpful to measure blood levels of the anticonvulsant drugs administered either to ensure that satisfactory blood levels have been achieved or if toxic side-effects are suspected.

The effectiveness of anticonvulsant drugs in idiopathic epilepsy usually remains constant. If variations do occur changes in dosage or type of drug are required.

Once the diagnosis of epilepsy is made and any treatable causative or pre- cipitatory factors are dealt with anticonvulsant therapy continued in full dosage for 3 or 4 years appears to offer the patient the best chance of lasting freedom from all manifestations of epilepsy (Eadie and Tyrer, 1974).

Status Epilepticus

MAJOR STATUS

A child is said to be in major status when tonic-clonic convulsions occur in succession without intervening periods of recovery. Major status presents an immediate threat to life on account of respiratory obstruction, hypoxic brain damage or cardiac arrhythmia. Serious sequelae may result from neuronal damage during prolonged seizures lasting 30 minutes or longer.

Aicardi and Chevrie (1970) reported the outcome of convulsive status in 239 infants and young children, three-quarters being under 3 years of age. In 77 per cent this was the first ictal manifestation. In one-half definite causes were found, the commonest being electrolyte disturbances, meningitis, encephalitis, chronic anoxic encephalopathy and degenerative disorders. In 30 per cent the clinical picture was indistinguishable from simple febrile convulsions except for the duration of fits. Prognosis was grave: 11 per cent died during their first status or later and of the survivors 37 per cent had permanent neurological sequelae such as hemiplegia, diplegia and microcephaly; 48 per cent were mentally retarded. It was noted that over one-half of these features could be directly related to the episode of status as patients were normal prior to this. This study underlines the importance of management as an acute medical emergency.

Management
    (1) Secure adequate airway, oxygen may be required.
    (2) Control the seizures by drugs (Table 17.2). If anticonvulsant drugs fail to control the seizures the only remaining course is to anaesthetize the patient and maintain until the seizures do not recur when anaesthesia is lightened. This should be done in an intensive care unit.

(3) Maintain fluid and electrolyte balance.

(4) Investigate for and treat any cause such as infection, tumour or sudden withdrawal of previous anticonvulsant therapy.

Immediate drug therapy is as described below for febrile convulsions.

MINOR STATUS

This term is used to describe a prolonged state of clouded mental activity ranging from a slowing of thought and expression to a confusional state and mental regression, frequently with myoclonic jerks, flickering eyelids, drooling of saliva and ataxia of arms and gait.

The EEG shows continuously occurring, bilaterally synchronous spike-wave complexes and multiple spike discharges (Fig. 17.4).

Drug therapy is detailed in Table 17.2. Prognosis depends on underlying cerebral pathology.

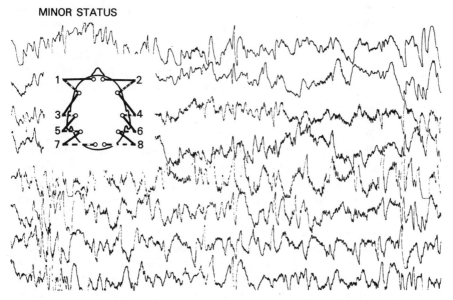

MINOR STATUS

FIG. 17.4. EEG shows continuously occurring generalized slow waves and spike-wave complexes in minor status.

Febrile Convulsions

Febrile convulsions are those occurring with fever excepting fever due to infections of the nervous system. They occur most commonly between the ages of 6 months and 5 years, affect about 5 per cent of all children and often show a familial tendency.

The convulsion is generalized and usually brief. Severe convulsions, defined as lasting longer than 30 minutes or being mainly unilateral, occur in up to 20 per cent of patients.

Thirty per cent of febrile convulsions in infants of 13 months or younger are severe, compared with 10 per cent in children over 3 years of age. Girls are more prone than boys to have severe convulsions because their peak incidence is in the first year.

Treatment

This consists of stopping the seizure as soon as possible. Drugs are detailed in Table 17.2. If it is difficult to give an intravenous injection in the younger child, intramuscular paraldehyde is the drug of choice. Intramuscular phenobarbitone and phenytoin are useless, as effective serum drug levels are not reached until 30 minutes or later.

Generalized measures are as described for major status.

Prophylactic therapy involves prompt treatment of new febrile episodes and immediate measures to prevent high temperatures, by tepid sponging and the administration of an anti-pyretic agent (e.g. paracetamol). Intermittent anti-convulsants given only during febrile illnesses are seldom of value since the fit may be the first sign of fever and adequate serum drug levels cannot be achieved quickly.

Long-term prophylactic therapy has been shown to be effective in preventing further episodes (Faero *et al.*, 1972). As medication must be taken continuously until the age of 4 years, those at highest risk of recurrence (as detailed below) should be selected for long-term therapy.

Prognosis

Risk of recurrence depends on age, sex and family history. When the child is 13 months or younger, a further febrile convulsion can be predicted in over one-half of girls and one-third of boys. Between 14 months and 3 years the chance of recurrence is 50 per cent if there is a positive family history and 25 per cent if there is not. When the child is over 3 years the chance of recurrence is 12 per cent (Lennox-Buchtal, 1973).

The outcome after febrile convulsions depends on how promptly the seizure is controlled. The risk of subsequent epilepsy is probably of the order of 3 per cent. The risk is increased when the patient has a prolonged or focal convulsion. In the majority of cases subsequent seizures are psychomotor or temporal lobe, with or without grand mal. Pathology consists of mesial temporal sclerosis (Falconer and Taylor, 1968).

Infantile Spasms

These seizures, variously described as infantile spasms, or as lightning, salaam and jack knife attacks, usually begin between the ages of 3–24 months with peak incidence at 5–6 months. Male: female ratio is 2:1.

The commonest clinical presentation is the flexor spasm, consisting of a sudden brief generalized myoclonic jerk, with flexion of neck and trunk and elevation of arms. Isolated flexion of the head or extension of trunk and legs (extensor spasm) are also seen. Typically the attacks occur as series of spasms, separated by a few seconds and sometimes lasting many minutes. From the onset of spasms rate of development usually slows or regresses. The infant may become so unresponsive that deafness and blindness are suspected.

The EEG pattern (hypsarrythmia) consists of a grossly chaotic mixture of slow waves and spikes and sharp waves which vary in amplitude, form, duration and site (Fig. 17.5).

HYPSARRYTHMIA
(Before Treatment)

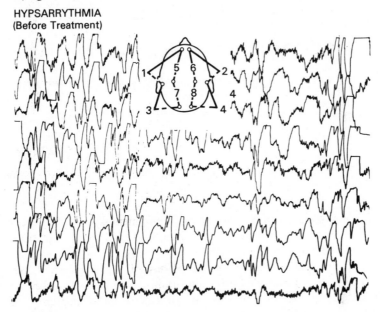

FIG. 17.5. EEG pattern (hypsarrhythmia) in 9-month-old consisting of a grossly chaotic mixture of slow waves and spikes which vary in amplitude, form, duration and site.

Aetiology

Spasms are classified as symptomatic when a cause is known and as idiopathic when there is no obvious cause and no abnormality is found on examination. In the latter group, which accounts for about 40 per cent of patients, development is normal up to the onset of spasms. In about 15–20 per cent of cases a temporal relationship exists between the onset of spasms and immunization, especially with diphtheria-pertussis-tetanus (DPT) vaccine.

A cause can be identified in symptomatic cases. Spasms may occur in children with neurological abnormality attributable to brain damage due to perinatal complications. Tuberose sclerosis may present with spasms, diagnosis being difficult as the typical skin rash does not appear before 3 years of age, though depigmented patches of skin appear earlier. Other rare causes are phenylketo-nuria, congenital viral infections and cerebral lipidoses.

Treatment and prognosis

High doses of adrenal cortical steroids offer the best hope of success in idiopathic and post-immunization cases. The spasms may be reduced or abolished and EEG features be improved (Fig. 17.6). There may also be an improvement in

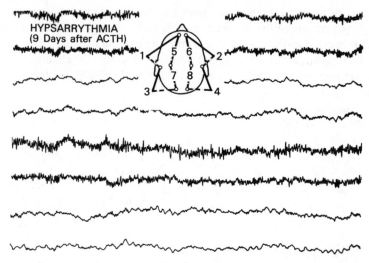

FIG. 17.6. EEG (same child as in Fig. 17.5) 9 days after treatment with ACTH showing normal pattern.

social responsiveness and a resumption of developmental progress. Later normal mentality is found in one-third. The earlier is steroid therapy instituted, the more favourable the outcome (Jeavons *et al.*, 1973).

In secondary spasms the immediate effects of steroid therapy are good. Nitrazepam is also useful in controlling spasms. Unfortunately later mentality is usually very poor, the majority of patients remaining severely mentally retarded.

Seizures of the Newborn

Although the newborn infant has a full complement of neurones, dendritic and synaptic connections and myelination are incomplete and glial elements have not formed their later relationships with neurones (Dobbing, 1970). Because of this immaturity typical grand mal seizures are not seen in the first year of life. In the newborn a multifocal erratic, shifting nature of both cerebral discharge and motor symptoms is characteristic.

Seizures consist of brief tonic extension of the body, clonic movements of a limb, sudden chewing movements, episodes of limpness or apnoea and vasomotor changes.

The symptomatic nature of neonatal seizures has been stressed (Brown *et al.*, 1972; Keen and Lee, 1973). There are two peak periods when fits occur. In the first 48 hours fits are most likely to be associated with cerebral birth injury and hypoglycaemia with a correspondingly poor prognosis. Between 4 and 7 days fits are mostly accounted for by hypocalcaemia and hypomagnesaemia with a good prognosis for survival and later status. Other causes of fits are intrauterine and postnatal infections, metabolic disorders, degenerative conditions and maternal addictions.

Treatment is that of the causative condition, supportive measures as indicated and anticonvulsant drugs.

Associated Disorders

Intellectual impairment

The mentality of children with idiopathic epilepsy is little different from that of the general population. Children with secondary epilepsy are more likely to be retarded as both intellectual impairment and epilepsy may be manifestations of the same underlying cerebral pathology.

Children with early onset of epilepsy tend to have lower intelligence test scores than those with later onset. This may be due to greater brain damage or the adverse effect of early injury on cerebral maturation and normal development of neurophysiological patterns of cerebral function.

Anticonvulsants may produce mental dulling and interfere with learning. In addition, the fits themselves may have an adverse effect on satisfactory educational placement.

Behaviour disturbances

Behavioural disorder is common in children with epilepsy particularly if fits are associated with other neurological defect (Rutter *et al.*, 1970). This could be due to the underlying epileptic condition, especially if fits are poorly controlled; to disturbance of the limbic system, which is associated with emotional responses and closely related to the temporal lobes; to the effect of anticonvulsant drugs; to a psychological reaction to domestic and social frustrations, or to a combination of these factors.

Neurological deficits

Secondary epilepsy is commonly associated with other neurological deficits, the type and severity depending on the portion of the brain involved. In spastic cerebral palsy two-thirds of children have fits as do between 17 and 34 per cent of dyskinetics. Perceptual motor problems and learning difficulties may also be associated with epilepsy (Stores, 1971; Yule, 1973).

Prognosis

Apart from simple biochemical fits and those associated with maternal diabetes, seizures during the neonatal period carry a poor prognosis, one-half either dying or surviving with moderate to severe neurological defect (Lombroso, 1974). Seizures starting in the first year also have a poor prognosis (Strobos, 1959). Seizures associated with structural brain lesions usually recur after treatment and require prolonged anticonvulsant therapy. In approximately one-half of children with idiopathic epilepsy, complete control of seizures is obtained and in one-quarter partial control.

Hollowach and colleagues (1972) showed that if seizures had been completely suppressed for 4 years, there was a 75 per cent chance of freedom from further seizures for at least 5 years after withdrawal of therapy. With an early age of onset and prompt control, the recurrence rate was 13 per cent but at least twice as high with late onset, prolonged duration and with neurological, psychological or continuing EEG abnormalities. Relapse rates by type of seizure were respectively: grand mal attacks, 8 per cent; petit mal attacks and febrile convulsions, 12 per cent; psychomotor attacks, 25 per cent; multiple seizure types, 40 per cent; and focal seizures, 53 per cent.

Rodin (1974) suggests the following variables as indicators of poor prognosis: a long duration of the epilepsy, a combination of several different seizure types, frequent seizures, and the presence of psychomotor seizures. Additional features in his own study were that injuries during seizures and a tendency for the seizures to come in clusters also carried a poor prognosis.

References

AICARDI J. and CHEVRIE J.J. (1970) Convulsive status epilepticus in infants and children. *Epilepsia (Amst.)*, **11**, 187.

BROWN J.K., COCKBURN F. and FORFAR J.O. (1972) Clinical and chemical correlates in convulsions of the newborn. *Lancet*, **i**, 135.

DOBBING J. (1970) Undernutrition and the developing brain. The relevance of animal models to the human problem. *American Journal of Diseases of Children*, **120**, 411.

EADIE M.J. and TYRER J.H. (1974) *Anticonvulsant Therapy: pharmacological basis and practice*. Edinburgh: Churchill Livingstone.

FAERO O., KASTRUP K.W., LYKKEGAARD NIELSEN E., MELCHIOR J.C. and THORN I. (1972), Successful prophylaxis of febrile convulsions with phenobarbitol. *Epilepsia (Amst.)*, **13**, 279.

FALCONER M.A. and TAYLOR D.C. (1968) Surgical treatment of drug resistant epilepsy due to mesial temporal sclerosis. *Archives of Neurology*, **19**, 353.

HOLLOWACH J., THURSTON D.L. and O'LEARY J. (1972) Prognosis in childhood epilepsy. *New England Journal of Medicine*, **286**, 169.

JEAVONS P.M., BOWER B.D. and DIMITRAKOUDI M. (1973) Long-term prognosis of 150 cases of 'West syndrome'. *Epilepsia (Amst.)*, **14**, 153.

KEEN J.H. and LEE D. (1973) Sequelae of neonatal convulsions. *Archives of Disease in Childhood*, **48**, 542.

LENNOX-BUCHTAL M.A. (1973) Febrile convulsions, a reappraisal. *Electroencephalography and Clinical Neurophysiology*, Supplement No. 32.

LOMBROSO C. (1974) Seizures in the newborn period. In *Handbook of Clinical Neurology*, eds. Vinken P.J. and Bruyn G.W. Vol. 15 Epilepsy, p. 189. Amsterdam: North Holland Publishing Co.

METRAKOS J.D. and METRAKOS K. (1972) *Genetic factors in the epilepsies: A workshop*. eds. Alter M. and Allen Hauser W. NINDS monograph No. 14, p. 97.

RODIN E.A. (1972) Medical and social prognosis in epilepsy. *Epilepsia (Amst.)*, **13**, 121.

RUTTER M., GRAHAM P. and YULE W. (1970) *A Neuropsychiatric Study in Childhood. Clinics in Developmental Medicine Nos. 35/36*. London: Heinemann.

STORES G. (1971) Cognitive function in epilepsy. *British Journal of Hospital Medicine*, **6**, 207.

STROBOS R.R.J. (1959) Prognosis in convulsive disorders. AMA *Archives of Neurology*, **1**, 216.

YULE W. (1973) Epilepsy; education and enigma. *Special Education*, **62**, 16.

CHAPTER 18

Spina Bifida Cystica

Incidence, Causes and Prevention

Spina bifida cystica is the commonest congenital defect of the central nervous system. In the 1970s its approximate incidence is 1 to 2 per 1000 babies, but this incidence varies in different parts of the country from higher figures in Ireland, South Wales and parts of the north-west to much lower figures in the south-east of England. Recent figures from Sheffield show that the incidence fell from 2 per 1000 to less than 1 per 1000 over the last 6 years. This fact, together with the nationally falling birth rate, suggests that the total number expected to be born in Great Britain at the present time is of the order of 1 per 1000 per year.

Spina bifida is much more common in the lower social classes and among the poorest sections of the community. There is only a slightly increased risk for very young or for older mothers.

The risk of a further spina bifida child is considerably increased for couples who have already had a spina bifida baby or an anencephalic fetus. The risk is about 5–8 per cent for one or other of these defects which are probably aetiologically identical, and about 4 per cent for spina bifida alone. If a couple have already had 2 infants affected by either condition, then the risk is even higher (Lorber, 1965; Laurence et al., 1968). The risk that a sibling of a spina bifida subject may have an affected child is higher than in the general population but is less than 1 per cent. Finally, the risk that a spina bifida mother or father may have a spina bifida offspring is about 4 per cent. Such increased risks are very important bearing in mind the severity of the condition in most of those affected. These and other data suggest that spina bifida is a polygenetically inherited predisposition, and that environmental factors may also play a part in the causation. However, we do not yet know the true cause or causes (Laurence, 1969).

Fortunately, within the last few years, antenatal detection of spina bifida has become possible by the quantitative determination of alpha fetoprotein (AFP) in the amniotic fluid (Brock and Sutcliffe, 1972). The optimum time to carry out amniocentesis is about the sixteenth week of pregnancy. This can be done on an out-patient basis, under local anaesthesia. The placenta should first be located by ultrasonic examination to ensure that it is avoided by the puncture and a blood free sample of amniotic fluid is aspirated. The AFP level is determined by immuno-diffusion technique (Stewart, Ward and Lorber, 1975) and the result is usually available within a few days. The normal AFP value of 6–35 μg/ml is usually greatly exceeded if the fetus is anencephalic or has open spina bifida and values of up to 900 μg/ml may be found. However, small or closed spina bifida lesions are not detected by this method. This is probably fortunate, because termination would not be advised if the baby was only slightly affected. In all other cases termination of pregnancy is usually carried out if the AFP level is unquestionably high.

This is a most encouraging recent advance and gives 'high risk' couples the chance to have as large a family as they wish, knowing that most abnormal pregnancies can now be detected and need not be continued. As a direct result of this technique many more normal, wanted babies will be born, because even in high risk families some 95 per cent of babies are normal. Before this test many parents did not dare risk a further pregnancy for fear of having another abnormal baby.

Unfortunately, because it is practically impossible and ethically unjustified to carry out this procedure on all pregnant women, amniocentesis can only prevent the births of some 5 per cent of cases of spina bifida, since 95 per cent of all cases occur in families who have not had an affected baby before.

However, in over half of abnormal pregnancies maternal serum AFP also rises to an abnormal level between the fifteenth and twentieth week of gestation (Wald *et al.*, 1974). A multicentre study is in progress to define precisely the place of serum tests in pregnant women. It is hoped that, subject to sufficient financial support, it will be possible to include such tests among routine antenatal blood tests in the future and so reduce the risk of spina bifida and especially of severe forms.

Clinical Presentation

There are two main types of spina bifida cystica. In both types the spinous processes of some vertebrae fail to develop and there may be abnormalities of other parts of the vertebrae. The subcutaneous tissues and the skin over the affected vertebrae do not develop and a cystic lesion, usually membrane-covered, is exposed in the midline on the infant's back. This is readily diagnosable immediately after the birth of the baby.

Meningocele
This is a mild condition in which the cystic swelling may be partly skin covered and consists only of a membrane (meninges) and cerebrospinal fluid (CSF). The spinal cord is normally formed and lies in its normal position. There are no motor or sensory defects. The incidence of hydrocephalus is a little higher than in the general population. Such lesions are usually cervical, upper thoracic or sacral and are rarely large. Treatment by excision is simple and presents neither technical nor ethical problems. Most babies recover without sequelae (Lorber, 1972). Unfortunately, this minor variety of spina bifida accounts for only about 5 per cent of all cases.

Myelomeningocele
In this lesion part of the spinal cord has failed to develop normally from an

early embryonic stage onwards and remains as a flat ribbon. The affected segments are exposed on the surface of the infant's back in the centre of the lesion and constitute the so-called 'neural plaque' (Fig. 18.1). In the newborn infant this looks like a kipper and the spinal nerve roots are clearly visible through the membrane.

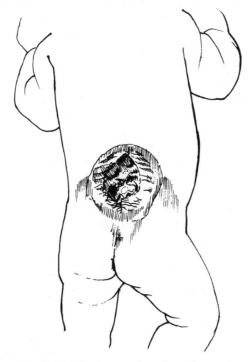

FIG. 18.1. A lumbo-sacral myelomeningocoele.

Myelomeningocele lesions are usually in the middle of the back (lower thoraco-lumbar or lumbosacral) and large, measuring some 6 × 9 cm. If the membrane ruptures during or after birth, there may be CSF leak which increases the ever present risk of meningitis.

These infants have variable degrees of paralysis of their legs (often with gross and complex deformities) associated with analgesia of the same neural segments. The level and degree of paralysis and the types of deformities depend on the upper level and the size of the myelomeningocele. High lesions, with an upper neurological level at the lower thoracic segments, are usually associated with total paraplegia and little or no leg deformity. Medium high (lumbosacral) lesions result in less severe paralysis but gross deformities, because some muscle groups acting on joints are paralysed whilst others are not. Prenatal deformities are common and frequently progress further after birth, up to any age, often in spite of much skilled orthopaedic care. One of the commonest problems is dislocation of hip joints due to acting hip flexors and adductors, but paralysed abductors and extensors as those derive their innervation from lower spinal segments. The various deformities of the legs may be asymmetrical and are predictable from the level of the lesion (Sharrard, 1962). Apart from paralysis of the legs there is almost invariably paralysis of the urethral and rectal sphincters, resulting in dribbling incontinence of urine and a patulous anus.

If the myelomeningocele is very low (i.e. purely sacral) then there may be little if any paralysis of the legs, but neurogenic incontinence remains a feature. Very rarely a myelomeningocele is upper thoracic or cervical. In such a case, weakness may affect the hands or arms and there may be spastic weakness of the legs. There are often gross vertebral anomalies, such as hemivertebrae, associated with such lesions which can only be detected radiologically.

In general, most infants have flaccid paralysis but this may be combined with spastic weakness and contractures of joints. An excellent description of the assessment of the newborn is given by Stark (1971).

Hydrocephalus is almost always present in myelomeningocele and occurs in virtually 100 per cent if the lesion is thoracolumbar or lumbosacral (Lorber, 1961). This hydrocephalus in young infants does not necessarily show itself by a large head or even by abnormal fontanelle tension, separation of the sutures or other characteristic signs. Hydrocephalus does not '*develop*' postnatally after closure of the spinal lesion or for any other reason, except for ventriculitis. It does, however, become *clinically evident* in most infants, within a short time. Hydrocephalus can only be excluded or diagnosed by specific investigations such as ventriculography, for which air or positive contrast media are used or, if available, computerized axial tomography, for which general anaesthesia is required. Hydrocephalus may be of variable degree from trivial to extreme. Milder cases (the majority of those spina bifida babies treated today) will have moderate hydrocephalus which does not necessarily require surgical treatment (p. 376). Such infants have an excellent chance of survival with normal sized heads and with normal intelligence, without surgery (Lorber, 1977).

Many severely affected infants suffer from kyphosis at birth which makes surgical treatment even more difficult (Sharrard, 1968). However, such infants are usually so grossly affected in every way that active treatment of any kind is contraindicated (Lorber, 1971).

Management

It is generally considered that the best results are obtained if closure of the spinal defect is carried out in the first 24 hours of life (Sharrard *et al.*, 1963). The principal reasons for early closure are to operate before the back becomes infected and possibly to prevent deterioration of the legs. However, even the earliest operation is no guarantee against ventriculitis or gross loss of muscle power.

Selective treatment

An accurate neonatal assessment (which does not necessarily need any radiological or other specific investigations) will clearly separate those patients who, subject to life-long skilful management, will have a chance of an acceptable quality of life, from those who will not.

The days of the 1960s, when in most units nearly all infants were operated on, are over. A policy of selection has been widely adopted following detailed analysis of the long-term results in a very large series (Lorber, 1971) but even before this there were units where selection was exercised in England (Hide *et al.*, 1972), Scotland (Stark and Drummond, 1973) and Australia (Smith and Smith, 1973). The results in these widely scattered units showed remarkable similarity and contraindications to active (other than palliative) treatment were based on similar criteria. These criteria were drawn up on the grounds that if a newborn infant had any one, or a combination, of the following easily ascertainable physical signs, then not only was the mortality high in spite of treatment but all the survivors had such gross combined handicaps that their quality of life was unacceptably poor. Their families underwent great and continuous privation and stress, including break-up of marriage and mental illness in the parents (Tew *et al.*, 1974).

The criteria against treatment are as follows:

a large thoracolumbar or thoracolumbosacral lesion,
severe paraplegia with no innervation below the L3 segment,
kyphosis or scoliosis clinically evident at birth,
gross hydrocephalus as shown by a head circumference exceeding the 90th
    centile by at least 2 cm,
other gross congenital defects, e.g. congenital heart disease, and
severe cerebral birth injury or intracranial haemorrhage.

In addition, if an infant whose spinal lesion is closed and who already has hydrocephalus develops meningitis, this infant should only be treated palliatively. Finally, the infant's social circumstances should be considered in detail. The fate of an abandoned or unwanted child is very grave even if his physical condition is a little better than those with major adverse criteria.

As the neonatal assessment should be carried out by an expert in this field, it is essential to refer all babies to a special centre, thus avoiding mistakes in either direction.

It is necessary in every case to have a detailed discussion with the parents, or at least with the father and a member of the mother's family, if the mother is not available or not fit for this discussion. The parents must be fully acquainted in every detail about their infant's condition and what would happen if he were given 'full active treatment' or if he were given supporting care, including mild sedation.

Such a discussion must be slow, long, in simple terms and must be conducted by a consultant with special knowledge, in the presence of at least one member of the junior medical staff and of the nurses who will be caring for the baby. At the end the doctor gives his recommendation for or against treatment and offers a second opinion if the family wishes.

Under such circumstances the parents usually come to the same conclusion as the doctor, and long before he has made his recommendation. In a consecutive series of 100 infants referred to this author, active treatment was not recommended in 63. All the parents agreed and most asked that something should be done quickly, to shorten the infant's life. Although this is not possible, all untreated infants are sedated gently, are given demand feeding, normal nursing care and no more. The baby is kept in hospital as long as he lives, unless the parents insist on taking him home. Tube feeding, the administration of oxygen, antibiotics or any other treatments which may prolong life are forbidden. Half-treatment is the worst of all possibilities and palliative operations (e.g. shunt operation for the hydrocephalus) are most unwise, because they prolong life. Anticonvulsants or any other drug that makes the baby more comfortable and free from pain are naturally given as needed.

The parents of infants not given active treatment must be fully supported as long as their infant lives. After the infant dies they must be seen again to reassure them that the birth of their severely handicapped infant was not their fault, to allay any guilt feelings they may have and to give full genetic advice. The parents' own doctor and health visitor or social worker should play an important part at this difficult stage.

Active treatment

Active treatment is recommended for, and is usually carried out on, babies who at birth do not have the adverse criteria given above.

Treatment begins with immediate closure of the spinal defect. Usually this is straightforward but meningitis or ventriculitis may develop in spite of early closure. A careful watch must be kept and if there is any suspicion a ventricular tap is carried out to diagnose or exclude infection. In mild cases of spina bifida adequate antibiotic treatment can lead to complete recovery without adding to the infant's handicaps.

During the immediate postoperative period the infant is assessed more fully from the point of view of hydrocephalus, the whole urinary tract and the orthopaedic problems, if any.

Hydrocephalus. If there is any doubt about hydrocephalus, and certainly if the infant's occipito-frontal head circumference increases at more than an average of 1 mm per day, then ventriculography is carried out and the degree of hydrocephalus is determined by measuring the thickness of the cerebral mantle, which in normal full-term newborns exceeds 35 mm (Lorber, 1961, 1971). Mild degrees of hydrocephalus (with considerable residual brain tissue) need no treatment; moderate degrees also frequently arrest spontaneously without physical or intellectual deficit and watchful expectancy is wiser than immediate operation. Isosorbide, an osmotic agent, can be given by mouth over several weeks or months and surgery can often be either avoided altogether (Fig. 18.2) or can be delayed, if the response is not fully satisfactory (Lorber, 1975). More severe degrees of hydrocephalus do not respond to medical treatment. Severe cases (where the cerebral mantle may only be a few millimetres thick) and those with moderate ventricular dilatation, whose hydrocephalus nevertheless is rapidly progressive, must be operated on using valve incorporated shunts.

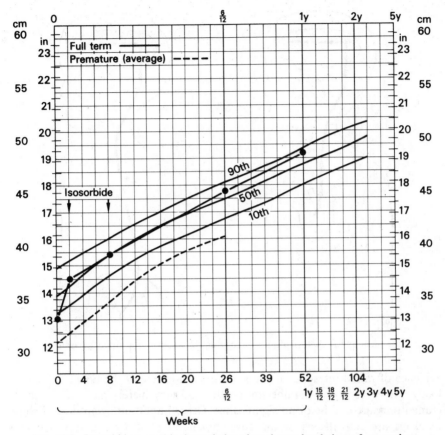

Fig. 18.2. Isosorbide treated hydrocephalus plotted on a head circumference chart.

There are many types of shunts available, the Pudenz-Heyer and the Holter being the most commonly used. The latter may be used with a Rickham reservoir interposed between the ventricular catheter and the valve chamber. With this device one can ascertain and relieve ventricular pressure without puncturing the brain, obtain samples of CSF to check for infection and inject antibiotic drugs.

The two main forms of drainage are ventriculoatrial and ventriculoperitoneal Fig. 18.3a and b). There is no conclusive evidence that either is superior to the other and often if one blocks the alternative route is used in the same patient.

Such shunts do not require to be pumped, but either the chamber between the two valves in the Holter system or the reservoir in the Pudenz system can be checked for patency by compression with the finger. Normally the chamber is full of CSF and not tense. It should compress easily and refill quickly. Blockage of the lower catheter (by blood clot in the veins or omental cysts in the peritoneum) is suspected if the chamber is stiff and hard to compress, and if the child has signs or symptoms of raised intracranial pressure, such as a bulging fontanelle in an infant, or headache, vomiting, drowsiness or papilloedema in an older child. If the chamber is flat, or very slow to refill, with accompanying

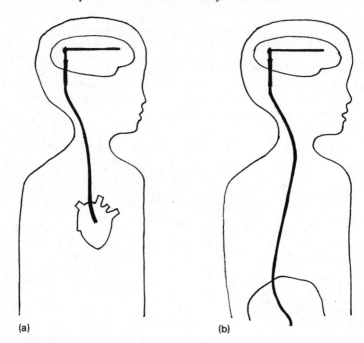

(a)   (b)

FIG. 18.3a and b. Ventriculo-atrial and ventriculo-peritoneal drainage systems.

evidence of raised intracranial pressure, then blockage of the upper catheter is likely. However, a flat chamber in a well child may merely mean a low intracranial pressure and be of no significance. Other important symptoms of shunt blockage are convulsions or the development of paralytic squint which may remain permanent.

Complications of shunt therapy are frequent and, if not promptly dealt with, may threaten life, intelligence and vision. These complications are principally blockages of the shunt at either end, detachment or breakage of catheters and infection. Colonization of the shunt system leads to ventriculitis or chronic septicaemia.

Once a patient has a shunt he must be under continuous supervision. After successful insertion the head may stop growing for a time and then start growing at a normal rate. The head circumference must be plotted on a chart. Any sudden increase is an indication of shunt blockage and must be dealt with by exploring the shunt and correcting the blockage. In older children blockage will rarely cause sudden enlargement of the head, but the symptoms and signs mentioned above must always be looked for at every clinic attendance or if the child is not well. Ophthalmoscopy is an essential routine part of the follow-up examinations.

Colonization of a ventriculoatrial shunt manifests itself as a chronic illness with low grade prolonged pyrexia, progressive anaemia, wasting, enlargement of the spleen and possibly petechial rash. The commonest organism responsible is the Staphylococcus albus, which may be cultured from the CSF or the blood.

Confirmation of the diagnosis may also be obtained by a high or rising antibody titre in the blood (Bayston, 1975). Occasionally more virulent organisms may cause septicaemia and a more fulminating illness. Antibiotic treatment alone can rarely eradicate shunt colonization. Continuous antibiotic treatment for years, e.g. with penicillin or co-trimoxazole, may keep the patient fully well but more often the shunt has to be removed and after antibiotic treatment a new one inserted, *if* the hydrocephalus is still active. One rare complication of colonization is shunt nephritis, with albuminuria, haematuria and casts in the urine.

Unfortunately shunt complications mean repeated operations. Some children are lucky and may need none in the first 5 years of life, others have many, even 10 or more. Late recognition of shunt complications is common, mortality is high and morbidity is even higher. Most patients who have a shunt will need it for a lifetime. It is for these reasons that a very conservative policy in dealing with the hydrocephalus is advocated. The institution of shunt therapy was the greatest advance in the treatment of hydrocephalus, but it is essential to use such an excellent though dangerous method of treatment with great caution. The decision whether or when to operate requires considerable clinical judgment in the light of all available evidence.

With proper management of the hydrocephalus, children with spina bifida born without adverse criteria should reach 5 years of age with normal intelligence, normal sight, no fits and a normal sized head.

Urological aspects. After closure of the back lesion the urinary tract is assessed. This includes clinical assessment by watching the pattern of the infant's spontaneous micturition and by expressing the bladder. It is not possible to express the bladder (by Credé's manoeuvre) in infants with normal bladder function. A manually expressible bladder and dribbling incontinence, with increased flow rate on crying (when the abdominal muscles contract and produce a form of bladder expression) are indications of neurogenic incontinence. Less often the bladder has autonomic innervation, the baby can pass a good stream but this will never become a conscious act, as there is no connection between the sacral bladder centre and the cerebral centres.

The urine is examined microscopically, cultured and any infection treated appropriately. Before the infant is discharged from hospital the parents should be taught how to obtain clean samples and culture the urine themselves, using the dip slide technique. Fresh urine must also be tested at each clinic visit. The prevention and adequate treatment of infection is of paramount importance.

Kidney structure and function are investigated by intravenous pyelography soon after birth and, if the child is incontinent, at approximately 2 yearly intervals thereafter. Micturating cysto-urethrography, isotope renography and cystometry are additional techniques which may add further valuable information for the management of the child.

The usual way to manage urinary incontinence is by bladder expression four to five times daily, to prevent residual urine and hence recurrent or chronic infections. If expression is difficult then dilatation of the urethra or operation on the bladder neck may be helpful. An alternative method, especially in girls, is catheterization, but this method is only suitable if the utmost cleanliness can be guaranteed. Catheterization may be intermittent (several times a day) or continuous. An indwelling catheter of rubber or silastic is attached to a plastic bag which should be frequently emptied and the catheter changed once a week. A daily bladder washout with 1 per cent hibitane solution is recommended and some clinicians also prefer to keep these children on permanent antibacterial prophylaxis. However, in some children leakage of urine occurs around the catheter, others develop sensitivity to the polythene or rubber and in some cases hygiene at home is poor. These children have to be kept in nappies till a later date.

Major surgery, i.e. the creation of an ileo-cutaneous ureterostomy ('ileal conduit' or 'loop'), is very rarely advocated now, especially for younger children and then only for major medical and not for social reasons. The complications of such an operation are many and serious and deterioration of the upper renal tract may occur in spite of it. However, if an ileal conduit is recommended, the parents should be given the manual on the care of such appliances published by the Association for Spina Bifida and Hydrocephalus (Smith *et al.*, 1976).

There is no convincing evidence that intravesical or other forms of electrical stimulation are of benefit for the control of incontinence and the use of new drugs, such as phenoxybenzamine, is still in the early stages of assessment. Nevertheless, by 5 years of age, in intelligent children with intelligent parents, bladder training can be attempted and is sometimes successful.

Unfortunately, urinary problems are frequent and can be serious even in the least severely affected children, with sacral myelomengingoceles and no other problems.

Orthopaedic aspects. Most children with myelomengingocele will have some paralysis and consequent deformities. It is essential to remember that in spina bifida all deformities are due to paralytic lesions and therefore cannot be permanently corrected by immobilization. Furthermore, plaster casts may be dangerous in children who are analgesic as sores can be produced. Prolonged immobilization also predisposes to the already considerable risk of almost spontaneous, and usually painless, fractures.

The orthopaedic surgeon must assess the newborn baby and prepare his plans with three main aims in mind (Sharrard, 1976): to correct deformity, to maintain its correction, to prevent recurrence, and to avoid production of other deformities; to obtain the best possible locomotor function; to prevent or minimize the effects of sensory and motor deficiency.

Much can be achieved by surgery but 'cure' is usually out of the question and even the best operations may fail to achieve their object fully or may be followed by further deformities. There is, therefore, a swing away from too active orthopaedic intervention and the aim now is to make the most of one or two operative sessions, when multiple relatively minor procedures are carried out (Menelaus, 1976).

With skill most children now being actively treated should be able to walk with minimal apparatus (such as below-knee calipers and a rollator) by 5 years of age. It is essential to ensure that the child's feet are plantigrade and that he can wear proper shoes.

The pressure points must be carefully looked after in children with analgesia. Sores can develop quickly as a result of pressure or exposure to heat or cold and such sores take a very long time to heal. Under 5 years of age problems of scoliosis rarely arise.

Ophthalmic aspects. There is a very high incidence of squints in spina bifida children, so that ophthalmic assessment and care is an essential part of the 'combined clinic' for most children. Furthermore, shunt complications in hydrocephalic children often manifest themselves as or lead to ophthalmic problems, so that the help of an ophthalmologist, especially in difficult cases, is valuable. The management of squint in spina bifida does not differ from that in other children (p. 422).

Social, economic and family aspects. It is impossible in a short text to do justice to these vitally important aspects. Fortunately, local and national spina bifida associations exist (Association for Spina Bifida and Hydrocephalus, and the Scottish Spina Bifida Association) and parents should be encouraged to belong to their nearest branch. The Associations are able to give all forms of advice as well as more practical help. Many branches, as well as ASBAH itself, have homes for holidays and temporary care. They publish a journal, *Link*, and booklets (see below) which should be given to parents on their child's discharge from hospital. Contact with other members of the Association is most valuable and of benefit to families.

Booklets for parents

Your Child with Spina Bifida. J. Lorber
Your Child with Hydrocephalus. J. Lorber
The Nursery Years. S. Haskell and M.E. Paul
Children with Spina Bifida at School. ed. P. Henderson
The Care of an Ileal Conduit and Urinary Appliances. E.D. Smith and others
Clothing for the Spina Bifida Child. B. Webster
Available from ASBAH, 30 Devonshire Street, London W1N 2EB

The Spina Bifida Baby (being revised). O.R. Nettles
Growing Up with Spina Bifida. O.R. Nettles
Available from the Scottish Spina Bifida Association, 190 Queensferry Road, Edinburgh EH4 2BW.

References

BAYSTON R. (1975) Serological surveillance of children with CSF shunting devices. *Developmental Medicine and Child Neurology*, **17**, Suppl. **35**, 104.

BROCK D.J.H. and SUTCLIFFE R.G. (1972) Alpha fetoprotein in the antenatal diagnosis of anencephaly and spina bifida. *Lancet*, **ii**, 197.

HIDE D.W., PARRY WILLIAMS H. and ELLIS H.L. (1972) The outlook for a child with myelomeningocele for whom early surgery was considered inadvisable. *Developmental Medicine and Child Neurology*, **14**, 304.

LAURENCE K.M. (1969) The recurrence risk in spina bifida cystica and anencephaly. *Developmental Medicine and Child Neurology*, *11*, Suppl. **20**, 23.

LAURENCE K.M., CARTER C.O. and DAVID P.A. (1968) Major central nervous system malformations in South Wales. I. Incidence, local variations and geographical factors. II. Pregnancy factors, seasonal variation and social class effects. *British Journal of Preventive and Social Medicine*, **22**. 146, 212.

LORBER J. (1961) Systematic ventriculographic studies in infants born with meningomyelocele and encephalocele. The incidence and development of hydrocephalus. *Archives of Disease in Childhood*, **36**, 381.

LORBER J. (1965) The family of spina bifida cystica. *Pediatrics*, **35**, 589.

LORBER J. (1971) Results of treatment of myelomeningocele. An analysis of 524 unselected cases with special reference to possible selection for treatment. *Developmental Medicine and Child Neurology*, **13**, 279.

LORBER J. (1971) Medical and surgical aspects in the treatment of congenital hydrocephalus. *Neuropädiatrie*, **2**, 239.

LORBER J. (1972) Spina bifida cystica: results of treatment of 270 consecutive cases with criteria for selection for the future. *Archives of Disease in Childhood*, **47**, 854.

LORBER J. (1975) Isosorbide in treatment of infantile hydrocephalus *Archives of Disease in Childhood*, **50**, 431.

LORBER J. (1977) In the press.

MENELAUS, M.B. (1977) Orthopaedic management of children with myelomeningocele: a plea for realistic goals. *Developmental Medicine and Child Neurology*, *18*, Suppl. **37**, 3.

SHARRARD W.J.W. (1962) The mechanism of paralytic deformity in spina bifida. *Developmental Medicine and Child Neurology*, **4**, 310.

SHARRARD W.J.W. (1968) Spinal osteotomy for congenital kyphosis in myelomeningocele. *Journal of Bone and Joint Surgery*, **50B**, 466.

SHARRARD W.J.W. (1976) General orthopaedic management and operative treatment. In *Spina Bifida for the Clinician*. eds. Brocklehurst G., Sharrard W.J.W., Forrest D. and Stark G. *Clinics in Developmental Medicine. No. 57*. London: Heinemann.

SHARRARD W.J.W., ZACHARY R.B., LORBER J. and BRUCE A.M. (1963) A controlled trial of immediate and delayed closure of spina bifida cystica. *Archives of Disease in Childhood*, **38**, 18.

SMITH G.K. and SMITH E.D. (1973) Selection for treatment in spina bifida cystica. *British Medical Journal*, **4**, 189.

SMITH E.D., MAGNUS R., SMITH E., LORBER J., ZACHARY R.B. and ESHELBY J. (1976) *The Care of an Ileal Conduit and Urinary Appliances in Children*. London: Association for Spina Bifida and Hydrocephalus.

STARK G.D. (1971) Neonatal assessment of the child with myelomeningocele. *Archives of Disease in Childhood*, **46**, 539.

STARK G.D. and DRUMMOND M. (1973) Results of selective early operation in myelomeningocele. *Archives of Disease in Childhood*, **48**, 676.

STEWART C.R., MILFORD WARD A. and LORBER J. (1975) Amniotic fluid alpha fetoprotein in the diagnosis of neural tract malformations. *British Journal of Obstetrics and Gynaecology*, **82**, 257.

TEW B.J., PAYNE H. and LAURENCE K.M. (1974) Must a family with a handicapped child be a handicapped family? *Developmental Medicine and Child Neurology*, *16*, Suppl. **32**. 95.

WALD N.S., BROCK D.J.H. and BONNAR J. (1974) Prenatal diagnosis of spina bifida and anencephaly by maternal serum alpha fetoprotein measurement. A controlled study. *Lancet*, **i**, 765.

Further Reading

STARK G.D. (1977) *Spina Bifida: problems and management*. Oxford: Blackwell Scientific Publications.

CHAPTER 19

Neuromuscular Disorders

Our knowledge and understanding of neuromuscular disorders of childhood has increased considerably over the last two decades. The application of modern techniques of investigation, in particular enzyme histochemistry and electron-microscopy, has led to a better delineation of the various clinical syndromes and to the discovery of many new muscle disorders.

Classification

Neuromuscular disorders can be classified by the anatomical site of the main lesion, as shown in Fig. 19.1. Not all the disorders fall neatly into this classification, e.g. some of the glycogen storage diseases can affect both muscle and anterior horn cell. Nevertheless, it is practical and ensures that all the possible conditions not immediately evident are considered.

Clinical Presentation

Most of the conditions listed in Fig. 19.1 will present either as a floppy infant with delayed motor milestones or with muscle weakness in later childhood.

Floppy infant syndrome
Assessment of tone. The floppy infant is hypotonic. Tone is assessed by observing posture in supine and prone, at rest and against gravity. The floppy infant lies with hips abducted and flexed, knees flexed and arms flexed or extended. With traction on the arms there is complete head lag and on ventral suspension the head, arms and legs hang down limply. Head lag can also be due to increased extensor tone in the neck muscles, but in this case the head will be extended in the prone position. Face and brow presentations at delivery may produce similar head posture, but this disappears within a few days of birth.

Tone is also assessed by feeling the resistance to passive movement, especially in the elbows, hips and knees, and by checking the range of movement, especially in abduction of the hips and extension of the knees. The joints show excessive mobility and the knee and elbow joints often hyperextend. Hyperextensibility is not always due to decreased muscle tone and may be due to lax ligaments.

Differential diagnosis of the floppy infant syndrome has been reviewed by Dubowitz (1969a).

A useful practical guide for distinguishing hypotonia due to a lower motor

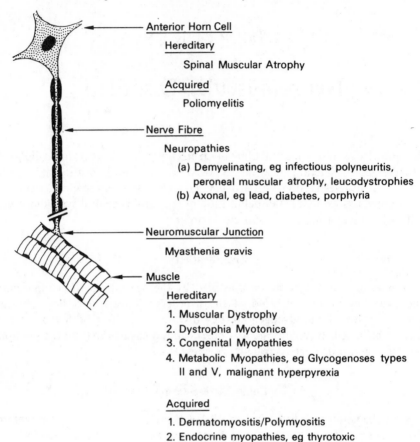

Anterior Horn Cell

Hereditary

Spinal Muscular Atrophy

Acquired

Poliomyelitis

Nerve Fibre

Neuropathies

(a) Demyelinating, eg infectious polyneuritis,
peroneal muscular atrophy, leucodystrophies
(b) Axonal, eg lead, diabetes, porphyria

Neuromuscular Junction

Myasthenia gravis

Muscle

Hereditary

1. Muscular Dystrophy
2. Dystrophia Myotonica
3. Congenital Myopathies
4. Metabolic Myopathies, eg Glycogenoses types
II and V, malignant hyperpyrexia

Acquired

1. Dermatomyositis/Polymyositis
2. Endocrine myopathies, eg thyrotoxic
3. Iatrogenic, eg steriod myopathy

FIG. 19.1. Classification of neuromuscular disorders of infancy and childhood based on the anatomical site of the main lesion.

neurone or muscle lesion from that due to a central nervous system lesion is to ask oneself the following question: is the child floppy and weak or is the child floppy but not significantly weak, as crudely judged by ability to lift up arms or legs against gravity? If hypotonia can be explained by weakness then one is dealing in most instances with a disorder of the lower motor neurone or muscle, e.g. spinal muscular atrophy or myopathy. If the infant is floppy but not significantly weak than one is probably dealing with a central problem.

Hypotonia may simply be a variation of normal as occurs in the pre-term infant. It also occurs in generalized disorders such as malnutrition, malabsorption, rickets, chronic renal disease, chromosomal abnormalities and non-specific primary mental retardation. Another important and often neglected cause of hypotonia and delayed motor development is maternal deprivation in the early months of life (Buda *et al.*, 1972). Hypotonia as an early manifestation of cerebral palsy is discussed elsewhere (p. 267).

Hypotonia and feeding difficulties in early infancy followed by stunting of growth, obesity, delayed skeletal maturation and mental retardation should suggest Prader-Willi syndrome. These children have small almond shaped eyes, triangular shaped mouth, fair hair and blue eyes, small hands and feet, and males have undescended testes.

In severe cervical cord injury, usually following difficult breech extraction, the child is paralysed from the neck down and may look like an infant with Werdnig-Hoffman disease. However, reflexes in the lower limbs are often brisk with ankle clonus.

Amongst floppy infants without significant muscle weakness are those with laxity of ligaments and others with variants of the Ehlers-Danlos syndrome, in both of which improvement occurs although hypermobility of joints may persist (McKusick, 1972). These infants often have blue sclera and there is frequently a positive family history of double jointedness.

Walton (1957) first used the term benign congenital hypotonia to describe a group of floppy infants with delayed motor control in whom improvement, and in some complete recovery, occurred. The application of modern techniques of investigation have led to a virtual disappearance of this entity; many causes of this syndrome are now recognized, all of which are relatively benign.

The floppy infant syndrome does not always carry a bad prognosis and every attempt should be made to arrive at an accurate diagnosis.

Muscle weakness
The older child with neuromuscular disorder usually presents with symptoms attributable to muscle weakness. Common are 'waddling' gait, difficulties in climbing stairs, inability to stand or hop on one leg, frequent falls, and difficulties in getting up from the supine position. The child with weakness of the trunk and pelvic girdle muscles will get up from the floor by rolling over from supine to prone, and pushing himself up on his legs with his arms until he is sufficiently erect to extend the trunk (the classical Gowers' sign). This manoeuvre is not pathognomonic of Duchenne dystrophy; it simply indicates weakness of trunk and pelvic girdle muscles and can be seen in other disorders such as spinal muscular atrophy or congenital myopathy. Sometimes the only evidence of weakness in the pelvic girdle muscles is the fact that on getting up from the floor the child momentarily uses one hand to push on his knee.

Investigation of Neuromuscular Disorders

The three investigations needed for accurate diagnosis are blood creatine phosphokinase estimation, electromyography and nerve conduction, and muscle biopsy (Moosa, 1974a).

Creatine phosphokinase (CPK)
The CPK levels usually encountered in various neuromuscular disorders are listed in Table 19.1.

TABLE 19.1. Serum CPK levels in neuromuscular diseases.

Disease	Serum CPK level iu/litre
Normal	8–60
Muscular dystrophy	
Duchenne type (sex-linked)	> 1000
Female carriers	10–500
Limb-girdle	10–500 but may exceed 1000
Facio-scapulo-humeral	10–200
Dystrophia myotonica	10–200
Congenital myopathies	10–200
Polymyositis/dermatomyositis	Normal but may be > 1000 in acute phase
Neurogenic atrophies	Normal
Benign Kugelberg-Welander type	10–200
Glycogenoses, e.g. McArdle's syndrome	Up to 1000
Malignant hyperpyrexia	
Acute	> 1000
Subclinical	10–200

Electrophysiology

Every floppy infant or child with muscle weakness should have nerve conduction and electromyographic studies done. This requires patience and understanding of children and is best done by a paediatrician with training in neuromuscular disorders. Satisfactory examinations can be made in almost all infants and young children without resort to general anaesthesia or sedation.

Nerve conduction studies. By stimulating a suitable superficial nerve (such as the ulnar or posterior tibial) and recording the evoked motor response from an appropriate muscle, the conduction velocity can be determined. This is contingent on the diameter and degree of myelination of the nerve's constituent fibres and is age dependent. Slow nerve conduction velocities usually indicate the presence of a peripheral neuropathy.

Electromyography (EMG) is best performed using a concentric needle electrode inserted into a suitable muscle (judged on clinical assessment of weakness). The electrical activity generated by contracting muscles is amplified and displayed audiovisually. A normal muscle at rest shows electrical silence but with activity motor unit potentials are generated. These are the electrical potentials produced by the group of muscle fibres stimulated by single motor neurones. With increasing activity they summate to produce the so-called interference pattern (Fig. 19.2).

Changes in EMG parameters help localize the lesion to the anterior horn cell, peripheral nerve or muscle.

Denervation produces fibrillation and fasciculation potentials at rest; the former are biphasic, of low amplitude and short duration and are generated by single muscle fibres. The latter are of high amplitude, are polyphasic and are

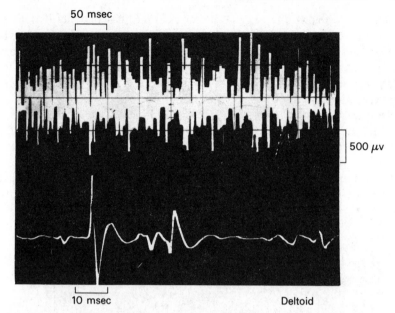

50 msec

500 μv

10 msec   Deltoid

FIG. 19.2. EMG of the deltoid muscle in a normal child. Above: normal interference pattern. Below: normal triphasic single motor unit potential.

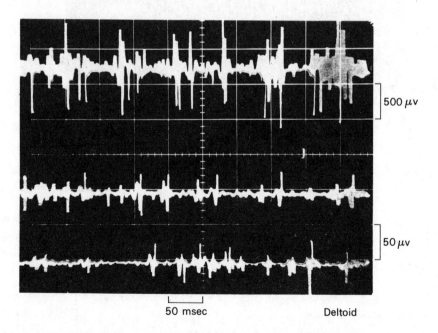

500 μv

50 μv

50 msec   Deltoid

FIG. 19.3. EMG of the deltoid muscle in an infant with Werdnig-Hoffmann disease. Above: reduced interference pattern. Below: fibrillation potentials indicating denervated fibres.

produced by lesions affecting the motor neurone. Whereas fibrillation is not visible to the naked eye, fasciculation potentials may be accompanied by visible contractions within the muscle. A decreased interference pattern is seen with activity. In chronic denervating processes the motor unit potentials are of higher amplitude and longer duration and more polyphasic than normal due to reinnervation (Fig. 19.3).

Because of random loss of muscle fibres in myopathies, the motor unit potentials are of smaller amplitude, shorter duration and more polyphasic than normal (myopathic EMG) (Fig. 19.4). The full interference pattern is usually maintained until the late stages of the disease. Fasciculation potentials at rest do not occur and fibrillation potentials are rare. When fibrillation potentials at rest are frequent with a myopathic EMG, then polymyositis is a strong possibility.

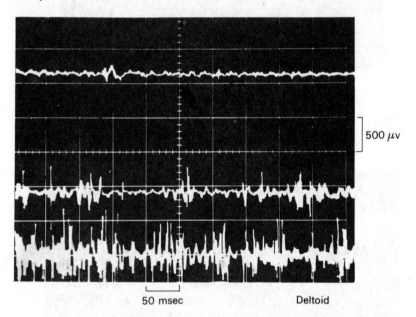

FIG. 19.4. EMG of the deltoid muscle in a boy with Duchenne dystrophy. Above: no spontaneous activity at rest. Below: typical myopathic pattern.

Myotonia, which is shown by delayed relaxation after voluntary contraction, produces a very typical EMG with characteristic after-discharges which wax and wane and produce a typical 'dive-bomber' sound (Fig. 19.5). Myotonic discharges occur in myotonia congenita and dystrophia myotonica.

Muscle biopsy

Most patients with a neuromuscular disorder will require a muscle biopsy to establish a definite diagnosis. It is best if the patient is referred to one of the centres specializing in muscle histochemistry, rather than sending a muscle sample which often arrives in an unsatisfactory state.

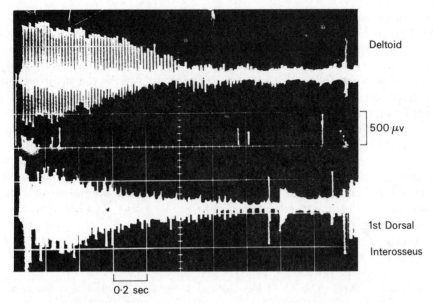

Deltoid

500 μv

1st Dorsal

Interosseus

0·2 sec

FIG. 19.5. EMG of the deltoid muscle in a child with dystrophia myotonica (above) and of the first dorsal interosseus muscle of her mother (below) showing characteristic after-discharges.

It is beyond the scope of this chapter to describe the histological and histo-chemical changes in detail; readers are referred to the text by Dubowitz and Brooke (1973). Briefly, histochemical studies show that muscle fibres consist essentially of two fibre types, those rich in oxidative enzymes (type 1) and those rich in glycolytic enzymes (type 2). In certain conditions there is predominant involvement of one or other type of fibre. Muscle biopsy will distinguish the denervating from the 'myopathic' disorders in most instances. Muscle histo-chemistry and biochemistry and electron microscopy are essential for the diagnosis of many of the congenital myopathies (p. 396).

Spinal Muscular Atrophy

Clinical features
Spinal muscular atrophy is a hereditary disease characterized by degeneration and loss of motor neurones in the spinal cord and brain stem.

Severe infantile form (Werdnig-Hoffman disease). The onset is *in utero* or within 2–3 months of birth. Quickening is felt at the normal time but there may be a cessation of fetal movement. The onset may be equally abrupt postnatally and a normally active infant suddenly become paralysed. Occasionally there is a preceding infectious illness but in the majority of cases there are no precipitating factors.

The infant is very hypotonic and virtually completely paralysed. Proximal muscles are more severely affected than distal, and lower limbs more than upper limbs. The infant lies in the frog-like posture with hips abducted and flexed.

The arms may show limitation of external rotation at the shoulders so that they lie in an internally rotated and jug-handle position with elbows flexed and hands pronated. The trunk muscles are also severely affected and the infant will be unable to control his head. Facial muscles are not usually involved and the infant smiles and follows with his eyes. Fasciculation of the tongue, if present, is diagnostic. Bulbar paralysis is almost invariable with difficulty in swallowing and accumulation of secretions. Respiratory muscles are involved and respirations are entirely diaphragmatic. The diaphragm is also involved, but to a lesser extent than the intercostal muscles. The cry is weak. The reflexes are all absent. There are no sphincter disturbances nor any obvious sensory impairment. Some infants sweat profusely and this may indicate involvement of the autonomic nervous system. The heart is not involved. Contractures are not conspicuous and the distal contractures of hands and feet that occur in arthrogryposis are not seen.

Prognosis is very poor and death usually occurs within the first year from recurrent respiratory infections.

Intermediate form. The child has normal early milestones and achieves the ability to sit unaided at the normal age of 8–9 months. Thereafter, no further motor progress occurs and he is unable to stand or walk (Dubowitz, 1964). Weakness is symmetrical but affects legs more than arms. The face is unaffected and usually bulbar muscles are spared. Fasciculation of the tongue is more frequently seen in this form and occasionally fasciculation of skeletal muscles may be observed. A characteristic but not pathognomonic sign observed in this and the mild form is a coarse tremor of the outstretched hands (Moosa and Dubowitz, 1973). The respiratory muscles may be involved but less so than in the severe form. Contractures may develop and are almost always due to faulty posture. Scoliosis will adversely affect prognosis because of further encroachment on the respiratory reserve, if not prevented by adequate bracing and ensuring that the wheelchair has a soft pliable back. Contractures of hips and knees are common because of wheelchair existence. They can be prevented by active physiotherapy, and this is particularly important in those children with sufficient power in their arms to cope with sticks and long leg calipers, who can be kept ambulant longer if assessed and treated early. These children are often of above average intelligence.

Prognosis depends on respiratory function. Those with good function will survive into adulthood, albeit in a wheelchair.

Mild form (Kugelberg and Welander, 1956). This type usually has a later onset, children are less severely affected and achieve the ability to walk unaided, although this may be delayed. They usually present with symptoms which are similar to those of muscular dystrophy (p. 393), with which the condition is often confused. If present, fasciculation of tongue and skeletal muscle and tremor of hands will distinguish it from muscular dystrophy. Another difference is the tendency for the feet to evert so that patients are flat-footed, whereas those with Duchenne muscular dystrophy tend to walk on their toes.

Legs are more affected than arms and tendon reflexes may be normal or absent. Respiratory involvement does not occur as a rule.

Prognosis is good, the weakness remains static and may even improve, probably because of reinnervation. Occasionally the weakness may be very slowly progressive.

Diagnosis
Serum enzymes. The serum CPK is usually normal except in the mild form in which it may be increased two- to three-fold.

Electrophysiology. The nerve conduction velocities are normal in the intermediate and mild forms. In the severe form consistently slow motor nerve conduction velocities have been found (Moosa and Dubowitz, 1976).

On EMG, regular fasciculation potentials are diagnostic of the severe form. Fibrillation potentials are also seen and on activity the interference pattern is reduced, the motor units being of higher amplitude, longer duration and more polyphasic than normal. In the mild and intermediate forms the changes in the motor units on activity are even more marked, producing the so-called giant units. These EMG changes will be found in all proximal muscles examined.

Muscle biopsy. The typical changes consist of atrophy of large groups of fibres (often bundles) with other groups of fibres remaining of normal size or hypertrophied. On histochemical staining the atrophic fibres will consist of both fibre types, whereas the hypertrophied fibres show uniform staining reaction. This fibre type grouping is indicative of reinnervation.

Genetics
All forms of spinal muscular atrophy are hereditary with an autosomal recessive mode of inheritance. Occasional families with dominant mode of inheritance are described but these usually have the milder form of the disease. As a rule there is concordance of severity within families but many instances of spinal muscular atrophy of varying severity, occurring within the same family, are recorded. This provides the strongest evidence in favour of a single genetic basis for the various clinical syndromes of spinal muscular atrophy. However, there is still debate about this and many consider the severe form to be genetically distinct from the others.

Heterozygotes are asymptomatic and do not show any abnormality in the serum enzymes, EMG or muscle biopsy.

Management
There is no effective treatment for this condition apart from the supportive measures described.

Peripheral Neuropathies

This diagnosis is often difficult in infants and young children. The application of motor nerve conduction studies, however, has greatly facilitated the diagnosis. Disorders of the peripheral nerve affect mainly the axon or the Schwann cell (Thomas, 1971).

Axonal neuropathies
Here the primary disturbance of function is in the axon. As this is an extension of the cell body, disorders of anterior horn cells may be considered as examples of axonal neuropathies. Other causes include thalidomide and vincristine toxicity, thiamine deficiency and genetic factors (the hereditary sensory neuropathies).

The motor nerve conduction velocities in axonal neuropathies are normal or slightly reduced.

Demyelinating neuropathies
Diseases of Schwann cell produce segmental demyelination which causes gross slowing of neural conduction. Segmental demyelination may be confined to the peripheral nervous system or may occur in association with a more widespread demyelinating disorder involving the CNS as well.

Neuropathies with CNS involvement. Demyelinating peripheral neuropathy occurs in metachromatic and globoid cell type leucodystrophy, and its detection by slow nerve conduction is a valuable screening test for distinguishing the leucodystrophies from other progressive degenerative disorders of the CNS. A similar neuropathy occurs in Cockayne's syndrome (Moosa and Dubowitz, 1970) and in some cases of subacute necrotizing encephalomyelopathy of Leigh (Moosa, 1975).

Neuropathies without CNS involvement. Segmental demyelination confined to the peripheral nerves occurs in the Guillain-Barré syndrome, peroneal muscular atrophy and hereditary hypertrophic polyneuropathy of Dejerine-Sottas syndrome. These conditions all produce marked slowing of nerve conduction. All may present with delay in reaching normal motor milestones and clumsiness in childhood. Weakness is predominantly peripheral and reflexes usually absent. Peroneal muscular atrophy is inherited as a dominant and one or other parent will have slow motor conduction, even in the absence of clinical symptoms. In early childhood wasting of peroneal muscles may not be obvious and the diagnosis made with nerve conduction studies only. This form of dominantly inherited polyneuropathy is the commonest form of chronic neuropathy encountered in paediatric practice.

Myasthenia Gravis

Myasthenia gravis is rare in paediatric practice (Millichap and Dodge, 1960). Nevertheless it is an important condition to consider in differential diagnosis of a floppy infant or a child with relapsing and remitting weakness, since it is one of the few neuromuscular conditions that can be effectively treated.

Myasthenia gravis can affect the offspring of a mother with the condition. Such infants become floppy and develop feeding and respiratory difficulty from accumulated secretions soon after birth. Congenital myasthenia is even rarer and usually presents either with episodic weakness of limbs, which may or may not be associated with ophthalmoplegia and ptosis, or with recurrent episodes of respiratory difficulties due to bulbar paralysis. An immediate improvement in muscle power following intravenous Tensilon (1 mg IV) confirms the diagnosis.

Muscular Dystrophy

The term muscular dystrophy refers to those inherited disorders in which there is progressive weakness and degeneration of skeletal muscle without apparent cause in either the peripheral or central nervous system (Moosa, 1974b). It is still not clear if the primary defect is in nerve, muscle or in blood (Dubowitz, 1971), although recent evidence suggests the muscle membrane as the primary site of abnormality.

Classification
The most practical classification is that suggested by Dubowitz (1969b), based in the first instance on the clinical distribution and severity of weakness and then subdivided on the basis of inheritance (Table 19.2).

TABLE 19.2. Classification of muscular dystrophies.

Clinical type	Inheritance
Duchenne type	
Pelvic girdle (severe form)	Sex-linked recessive (usual)
	Autosomal recessive (rare)
Limb-girdle	
Pelvic girdle (mild form)	Autosomal recessive (usual)
	Sporadic
	Sex-linked recessive (Becker type)
	Autosomal dominant (rare)
Scapulo-humeral	Autosomal recessive
	Sporadic
Facio-scapulo-humeral	Autosomal dominant (usual)
	Autosomal recessive (rare)

Duchenne muscular dystrophy
This is the commonest form of muscular dystrophy and the commonest neuro-muscular disorder of early childhood. The incidence varies from 1 in 3000 male live births (Zellweger and Antonik, 1975) to 1 in 50 000 (Pearson, 1973). The prevalence in the UK is about 3 per 100 000, of which one-third are new mutants (Gardner-Medwin, 1970).

Clinical features. Duchenne dystrophy characteristically affects boys. Symptoms (p. 383) are usually noted within the first 3 years of life. Prominence of the calves is an early feature. Other muscles such as deltoid, brachio-radialis and quadriceps may also show this prominence. The tongue is frequently enlarged; this 'pseudohypertrophy' can occur in other types of muscular dystrophy.

The proximal muscles are always affected before the distal ones; the pelvic girdle muscles more than the scapulo-humeral. Facial muscles are unaffected except in the terminal stages. Sphincter control and swallowing are usually normal. The upper arm reflexes and the knee jerks are lost early while the ankle jerks are retained and may even be brisk. The plantar responses are flexor.

A proportion of children with muscular dystrophy have marked intellectual impairment which may precede the onset of weakness. The cause is not known, but it appears to run in certain families of dystrophics.

The muscle weakness gradually increases but there may be periods of apparent arrest for 6–12 months. At other times there may be rapid deterioration, especially following immobilization in bed, even for short periods. In these circumstances the ability to walk may be lost much earlier than at the usual 9–12 years.

Deformities. These do not occur whilst the child is ambulant, except for shortening of the tendo-achillis which causes the child to walk on his toes. This is probably due to imbalance between the stronger gastrocnemius and weaker anterior tibial muscles. Once the child loses the ability to walk and is confined to a wheelchair, he rapidly develops contractures of the hip and knee flexors and, unless prevented, scoliosis and equinovarus deformity of the feet. These are all related to the habitual posture of the child. Intensive physiotherapy with passive movement of joints may prevent contractures. Whilst the child is ambulant, particular attention should be paid to the ankles. When the child can still stand but barely walk, the fitting of light-weight calipers may keep him ambulant for a few more years. Once he becomes chair-bound, a rigid seat and adequate postural support for the spine are essential to prevent scoliosis. A wheelchair with a pliable back-rest which moulds to the child's back is preferable to one with a firm back support. Appropriate posture of the feet is important to prevent equinovarus deformity.

These children usually die of pneumonia in their late teens. Cardiac involvement is common and some die in a manner similar to myocardial infarction.

Diagnosis. The following investigations are required:

Serum enzymes. In early stages of the disease the CPK may be increased 100-fold or more but the level decreases as the disease progresses and muscle bulk diminishes. A normal CPK value in infancy excludes the diagnosis.

Grossly elevated CPK may occur in other conditions such as limb-girdle muscular dystrophy or dermatomyositis, so the diagnosis of Duchenne muscular dystrophy cannot be made on the CPK levels alone.

Nerve conduction and EMG. The conduction velocities of nerves in individual patients with Duchenne dystrophy are usually within the normal range. EMG shows a characteristic pattern consisting of low amplitude, short duration, polyphasic motor unit action potentials (Fig. 19.4). This myopathic picture is common to all forms of myopathies.

Muscle biopsy. Routine histological stains show increased variability in fibre size, rounded and 'opaque' fibres, degenerating fibres and phagocytosis, and basophilic regenerating fibres. Endomysial and perimysial connective tissue proliferation occurs early and, in the later phases, is replaced by adipose tissue. Similar changes are seen in other myopathies and histochemical studies are essential to exclude the various congenital myopathies. Histochemically there is loss of the clear-cut subdivision into fibre types with a tendency to type 1 fibre predominance.

Management. There is still no effective therapy for muscular dystrophy. Supportive therapy, as described (p. 394) is important. These children are prone to respiratory infection and will need intensive physiotherapy and antibiotics.

The parents, like those of any handicapped child, will need constant help and support in coming to terms with this disease and its ultimate prognosis and in coping with practical problems at home and school.

Carrier detection. Duchenne dystrophy is inherited by an X-linked mechanism. The female carriers of the gene are usually symptom-free but may occasionally complain of cramps or show prominent calves.

Elevated CPK levels (usually up to a two- to five-fold increase) are found in about 70 per cent of known carriers. If the CPK level is consistently elevated it provides presumptive evidence of the carrier state, but if it is consistently normal there is still a 30 per cent chance of an individual being a carrier. Histological and electron microscopic changes of muscle provide further means of carrier detection. Quantitative electromyography is also of value (Moosa *et al.*, 1972).

Genetic counselling. In a known carrier there is a 50 per cent risk of a male child being affected and a female child being a carrier. Using all the criteria mentioned above, about 90 per cent of carriers can be identified. This will leave a risk of 1 in 10 of a female being a possible carrier. The risk of such a female producing an affected son is 1 in 40, a risk which many are prepared to take (Bundey, 1977).

Antenatal detection of an affected fetus is not yet possible. The technique of sexing the fetus from amniotic fluid cells is now well developed and if a male fetus is present therapeutic abortion may be recommended.

Limb-girdle and facio-scapulo-humeral dystrophy

These forms of muscular dystrophy are rarely seen in early childhood. They present in late childhood and adolescence and are much more benign than Duchenne dystrophy and compatible with a survival into adult life. Limb-girdle dystrophy is inherited by the recessive mode of inheritance and facio-scapulo-humeral dystrophy usually by the dominant mode. Dubowitz (1965) classifies benign X-linked (Becker type) muscular dystrophy as an X-linked form of limb-girdle dystrophy.

Dystrophia myotonica

This condition is usually classified with the muscular dystrophies because it is genetically determined and the primary abnormality is in the muscle itself. However, other features of the disease suggest a multi-system involvement. Although previously considered a disease of adult life, starting in adolescence, it is now well recognized that it can occur in infancy and childhood and may even be present at birth.

The presenting features include generalized hypotonia, poor sucking and swallowing, deformities of feet, facial paresis, ophthalmoplegia, gastrointestinal symptoms such as constipation, dysphagia and malabsorption, conduction defects of the heart, and severe intellectual retardation. Muscle weakness is generalized, affecting facial, sternomastoid and limb muscles. It may be asymmetrical and distal muscles may be affected more than proximal. Myotonia may be difficult to detect clinically but may occasionally be recognized by delayed opening of eyes after crying.

Inheritance is by an autosomal dominant mechanism with incomplete penetrance (Harper, 1975). Some patients within the same affected family may have minimal weakness and marked myotonia while in others the weakness is marked and myotonia is elicited on EMG only.

Diagnosis. This is made by eliciting myotonia and detecting facial weakness in the *mother*. The finding of characteristic myotonic after-discharges on EMG in mother or child confirms the diagnosis (Fig. 19.5). The serum CPK level is usually normal or mildly elevated. Routine muscle histology may show variation of fibre size with central nuclei and histochemical stains show type 1 fibre atrophy.

The conditions most often confused with dystrophia myotonica are the Möbius syndrome and facio-scapulo-humeral dystrophy. Myotonia is also found in myotonia congenita which is benign and does not cause muscle weakness.

Treatment with quinine, procainamide or steroids may alleviate the myotonia but has no effect on the weakness, which is often the patient's major disability.

Congenital myopathies

The congenital myopathies fall broadly into three groups.

(1) Those in which specific biochemical abnormalities have been identified. Examples of these include glycogen storage diseases which affect muscle (Dubowitz, 1966). Types II and III (acid maltase deficiency and debranching enzyme deficiency) usually present in infancy with a floppy infant syndrome, hepatomegaly and cardiac involvement with a characteristic ECG abnormality (short PR interval). All types can only be accurately diagnosed by detailed biochemical analysis of muscle obtained by biopsy.

(2) Those in which modern staining techniques have identified specific

structural abnormalities. Examples include central core disease, in which the centre of the muscle fibres are devoid of enzymatic activity; nemaline myopathy, in which rod-like structures are present arising from the Z-line material of muscle fibres; centronuclear myopathy, in which the nuclei are central rather than peripherally placed; congenital fibre disproportion, in which there is a disproportion in the size and number of the histochemical fibre types, and mitochondrial myopathies, in which various mitochondrial abnormalities are present.

(3) Those infants who are hypotonic and weak and have multiple contractures and myopathic EMG and whose muscle biopsy shows changes very similar to those seen in muscular dystrophy (particularly the fibrosis) hence the name congenital muscular dystrophy. However, unlike the usual forms of muscular dystrophy, the congenital form tends to be non-progressive with a good prognosis (Donner *et al.*, 1975).

All these conditions present either as the floppy infant syndrome or with proximal muscle weakness in childhood; the latter may be confused with muscular dystrophy. However the weakness is non-progressive or only slowly progressive. Some of these conditions, in particular nemaline and myotubular myopathy, may be life-threatening because of respiratory difficulties.

The CPK is usually normal in the congenital myopathies and the EMG is normal or myopathic. Accurate diagnosis is possible only with detailed histochemical and electron microscopic studies of muscle. Most of the congenital myopathies are dominantly inherited with variable penetrance so that the parent may be asymptomatic.

Dermatomyositis

This condition is not common in the under-fives and is seen mainly in later childhood. Nevertheless it is an important condition to consider in any child with weakness, especially where such weakness is intermittent, because it is potentially curable. An aphorism which has been found most useful is: weakness + misery = dermatomyositis. There is a characteristic violaceous discolouration of the skin especially over the butterfly area of the face, the eyelids, elbows, knees and knuckles, which may be fairly inconspicuous and readily missed. The course is usually one of remissions and relapses but, with steroids, a permanent remission is often obtained. The longer the delay in starting steroids, the greater the chance of complications such as contractures.

CPK level may be elevated or normal. EMG shows a mixed picture of fibrillation potentials at rest (indicating denervated fibres) and myopathic potentials on activity. Muscle histology often shows myopathic changes but may be normal. The erythrocyte sedimentation rate (ESR) may be normal or raised.

Conclusion

The last two decades have seen tremendous advances in our understanding of neuromuscular disorders of childhood and we have come a long way to realize that 'all that waddles is not dystrophy'. We now know that several neurogenic and myopathic syndromes can have similar clinical presentation, either as the floppy infant syndrome or with muscle weakness. For accurate diagnosis and prognosis full investigation is essential. This consists of CPK, EMG and nerve conduction studies, and muscle biopsy, all of which can be done on an outpatient basis. These, however, must be undertaken by those experienced in interpreting the results and in centres where proper facilities for detailed studies exist. In so doing we will ensure that the patient receives the maximum benefit from available facilities and misdiagnosis is avoided.

References

BUDA F.B., ROTHNEY W.B. and RABE E.F. (1972) Hypotonia and the maternal child relationship. *American Journal of Diseases of Children*, **124**, 906.

BUNDEY S. (1977) Genetic counselling in disorders of muscle. *British Journal of Hospital Medicine*, **17**, 342.

DONNER M., RAPOLA J. and SOMER H. (1975) Congenital muscular dystrophy: a clinico-pathological and follow-up study of 15 patients. *Neuropädiatrie*, **6**, 239.

DUBOWITZ V. (1964) Infantile muscular atrophy: a prospective study with particular reference to a slowly progressive variety. *Brain*, **87**, 707.

DUBOWITZ V. (1965) Muscular dystrophy and related disorders. *Postgraduate Medical Journal*, **41**, 332.

DUBOWITZ V. (1966) The muscle glycogenoses. *Developmental Medicine and Child Neurology*, **8**, 432.

DUBOWITZ V. (1969a) *The Floppy Infant. Clinics in Developmental Medicine, No. 31*. London: Heinemann.

DUBOWITZ V. (1969b) Muscle disorders in childhood. *British Journal of Hospital Medicine*, **2**, 1627.

DUBOWITZ V. (1971) Muscular dystrophy: where is the lesion? *Developmental Medicine and Child Neurology*, **13**, 238.

DUBOWITZ V. and BROOKE M.H. (1973) *Muscle Biopsy: A Modern Approach*. Philadelphia: W.B. Saunders.

GARDNER-MEDWIN D. (1970) Mutation rate in Duchenne type of muscular dystrophy. *Journal of Medical Genetics*, **7**, 334.

HARPER P.S. (1975) Congenital myotonic dystrophy in Britain. A. Clinical aspects. *Archives of Disease in Childhood*, **50**, 505.

KUGELBERG E. and WELANDER L. (1956) Heredofamilial juvenile muscular atrophy simulating muscular dystrophy. *Archives of Neurology and Psychiatry*, **75**, 500.

McKUSICK V.A. (1972) *Hereditable Disorders of Connective Tissue*, 4th Edition. Saint Louis: C.V. Mosby.

MILLICHAP J.G. and DODGE P.R. (1960) Diagnosis and treatment of myasthenia in infancy, childhood and adolescence. *Neurology*, **10**, 1007.

MOOSA A. (1974a) Investigation of neuromuscular disease in early childhood. *British Journal of Hospital Medicine*, **12**, 166.

MOOSA A. (1974b) Muscular dystrophy in childhood. *Developmental Medicine and Child Neurology*, **16**, 97.

MOOSA A. (1975) Peripheral neuropathy in Leigh's subacute necrotising encephalomyelopathy. *Developmental Medicine and Child Neurology*, **17**, 621.

MOOSA A., BROWN B.H. and DUBOWITZ V. (1972) Quantitative electromyography: carrier detection in Duchenne type muscular dystrophy using a new automatic technique. *Journal of Neurology, Neurosurgery and Psychiatry*, **35**, 841.

MOOSA A. and DUBOWITZ V. (1970) Peripheral neuropathy in Cockayne's syndrome. *Archives of Disease in Childhood*, **45**, 674.

MOOSA A. and DUBOWITZ V. (1973) Spinal muscular atrophy in childhood: two clues to clinical diagnosis. *Archives of Disease in Childhood*, **48**, 386.

MOOSA A. and DUBOWITZ V. (1976) Motor nerve conduction velocity in spinal muscular atrophy of childhood. *Archives of Disease in Childhood*, **51**, 974.

PEARSON C.M. (1973) Childhood pseudohypertrophic muscular dystrophy. In *Birth Defects Atlas and Compendium*, ed. Bergsma D. p. 257. Baltimore: Williams and Wilkins.

THOMAS P.K. (1971) The morphological basis for alterations in nerve conduction in peripheral neuropathy. *Proceedings of the Royal Society of Medicine*, **64**, 295.

WALTON J.N. (1957) The limp child. *Journal of Neurology, Neurosurgery and Psychiatry*, **20**, 144.

ZELLWEGER H. and ANTONIK A. (1975) Newborn screening for Duchenne muscular dystrophy. *Pediatrics*, **55**, 30.

CHAPTER 20

Child Abuse and Child Neglect

Child abuse is manifest in many forms and results in a variety of clinical syndromes at the time it occurs. The long-term psychological damage is equally or more severe than the physical trauma, affecting the child's whole personality, his learning ability and his later capacity as a parent; abused children often have parents who were themselves abused.

The abusive environment may be indifferent and cold without concern for the child's basic needs and without the warm understanding, affection, security and encouragement, which characterize good parenting and stimulate growth and development. The environment may be hostile some or most of the time, but physical injury is only one facet of this and does not occur in every hostile family. Parents who use verbal aggression, sarcasm and ridicule, who shame and belittle their children, who frighten and threaten them verbally or use cruel and frightening punishments, are no less abusive than those who cause physical injury. Indeed some parents who have impulsive outbursts of violence really love their child and provide some degree of adequate parenting for part of the time. The fracture or contusion will heal but the psychological scars from a cold or hostile environment do not, unless the child is rescued at an early age and placed in a therapeutic setting with warm parenting. All professionals concerned with children must learn to recognize psychological as well as physical injury so that help may be given to protect the child and assist the parents with their problems.

Physical Abuse

On suspicion of inflicted injury, examination of the skin and bones of the naked child should be followed by fundoscopy and a skeletal x-ray survey. If physical findings provide further confirmation a full psycho-social study of the family is needed by a multi-disciplinary team. In some cases this can be a most taxing diagnostic exercise which should not be undertaken except by senior and experienced practitioners.

Many types of injury may be sustained by battered children. With some the diagnosis is obvious at a glance. In others a careful study of the injuries and the history, of the parents and their backgrounds and of the family's social setting will be needed to arrive at a correct diagnosis.

The history
In all cases of accident and injury, mild or severe, a detailed history of the family events leading up to the accident must be obtained. Even genuine accidents are

often due to family stress of one sort or another (Burton, 1968). Then come the questions, 'Who was present and saw it happen?' 'Who was nearby?' 'What happened next?' The details should be gently and quietly discussed with the worried parents and carefully recorded.

Abusing parents often become confused when asked for details of an apparently plausible story and may contradict each other, although allowance should be made for semantic problems in relatively inarticulate individuals. In many types of disorder doctors learn through experience to listen for the unspoken anxiety, the hesitation, the embarrassment in revealing certain details, and in no case is this more necessary than in talking to parents of a child suspected of non-accidental injury.

Particular note should be taken of incongruous or discrepant histories. It is disturbing how some doctors will unthinkingly accept that serious injuries can result from the trivial incidents reported. Babies under about 4 months cannot bruise themselves or roll off beds. In injuries to young babies it is not uncommon for parents to deny any accidents or injury at all, even in the face of multiple fractures, bruises and subdural haemorrhages. Delay in reporting injuries, an obviously false history as judged by the age of bruises, grazes or fractures and the presence of multiple injuries of different ages, perhaps trivial in themselves, should alert the doctor to the likelihood of child abuse.

The injuries

Details of how injuries inflicted on children may be recognized and how they are caused have been described (Hall, 1974; Cooper, 1975). The injuries are of infinite variety but may be grouped into nine categories and more than one type of injury is often present.

Bruises, lacerations, wheals and scars. Skin signs of one kind or another are present in over 90 per cent of all children with recognized non-accidental injury. Many battered children are dirty or badly cared for and it is easy to miss the significance of infected scratches, small burns or pressure marks, especially when they are healing and in no need of treatment.

The importance of injuries to the face, mouth and region of the ear cannot be over-stressed. Petechial haemorrhages into the auricle, a torn frenulum of the tongue or upper lip and cheek bruises almost never occur in ordinary accidents. Pressure marks from grasping and finger-tip bruises are frequently missed. Petechial haemorrhages on babies from pressure or slapping may be seen. A black eye in a young child should arouse suspicion and two black eyes even more. Ligature marks around the neck, or sometimes round the limbs or trunk, may be overlooked or called intertrigo. Old scars should be carefully looked at in number and kind and a history of the supposed injuries obtained.

Burns and scalds. Attention to the detailed history and examination will reveal if the child could have burnt himself in the way described. A story that sparks from the fire caused a burn is almost always false.

The position of splash marks relative to a main scald should be noted. To explain a mild fresh scald above the left nipple and four smaller areas of milder reddening above this, a mother maintained that her 13-month-old daughter pulled a cup of hot tea over herself. The following day a sibling told her teacher that 'Our baby's gone to hospital 'cos me mam threw a cup of tea at her', thus confirming suspicions of upward splashing by the tea and distrust of the mother's glib account and quarrelsome personality.

Small cigarette burns in various stages of healing should always be carefully sought. 'Dunking' injuries of limbs into hot liquid or the fire, and of the buttocks with the child held flexed, should be remembered. Hot liquid poured on to a child's legs and feet while he is standing spares the soles and shows maximum scalding on the front of the legs or dorsum of the feet. When a child pulls over a vessel of hot fluid, scalds on the back only are extremely unlikely and a 'pouring' injury should always be considered.

Bone and joint injuries. A single fracture in a baby, whatever the history, should arouse suspicion. Some 10 per cent or more of all fractures in children under 3-years-old are due to abuse. Multiple unsuspected fractures in different stages of healing are often found, usually in the ribs or long bones, in babies or preschool children, but are less often seen, unsuspected, in older children.

Joint injuries from jerking or wrenching by grabbing the young child by a limb are often diagnosed as a sprain, as at first the x-ray may be normal apart from soft tissue swelling and perhaps slight joint effusion. Repeat x-ray in 2 weeks will reveal metaphyseal or epiphyseal injury and periosteal reaction around the shaft. Metaphyseal injuries and epiphyseal fragmentation or separation are extremely important signs of inflicted injury and must be carefully sought. A hair-line or spiral fracture can be missed when fresh but the repeat x-ray will show it more clearly and also the periosteal reaction around it. Joint effusions must be noted clinically and radiologically, comparing the two sides.

A baby with a haematoma around a bone or joint may present as a case of osteitis, with redness, swelling, heat and pain. Very careful x-rays are needed to reveal the 'bucket handle' metaphyseal injury or tiny chips of separated bone. If found, antibiotics should not be used immediately unless overwhelming evidence of infection is present. Repeat x-rays will show the further signs of abuse, but if antibiotics have already been used it will be difficult to differentiate from the appearance of treated osteitis. The differential diagnosis is seldom a problem but occasionally osteogenesis imperfecta, Caffey's disease, rickets, scurvy and syphilis, as well as osteitis, must be considered.

Brain, eye and ear injuries. Head injury is the principal cause of death in battered children. Subdural haemorrhages, often bilateral, are the most frequent brain lesions found and are usually accompanied by retinal haemorrhages. They are commonly caused by shaking rather than by direct trauma. Sometimes a fracture of the skull is present. The haematomas may be small and soon cleared by needle aspiration or may be larger and need drainage. They may present as acute and life threatening or with a slow, insidious onset with vomiting, failure to thrive and an enlarging head.

Signs of neurological damage may or may not be present at the time. If absent, this is no guarantee that neurological deficit will not be apparent later on. Shaking injury in young children is a cause of unrecognized brain damage, with minute areas of damage presenting more as specific defects in learning or as foci for epileptic attacks rather than as neurological deficit on formal testing (Caffey, 1972).

The ophthalmic manifestations of child abuse and their sequelae have been described (Harcourt and Hopkins, 1971; Mushin, 1971). A search for retinal haemorrhages by a doctor experienced in looking at infants' fundi is essential in the proper examination of a child suspected of inflicted injury. Although hearing defect due to child abuse has seldom been reported, it seems probable that it may sometimes occur. This could only be confirmed by adequate follow-up studies.

Visceral injuries. These include intra-abdominal and intra-thoracic injuries and trauma to the larynx and trachea in the neck. Intra-abdominal haemorrhage (usually from a ruptured liver) is the second most common cause of death in battered children. Tears in other viscera, especially the gut, may also occur and peritonitis can result if the injury remains untreated. It is important to remember that the relaxed abdomen may show no bruising or marks of trauma following a violent thump or kick. There may or may not be other signs of inflicted injury.

Injuries to the heart or lungs may occur, with haemorrhage and sometimes infection. Fractures of the ribs will usually be seen and special oblique films of the necks or angles of the ribs may reveal these when ordinary antero-posterior views fail to do so. Careful inspection of the infant's neck for faint ligature marks is mandatory and at post-mortem these may show better on the trachea or larynx than on the skin.

Poisoning. Pills and potions are more often administered feloniously to young children than most doctors realize. It is very hard to prove that the tablets were not 'taken from Gran's handbag on the kitchen table'. Casualty officers, family doctors and paediatricians should be much more alert to the possibility of deliberate poisoning, although this is complicated by the large numbers of young children seen with accidental ingestion.

Emphasis on a careful and detailed history will be helpful. When toddlers take pills accidentally they are usually discovered in the act or they give up after only a few have been sampled, and in general minimal symptoms result. When severe poisoning occurs from ingesting a large number of pills, where repeated ingestions occur, deliberate poisoning should be considered. Repeated poisonings can occur in hospital during visiting (Rogers *et al.*, 1976). The author has experience of cases where the deliberate administration of salt in the feeds resulted in severe hypernatraemic dehydration masquerading as gastroenteritis.

Children with repeated accidental ingestions can be differentiated from control subjects several years later by their deviant behaviour. The poisoning and subsequent behaviour signify a disturbance in parent/child relationships and attention to this at the time of the poisoning might prevent some of the later difficulties (Margolis, 1971).

Cot death. Recent studies (Emery, 1976) have confirmed clinical impressions that, in the majority of cases, families with cot deaths have a similar background to those with non-accidental injury, and that children with inflicted injuries have a family history of cot death more often than would occur by chance.

Children who later are shown to have been smothered with pillows or plastic bags are sometimes passed off as cot deaths. Experienced pathologists admit that, at times, it can be impossible to distinguish the two. In some cases elements of carelessness and neglect are present which make the diagnosis even more difficult. A careful history of the earlier care and attitudes of the parents may give clues to the proper diagnosis. Every case of cot death requires a careful psycho-social history. When sympathetically done this should also be a form of therapy for parents anguished by a genuine cot death, and in abusing families it may prevent the deaths of other children.

Drowning. Inflicted injury by drowning occurs in three types of situation. The child who 'fell into the canal' may have been pushed or dropped there. The story that a baby of a few weeks old 'slipped down under the water while I went to the front door' clearly demonstrates a threat, possibly unconscious, to his life and also a cry for help from the mother. Parents sometimes punish or frighten a child by pushing its face into a bowl of water. So far inflicted injury of this sort has been rarely recognized but increasing study may show its true prevalence.

Sexual abuse. Sexual provocation and mistreatment of children is another facet of child abuse needing early recognition and prevention. Affected children are more often girls in the middle school years or in early adolescence, but sexual abuse of preschool children is not unknown. Much sexual abuse has little evidence to identify it, but examination of the anus and vulva for bruising due to attempted intercourse should be a more frequent practice of physicians who see children, especially those with other forms of trauma or from disturbed families (Schecter and Roberge, 1976).

Failure to Thrive from Neglect and Deprivation of Mothering

The frequency of failure to thrive in children with inflicted injuries varies from 10 to 25 per cent. In Britain, MacCarthy (1974) has studied the maternal deprivation and rejection syndrome. Milder forms are often missed because growth charts are not used (Figs. 20.1, 20.2a).

In the full-blown clinical syndrome the child, usually a baby or toddler in its parents' care, fails to grow and develop. He is suffering from a profound degree of psychological rejection, sometimes subtle, which has permanent effects on growth, development and learning.

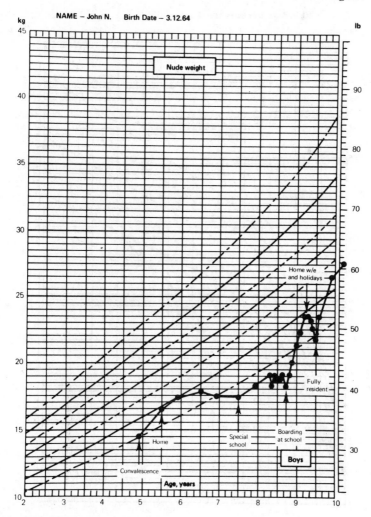

FIG. 20.1. Growth chart for John N.

John N.

5 years	Referred to Paediatric Clinic for asthma; disturbed home. Child in convalescent home for 3 months and gained weight.
5½ years	Returned home and slow gain for the next 5 months, then stationary weight for 1½ years.
7½ years	To special school as day boy; slow gain in weight and some improvement for eight months.
8¼ years	Much trouble with asthma and with family problems; gradual weight loss.
8¾ years	Became boarding pupil at the same school; immediate rapid gain in weight, 1 st. in 5 months.
9¼ years	Social Services suggested a trial at home for week-ends and holidays; weight loss half a stone in the next three months.
9½ years	Fully resident at boarding school again, immediate rapid weight gain.
10 years	Care Order in Court since family problems persisted. Child in Children's Home for holidays and visits his family when he chooses.

NAME – **P.C.** Birth Date – 20.6.72

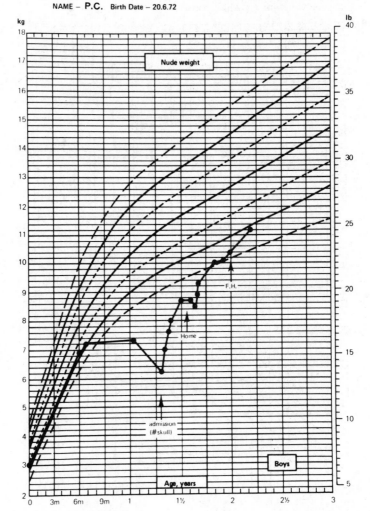

FIG. 20.2a. Growth chart for Paul C.

Paul C. middle of three boys from Social Class 5 family. Gained weight adequately first 7 months and then parents' marriage broke up after weeks of severe discord.

13 months	Seen at Child Health Clinic having had stationary weight for previous 6 months, together with some bronchitis. Clinic doctor thought poor weight due to bronchitis but, in fact, it was too severe to be wholly due to this and needed investigation. The Health Visitor was asked to call to help the mother but the mother refused entry to Health Visitor and Social Worker.
16 months	Neighbour called Health Visitor and asked her to rescue the child as the neighbour thought the child would die otherwise. Admitted immediately to hospital. Extremely wasted, miserable, unable to sit up. Immediate improvement and gained 6 lb in 6 weeks.
18 months	Trial at home with further loss of weight.
19½ months	Returned to hospital. Immediate gain in weight and sent for convalescence while further plans made.
2 years	Care Order in the Juvenile Court and fostered. Since then thriving and well.

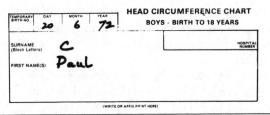

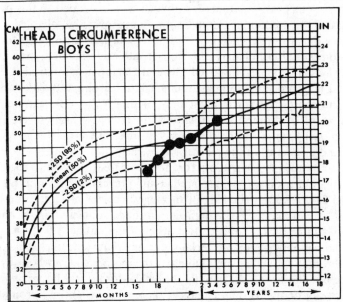

FIG. 20.2b. Skull chart (Paul C.) shows rapid increase in skull circumference from 16 to 20 months during rapid weight gain. Thereafter normal curve.

The baby is floppy (p. 384), apathetic and looks depressed and forlorn. He shows alterness in his eyes but the normal lively exploration and head turning with vigorous body movements and noisy vocalizations are absent.

Height and weight are at or below the third centile and the skull circumference may also be low. Often the child is thin as a baby. When a little older he may appear adequately nourished, although short stature with infantile proportions and very short legs is characteristic. The child looks pale with dull, cold, mottled skin. In severe cases the extremities may present with a red 'raw-beef' appearance or purplish cold oedema from vascular stasis. The hair is dull and may be sparse and dry with areas of a'opecia. A pot belly is common, sometimes accompanied by loose stools (often mis-diagnosed as gastroenteritis) or the pale bulky stools of malabsorption due to states of tension and frustration. Periodic intercurrent infections may complicate the picture.

In spite of a history of good appetite, lack of calories is the main cause of poor growth (Whitten *et al.*, 1969) although secondary hormonal disturbances occur in some children with long-standing starvation. These clear up spontaneously as soon as good nutrition is restored. A voracious appetite with greedy gorging is a striking feature of many of these children during recovery. Pica and a perverted appetite with scavenging from gutters or dustbins may be reported, and the mother often considers the child greedy, which increases her frustration and annoyance.

Depression and apathy may progress to a stage of inertia with inability to play, either alone or with others. The child is solitary. He may stand still for minutes or hours on end, immobile and staring, and the mother feels he is defying her. Sometimes catatonia (flexibilitas cerea) is added to this passivity.

Such a child is indifferent to separation but recovers his physical well-being quickly in a nurturing environment. His behaviour then gives cause for concern as he becomes indiscriminately affectionate, attention seeking and demanding and easily flies into a rage if thwarted. General development is retarded, especially speech and language, and permanent damage to learning capacity occurs.

From the neuro-psychiatric point of view this is the most extreme form of disturbance in the mother/child relationship. In a few cases severe puerperal depression is the cause of the problem, but most often it is due to a character disorder and originates in the mother's own early life.

Attention to adequate nurturing care for the parents as well as for the infant in the perinatal period will help to predict and prevent failure to thrive in many cases. The Court Report (DHSS, 1976) suggests means of monitoring and preventing these problems. Early signs of probable difficulty in mother/infant interaction can be picked up by observation of the mother's feelings about the baby in the perinatal period, especially during labour and the hours following delivery. Promoting immediate bonding of the mother and newborn by keeping them together and giving the parents their baby for several hours private study in the first day or two of life, enhances their relationship and promotes good development, while diminishing future problems in feeding, sleeping and behaviour (Kennell *et al.*, 1974; Greenberg and Morris, 1974). Environmental stresses in the mother's life can affect her handling of her baby, resulting in modification of mood, activity and alertness of the child. Such impairments may reciprocally and permanently alter the mother's responses and so the child's developmental level (Robertson, 1965).

With the established syndrome it is seldom possible to restore the relationship and foster care is needed with an accepting and warm family, who can put up with erratic and difficult behaviour for a few weeks or months while the child's sense of trust and self-confidence is developing. Moving the child from one home to another is extremely detrimental and in the long-term adoption should be considered for these children.

A rejecting mother may do better with her other children as perhaps the affected child is particularly vulnerable to subtle as well as overt patterns of parental malfunction. However, when one is removed another may be scapegoated.

Factors Contributing to Neurological Dysfunction

The importance of neurological problems in the development of battered and deprived children has been under-estimated and the importance of considering *functional* abnormalities too little understood. Traditional neurological examination may fail to reveal abnormal signs, or minor signs only may be present with increased clumsiness and poor coordination in gait and hand function.

The neurological dysfunction is probably compounded by some or all of the following factors.

Ante-natal hazards. Abused children tend to come from families where deficient antenatal care, heavy smoking, alcohol excess, nutritional neglect and accidents are all common problems. Unwanted pregnancy and attempted abortion have occurred in some cases.

Delivery problems. Problems during labour, with less well-prepared mothers, needing more drugs and more assisted deliveries, may also be a compounding factor. Drugs may contribute to impairment of the fragile mother/infant relationship by making the sleepy baby and the sedated mother less receptive to each other.

Low birth-weight. Prematurity and poor intrauterine growth are common in battered children. Medical problems in the perinatal period may result in neurological damage. Because of the special care needed by low birth-weight infants the tenuous mother/infant relationship may be affected even when steps to avoid separation are taken.

Early nutritional defect. Up to 25 per cent of physically abused children show malnutrition and many others fail to thrive without obvious assault. These are at risk of early nutritional deprivation of the brain which may affect neurological and intellectual function (Dobbing, 1974; Crawford and Sinclair, 1972). It is interesting that the skull circumference shows rapid catch-up growth (Winick, 1969; De Levie and Nogrady, 1970; Pearl *et al.*, 1972) when severely deprived children are treated in the first 12 to 18 months of life (Fig. 20.2b).

Poor medical care. In many of these children a significant amount of untreated intercurrent illness occurs with periods of ill-health impeding development. Squints and visual defects are also common.

Damage to the brain. This has been described (p. 402).

Poor mother/child relationship. This can damage or delay development in many ways causing neurological dysfunction (Martin and Kempe, 1976).

The inter-relationship of organic factors with psychological and environmental factors must be constantly appreciated in assessing the neurological function of battered or deprived children.

Characteristics of Abused and Deprived Children

Inhibition of early development

Gross motor and language performance suffer most delay while fine motor, adaptive and personal social skills are much less affected (Martin and Kempe, 1976). The discrepancies found in developmental testing results could be due either to absence of environmental stimulation and support necessary for furthering development, or to the child's unconscious adaptation to external danger. The two hypotheses are not mutually exclusive and it seems probable that abused children are affected by both. Abusing parents often fail to stimulate and encourage normal development in infants and toddlers and when the child is mobile he is likely to be hit for exploratory behaviour, for 'getting into things' or merely for the normal running about and climbing activity small children indulge in while developing locomotor skills. Some parents restrict opportunity by shutting children in cots, prams or playpens alone for hours on end. Thus the children fail to acquire normal agility and remain somewhat clumsy with rather immature movements.

The causes of delayed language development are probably also multiple, the two main ones being lack of verbal stimulation through talking, singing and play in a loving relationship at home, and verbal inhibition. The battered child tends to be struck when he develops negativism and the ability to say 'no' early in the second year. Noisy chatter and interminable questioning are part of normal language development in the preschool years. Abused children get hit for talking and so learn to remain silent just as they learn not to run about. In addition, subtle differences in early mother/infant bonding have been shown to affect the style of verbal communication between mothers and their children at 2 years (Klaus *et al.*, 1972; Ringler *et al.*, 1975).

Later speech and language disorders

As language improves with treatment or increasing age, careful assessment of syntax and vocabulary is needed because the ability to communicate, perhaps largely by gesture and immature speech, may confuse the adult as to the real deficit in language development.

Older children who, with various forms of intervention, seem to have caught up in vocabulary and articulation may be shown to be expressing themselves as younger children would on detailed examination of the form and complexity of their language on tapes. They are less well able to use language in a creative way as a tool for intimate communication or to express ideas, knowledge and feelings. Abstract conceptualization is impaired and they remain at a concrete and immature level in language development, showing up as inconsequential chatter often used to avoid tasks or to ingratiate themselves.

The degree of language delay and distortion depends much on the child's age when abuse occurs and on the type of intervention he receives. For the development of normal speech and language a child requires social and emotional interactions, stimulation and neurological and intellectual integrity, as well as encouragement and self-confidence for him to practice and mature these skills.

With malfunctioning parents in an abusive environment speech is a particularly sensitive skill which may be severely damaged.

Personality characteristics
The outstanding work of Martin and his colleagues in following up abused children in Denver (Martin and Kempe, 1976) and the more limited but important NSPCC study (1976) confirm that the abused child's personality and problems are shaped by the multiple adverse family factors in his total environment. Sometimes the results of intervention such as prolonged hospitalization and frequent changes of home, school and peer groups, may further affect the child's development.

In a detailed study of 50 abused children 5 years or more after the diagnosis, Martin listed nine characteristics seen in various combinations in these children. These were (percentages in parentheses): impaired capacity to enjoy life (66); psychiatric symptoms, e.g. enuresis, tantrums, hyperactivity and bizarre behaviour (62); low self-esteem (52); school learning problems (38); withdrawal (24); opposition (24); hypervigilance (22); compulsivity (22), and pseudo-mature behaviour (20).

No single personality pattern emerged but a variety of disturbances and behaviour traits were seen which were maladaptive to development and limited the capacity of the child to learn and mature. This list of traits can be equally well applied to the parents, most of whom show several of these features, limiting their own development and functioning.

Intelligence and learning problems
The learning problems of abused and deprived children are often out of proportion to any apparent intellectual impairment or to the results of standard IQ tests, and occur in children without overt neurological defect or sensory loss. Martin and his colleagues analysed the many contributory factors and pointed out that by his behaviour (which is adaptive to the abusive factors in the environment) the abused child demonstrates his intelligence. However, this behaviour becomes an impediment to learning, since the child's energy and attention are devoted to monitoring his environment and keeping it safe, e.g. by hypervigilance and role reversal attitudes to parents (Morris and Gould, 1963). Hyperactivity and distractability (common symptoms in a chaotic or abusive home) further impair learning. The child may also show symptoms of conflict and anxiety.

The normal baby exists in alternating states of tension and pleasure. As discomfort from hunger or other causes occurs tension rises and his cry summons relief. Thus he learns to control his environment which .gradually becomes predictable. He begins to learn cause and effect and that the world is a safe and mostly happy place and so trust and self-confidence begin to grow. The unpredictable world of the abused baby (when a cry may bring comfort one moment, neglect another and injury another) does not offer him the chance to develop trust, self-esteem or a sense of causality. Normal cognitive development needs an ordered, structured environment on which the young child can rely.

Abusing parents do not usually provide adequate play, stimulation and reciprocal verbal exchanges with their babies and lack patience and pleasure in teaching their children ordinary skills. Instead of viewing adults as sources of information and fun, they are seen by the child as impulsive, unpredictable individuals from whom he must protect himself. The child's mental energies are largely dispersed on survival techniques and his intelligence is effectively used in trying to gain some nurturing from his environment (Malone, 1966).

Academic learning at school and behaviour with peer groups is seriously impaired. Some children develop rigid obsessional traits or become perfectionists, having had to master certain tasks too early in an attempt to please demanding parents. Unrealistic expectations from parents result in the child gradually failing to satisfy their demands and their critical, denigrating attitudes further damage his self-esteem. Anxiety, fears and dreamy inattention from dwelling too much in a fantasy world, are other features which inhibit learning in spite of good intelligence.

Abused children are often quietly manipulative and subtly undermine attempts to investigate them and their problems. They are unable easily to show trust or form reciprocal relationships, which further depresses their capacity to learn. Their adaptive behaviours can be aggravating and extremely frustrating to teachers and hard to understand.

Much care and experience is needed in the assessment of these behavioural and learning problems. Notice should be taken of attention, attitudes and behaviour in test situations as well as in the schoolroom, playground and home. Evaluation is difficult and time-consuming.

Management and Treatment

In the early 1970s considerable alarm and concern was expressed in Britain, both in professional circles and in government departments, at the increasing number of children being reported killed or severely injured by their parents. Several public inquiries on dead children showed up deficiencies in the quality and organization of services and in communication between the professionals concerned.

The British Paediatric Association and the British Association of Paediatric Surgeons Comments and Guidelines for Immediate Management (1973) and the Tunbridge Wells Study Group Meeting (Franklin, 1975) were followed by a series of guidelines from the DHSS to area health authorities and to local authority departments of social services (CMO, (74)8; LASSL, (74)13; CMO, 6/75; CMO, (76)2 and 3; LASSL, (76)2). The NSPCC has also set up special units to study and help affected families (NSPCC, 1976).

Most areas have now set up a multi-disciplinary Area Review Committee to oversee the organization for immediate management of this difficult problem and each Committee has issued guidelines for the professional workers in all departments concerned with children and families. Any doctor, health visitor, midwife, teacher, social worker or other professional who is concerned about possible non-accidental injury should immediately consult with a senior colleague and if doubt continues, the child should usually be admitted to hospital the same day for full examination and investigation. A paediatric unit with full consultation facilities is usually the best place for the investigations to be made and for the psycho-social study of the family to begin through a multi-disciplinary team.

Studies of abusing families have so far concentrated more on understanding and helping parents than on assessing results of intervention for the children. Undoubtedly the difficult lives of the parents can be improved with support and help for such things as overcrowding, debts, ill-health, loneliness, frequent child-bearing and other social evils. Psychotherapy, casework help, group counselling, self-help groups, role playing and other forms of treatment will help many parents to mature and play a more effective role in the family, but attitudes to children are harder to change. As one mother said, 'I may not hit him any more but I don't like the little bastard any better'. It may be that the child's early perception of parental attitudes is also hard to change (Gray *et al.*, 1976).

Children remaining with their parents need experiences of adequate nurturing which can often be achieved through day care, either with a foster mother or in a well-run day nursery. These are more effective when the parents are also involved. Mothers may function better with their children if they have some diversion and companionship in a job outside the home for several hours a day.

Other children are best removed from the family temporarily or permanently. Children can find happy homes through fostering and adoption (Kadushin, 1970) and undoubtedly many need this care. However, fosterings frequently break down. Assessment of and help for the child may have been inadequate and the foster parents may not have been prepared for or guided through the difficult early months (Martin and Kempe, 1976).

Residential family therapy is expensive but very effective in certain cases (Ounsted, 1974). This has the advantage of keeping the family together and involving both parents and the siblings in the therapeutic regime. The parents benefit from observing healthy models of interaction and of reactions to pleasure and to stress, between staff and children and between staff and parents. Some parents have known no adult relationships except the highly pathological ones of their own parents. Much needed friendship, encouragement and warm nurturing for the parents can be given during this period, as well as attention to the mother's fatigue and health problems.

Prediction and Prevention

The importance of early mother/infant bonding in the prevention of physical abuse and deprivation has been discussed (p. 408). Reciprocal behaviour is in delicate balance in the early hours and days after delivery. Attendants need sensitivity and willingness to modify hospital ward routines in promoting this reciprocal relationship. Any separation of mother and baby after delivery should be avoided unless the baby is ill, and even then the mother should see and touch her baby frequently and as far as possible be closely involved with his care.

In Oxford, studies have shown that combinations of abnormal pregnancy and labour, illness of mother or baby and separation of baby from mother predispose to abuse. Mothers under 20 when their first baby is born, those who have known emotional or social problems and those for whom the maternity staff have anxieties about mothering were over-represented among abusing families (Lynch, 1975; 1976). These studies are now being repeated with more sophisticated methods to refine the instruments for prediction. Obviously health and social workers in touch with young families should be well-informed about mother/child interactions and problems and able to offer support and help. Regular developmental surveillance of the under 5's, as in a screening programme, can provide an effective early warning system (Pringle, 1976).

References

BRITISH PAEDIATRIC ASSOCIATION AND BRITISH ASSOCIATION OF PAEDIATRIC SURGEONS (1973) Non-accidental injury to children; introductory comments. *British Medical Journal* 4, 656.

BURTON L. (1968) *Vulnerable Children.* London: Routledge and Kegan Paul.

CAFFEY J. (1972) On the theory and practice of shaking infants. *American Journal of Diseases of Children* 24, 161.

COOPER C.E. (1975) In *Concerning Child Abuse*, ed. Franklin A.W., p. 21 London: Churchill Livingstone.

CRAWFORD M.A. and SINCLAIR A.J. (1972) In *Lipids, Malnutrition and the Developing Brain.* Ciba/Nestle Symposium., eds. Elliot K. and Knight J. Amsterdam: Elsevier.

DE LEVIE M. and NOGRADY M.B. (1970) Rapid brain growth upon restoration of adequate nutrition, causing false radiological evidence of increased intracranial pressure. *Journal of Paediatrics* 76, 523.

DEPARTMENT OF HEALTH and SOCIAL SECURITY (1974) *Non-Accidental Injury to Children* LASSL (74) 13; CMO (74) 8. London: Her Majesty's Stationery Office.

DEPARTMENT OF HEALTH AND SOCIAL SECURITY (1975) *Model Instructions for Accident and Emergency Departments* CMO 6/75. London: Her Majesty's Stationery Office.

DEPARTMENT OF HEALTH AND SOCIAL SECURITY (1976) *Non-Accidental Injury to Children: Area Review Committees* LASSL (76) 2; CMO (76) 2; CMO (76) 3 London: Her Majesty's Stationery Office.

DEPARTMENT OF HEALTH AND SOCIAL SECURITY (1976) *Fit for the Future.* Report of the Committee on Child Health Services Vol. 1. pp. 141, 274. London: Her Majesty's Stationery Office.

DOBBING J. (1974) The later development of the brain and its vulnerability. In *Scientific Foundations of Paediatrics*, eds. Davis J.A. and Dobbing J. London: Heinemann.

EMERY J.L. (1976) Unexpected death in infancy. In *Recent Advances in Paediatrics*, ed. Hull D. London: Churchill Livingstone.

GRAY J., CUTLER C., DEAN J. and KEMPE C.H. (1976) In *Child Abuse and Neglect* p. 377, eds. Helfer R.E. and Kempe C.H. Cambridge, Massachusetts: Ballinger.

GREENBERG M. and MORRIS N. (1974) Engrossment: the newborn's impact upon the father. *American Journal of Orthopsychiatry* 44, 520.

HALL M.H. (1974) The diagnosis and early management of non-accidental injury in children. *The Police Surgeon* No. 6, p. 17.

HARCOURT R.B. and HOPKINS D. (1971) Ophthalmic management of the battered baby syndrome. *British Medical Journal* 3, 398.

KADUSHIN A. (1970) *Adopting Older Children.* New York: Columbia University Press.

KENNELL J.H., JERAULD R., WOLFE H., Chesler D., KREGER N.C., MCALPINE W., STAFFA M. and KLAUS M.H. (1974) Maternal behaviour one year after early and extended post-partum contact. *Developmental Medicine and Child Neurology* 16, 172.

KLAUS M.H., JERAULD R., KREGER N.C., McALPINE W., STAFFA M. and KENNELL J.H. (1972) Maternal attachment: importance of the first post partum days. *New England Journal of Medicine*, **286**, 460.

LYNCH M. (1975) Ill health and child abuse. *Lancet*, **2**, 317.

LYNCH M. and ROBERTS J. (1977) Predicting child abuse: signs of bonding failure in the maternity hospital. *British Medical Journal*, **1**, 624.

MacCARTHY D. (1974) Effects of emotional disturbance and deprivation on somatic growth. In *Scientific Foundations of Paediatrics*, eds. Davis J.A. and Dobbing J. London: Heinemann.

MALONE C.A. (1966) Safety first: comments on the influence of external danger in the lives of children of disorganised families. *American Journal of Orthopsychiatry*, **36**, 6.

MARGOLIS J.A. (1971) Psychosocial study of childhood poisoning: a 5 year follow-up. *Pediatrics*, **74**, 439.

MARTIN H. and KEMPE C.H., eds. (1976) *The Abused Child*. Cambridge, Massachusetts: Ballinger.

MORRIS M.G. and GOULD R.W. (1963) Role reversal: a necessary concept in dealing with the battered child syndrome. *American Journal of Orthopsychiatry*, **33**, 298.

MUSHIN A.S. (1971) Ocular damage in the battered baby syndrome. *British Medical Journal*, **3**, 402.

NATIONAL SOCIETY FOR THE PREVENTION OF CRUELTY TO CHILDREN. BATTERED CHILD RESEARCH TEAM (1976) *At Risk*. London: Routledge and Kegan Paul.

OUNSTED C., OPPENHEIMER R. and LINDSAY, J. (1974) Aspects of bonding failure: the psychopathology and psychotherapeutic treatment of families of battered children. *Developmental Medicine and Child Neurology*, **16**, 447.

PEARL M., FINKELSTEIN J. and BERMAN M.R. (1972) Temporary widening of cranial sutures during recovery from failure to thrive. *Clinical Pediatrics*, **11**, 427.

PRINGLE M.K. (1976) Antidotes for the battering disease. *Community Care*, Oct. 13, p. 14.

RINGLER N.M., KENNELL J.H., JARVEILA R., NAVOJOSKI B.J. and KLAUS M.K. (1975) Mother to child speech at 2 years: effects of early post-natal contact. *Journal of Pediatrics*, **86**, 141.

ROBERTSON J. (1965) Mother–infant interaction from birth to twelve months. In *Determinants of Infant Behaviour III*, ed. Foss B.M. London: Methuen.

ROGERS D., TRIPP J., BENTOVIM A., ROBINSON A., BERRY D. and GOULDING R. (1976) Non-accidental poisoning: an extended syndrome of child-abuse. *British Medical Journal*, **1**, 793.

SCHECTER M.D. and ROBERGE L. (1976) In *Child Abuse and Neglect* eds. Helfer R.E. and Kempe C.H. p. 127. Cambridge, Massachusetts: Ballinger.

TUNBRIDGE WELLS STUDY GROUP (1975) *Concerning Child Abuse*, ed. Franklin A.W. London: Churchill Livingstone.

WHITTEN C.F., PETTIT M.G. and FISCHOFF J. (1969) Evidence that growth failure from maternal deprivation is secondary to undereating. *Journal of the American Medical Association*, **209**, 1675.

WINICK M. (1969) Malnutrition and brain development. *Journal of Pediatrics*, **74**, 667, 774.

Further Reading

The Battered Child Syndrome

CARTER J. (1974) *The Maltreated Child*. London: Priory Press.

DEPARTMENT OF HEALTH AND SOCIAL SECURITY (1975) *Report of the Committee of Enquiry into the Provision and Co-ordination of Services to the Family of John George Auckland*. London: Her Majesty's Stationery Office.

DEPARTMENT OF HEALTH AND SOCIAL SECURITY (1976) *Non-Accidental Injury to Children: The Police and Case Conferences* LASSL (76) 26; HC (76) 50; Home Office Circular 179/76. London: Her Majesty's Stationery Office.

HELFER R.E. and KEMPE C.H. (1974) *The Battered Child*, 2nd Ed. Chicago: University of Chicago Press.

KEMPE C.H. and HELFER R.E. (1972) *Helping the Battered Child and His Family*. Philadelphia: J.B. Lippincott.

SMITH S.M. (1975) *The Battered Child Syndrome*. London: Butterworth.
STORR A. (1970) *Human Aggression*. Harmondsworth, Middlesex: Pelican Books.
STORR, A. (1972) *Human Destructiveness*. London: Heinemann.

Parenthood and Child Development
ANTHONY E.J. and BEDEKEK T., eds. (1970) *Parenthood: its psychology and psychopathology*.
Boston: Little, Brown & Co.
CIBA FOUNDATION (1975) *Parent–Infant Interaction*. Amsterdam: Elsevier/Excerpta Medica.
DEPARTMENT OF HEALTH AND SOCIAL SECURITY (1974) *The Family in Society: Dimensions of Parenthood*. London: Her Majesty's Stationery Office.
LYNN D.B. (1974) *The Father: his role in child development*. Monterey, California: Brooks/Cole Publishing Company.
MAHLER M.S., PINE F. and BERGMAN A. (1975) *The Psychological Birth of the Human Infant*.
London: Hutchison.
RICHARDS M.P.M. (1974) *The Integration of a Child into a Social World*. Cambridge: Cambridge University Press.

New Aspects of Pregnancy and Childbirth
BREEN D. (1975) *The Birth of a First Child*. London: Tavistock Publications.
BROOK D. (1976) *Naturebirth*. Harmondsworth, Middlesex: Penguin Books.
COLMAN A. and COLMAN L. (1973) *Pregnancy: the psychological experience*. New York: The Seabury Press.
LEBOYER F. (1974) *Childbirth without Violence*. Obtainable from Wildwood House, 29 King Street, London.
LENNARE J. and LENNARE J. (1977) *Hard Labour*. London: Gollancz.
MACFARLANE A. (1977) *The Psychology of Childbirth*. London: Fontana.

CHAPTER 21

Visual Disability and Visual Handicap

Severely defective vision is one of the gravest handicaps in childhood, not only for the tragic isolation in society which it tends to induce, but also on account of the serious educational problems it poses, especially when, as is now so often the case (in industrialized countries at least), the visual defect is associated with other physical and mental handicaps. The association of deafness and blindness, as is seen in some cases of the expanded rubella syndrome, in Usher's syndrome (deafness and retinitis pigmentosa) and in other neurological disorders, is particularly grave; the problems of communication are extremely difficult to overcome and require great skill and patience from dedicated teachers over prolonged periods of time. This is such a unique problem that it is discussed in greater detail elsewhere (Chapter 23).

Degrees of Visual Handicap

It is important to differentiate between visual disabilities which are due to refractive errors and which can be corrected optically with appropriate spectacles and visual handicaps which are incapable of full optical correction. It is of course very important that the former should be diagnosed at an early age; for example, congenital or infantile myopia may slow down a child's development and limit his appreciation of his surroundings until appropriate spectacles are prescribed. Again, uncorrected unilateral refractive errors in young children are a potent cause of amblyopia when undiagnosed and untreated in the pre-school years.

The incidence of refractive errors is higher in many groups of handicapped children than in the normal child population (Gardiner et al., 1969). When this is so in the case of deaf children, poor vision due to undiagnosed and uncorrected refractive errors can lead to unnecessary additional disability, particularly in learning lip-reading and sign language. Nevertheless, these correctable optical defects (including squint which is discussed below) are in quite a different category from severe disorders of the eyes themselves, the afferent visual pathways and the visual cortex.

Serious visual handicaps in childhood are now rare in Great Britain. In most cases children who will need special education because of defective vision already suffer from their visual disorder in the preschool period, although in some cases the disorder is static and in others of a progressive nature. When dealing with very young children it is impossible to make a subjective assessment of visual acuity but it is helpful to consider the degree of any visual handicap as nearly as possible in terms of known visual standards, based on previous observations of other similarly affected children throughout their childhood. Early judgement of any child's visual acuity is most important, for decisions about treatment and future school placement are essentially based on those observations, and a rough assessment can often be surmised with practice even when the subject is extremely young.

In terms of later potential it is worth noting that if the best corrected vision with the two eyes together is less than 3/60 for distance and N.36 for near in Snellen and Times Roman equivalents, then academic education will be impossible without the use of Braille and the child will have to be taught by methods not involving the use of sight. This is the basis of the present statutory definition of blindness in childhood which is related to educational needs. It is hoped eventually to replace the term 'blind' with 'severely visually handicapped' in the definition, as in lay terms blindness suggests that vision is entirely absent, which is so in only a very small minority of cases. The definition of 'partially sighted' infers that some form of special education using modified sighted methods will be required, e.g. large print, extra illumination and magnifying aids. This category comprises children with best corrected vision with both eyes together of between 6/24 and 6/60 and near vision of N.14 or less. If the fields of vision are also constricted a child may be seriously visually handicapped even if central visual acuity is considerably better than this.

Squint

Squint and strabismus are synonymous terms used to describe conditions in which the two eyes are not simultaneously directed towards the object of regard; in all cases such ocular deviations can be looked upon as derangements of the binocular fixation reflexes. The macular regions of the retinae, and in particular the central foveae, have the highest resolving power and thus the greatest visual acuity potential. Each eye is normally directed by the tone of the extrinsic ocular muscles so that the image of the object of regard (i.e. the object of greatest interest in the visual panorama) falls upon the foveal area and is thus most capable of being inspected in detail.

The uniocular fixation reflex involves an input of visual sensation from the retina to the visual cortex in the occipital lobes of the cerebral hemispheres, linked to a motor response mediated through the oculo-motor centres in the brain stem and the oculo-motor nerves to the individual ocular muscles. These nerves are the oculo-motor (third cranial), trochlear (fourth cranial) and abducent (sixth cranial).

Although the two eyes can normally be observed to be moving in a co-ordinated manner over quite a wide range of directions within the first few weeks of birth at term, the more complex binocular fixation reflexes are gradually established over the first 6 years of life. When fully developed, the object of regard is visualized by the foveal area of each eye and the two sensory images are fused together so that the mind perceives a single image of the visual panorama as if from a single 'cyclopean' eye placed in the centre of the forehead. In addition, as each eye perceives the object of regard from a slightly different angle (particularly when the object is close to) and these two dissimilar images are fused together, a three-dimensional visual perception is achieved, termed stereopsis. These complex acquired reflexes are capable of being quite easily deranged particularly during the first 2 years.

During the first few months of life infants also learn to adjust the focusing point of their eyes over a large range of distances by the action of accommodation, the visual axes adjusting by the action of convergence so that the image of the object of regard continues to fall on the foveal area of each eye regardless of its distance from the child.

Types of squint

Derangements of the binocular fixation reflexes producing squint may affect the afferent visual pathways, the motor side of the reflexes or the central connections.

Motor (incomitant) squint. Squint affecting the oculo-motor nerves or muscles is termed paralytic, motor or incomitant squint. Characteristically the angle of squint differs in different directions of gaze, as only certain of the ocular muscles are likely to be affected. For example, if there is a right abducent nerve palsy the right lateral rectus muscle will be paralysed. As a result there will be a slight tendency to convergent squint when the eyes are directed straight ahead in the primary position; on looking to the left side the eyes will move normally together, but on right lateral gaze there will be an increasing angle of convergent squint of the right eye. Because the eyes are parallel in left gaze the affected child may learn to adopt a compensatory abnormal head posture, in this case turning the face towards the right side to keep the eyes parallel in the primary position. In young children this ocular torticollis has to be differentiated from true torticollis and its presence is an indication of a paralytic squint.

Trochlear palsy induces superior oblique weakness, which shows itself mainly by a tilting of the visual image as the obliques control the tortion or rolling movements of the eyes. A complete third nerve palsy produces a marked defect in all ocular movements except abduction and also a drooping of the upper eyelid (ptosis) and sometimes a dilated fixed pupil.

Acquired neurological disease may present first with paralytic squint either as a localizing sign (e.g. a partial third nerve palsy in a mid-brain lesion) or more frequently without localizing value, the most important example being an increasing bilateral lateral rectus paresis due to raised intracranial pressure (p. 381).

Sensory (concomitant) squint. A sensory squint will develop when the vision of one or both eyes is defective, for in that case there is insufficient stimulus to keep the eyes parallel for the sake of maintaining binocular vision. For this reason blind children often develop squint in addition to pendular nystagmus or roving eye movements. More commonly a constant uniocular squint develops when only one eye has poor vision and this finding in young children may be the first external indication of serious ocular disorder such as retinoblastoma. An adult with a blind eye usually develops a divergent squint but in young children, in whom accommodation is very strong, a convergent squint is more commonly seen. Severely retarded children who have defective visual acuity with poorly developed visual cortex and visual association areas commonly exhibit squints, as they lack the ability to develop the complex central mechanisms necessary for the normal development of binocular vision.

Sensory squints differ from motor squints in that the angle of squint remains the same in all directions of gaze as the ocular muscles are not affected; such squints are termed concomitant. However, the angle of the squint may vary considerably depending upon the distance of the fixation object. Such accommodative convergent squints are by far the most common variety in childhood and they are usually associated with significant refractive errors particularly hypermetropia. When the eyes exert accommodation to view near objects in clear focus there is an equivalent amount of convergence of the eyes exerted so that the binocular vision (bifoveal fixation) is maintained. Hypermetropic children can overcome their refractive error to a great extent by an additional effort of accommodation. However, this may induce a tendency to convergent squint from associated excessive convergence, particularly when viewing near objects and more so when the child is tired or ill. Similarly, but much more rarely, myopia in childhood may be associated with a tendency to divergent squint.

Uniocular concomitant convergent squint may be the result of local ocular disorder, either a unilateral refractive error (anisometropia) or defective ocular development such as coloboma or hypoplasia of the optic nerve head. Retinoblastoma is the most sinister cause of uniocular squint in childhood and some 25 per cent of cases of this second most common malignancy in children present in that way.

Latent squint. Latent squint is a tendency to significant imbalance between the positions of the two eyes which is normally controlled for the sake of maintaining binocular vision but which can be revealed when the eyes are dissociated.

Apparent (pseudo) squint. Many young children have broad nasal bridges and folds which cover the medial canthi of the eyelids. When such a child is tired with half-closed eyes (and particularly in the lateral gaze positions) there is often a marked illusion of convergent squint, since the epicanthic folds cause partial obscuration of the sclera nasal to the cornea as compared with the sclera lateral to the cornea. This is often termed 'apparent squint' and can be differentiated from real squint by the tests described below.

Incidence of squint
If latent forms are included squint affects between 4 and 6 per cent of children at the age of 5–6 years. The great majority of these squints are concomitant and about 75 per cent of them are convergent, many with an accommodative element. Motor as well as sensory squints are more common in neurologically

handicapped children than they are in the general population; in particular, squint is commonly associated with cerebral palsy and hydrocephalus.

The effect of squint

The initial effect of a squint is to produce double vision (diplopia) and confusion between the real and the false image. Adults cannot compensate for such symptoms apart from closing one eye, but children younger than 6 years of age quickly learn to suppress the false image from the squinting eye to overcome diplopia. At first this is a facultative process and the vision of each eye remains normal when the other is occluded. With the passage of time, however, the process becomes constant and the suppression leads on to amblyopia (or 'lazy eye'), a condition in which the eye is healthy but has defective central visual acuity. When a squint is constant but alternating, so that fixation varies freely between one eye and the other, amblyopia does not develop but neither does binocular vision. Up to the age of 6–8 years amblyopia can usually be overcome by appropriate treatment but after that age it becomes permanent and this unnecessary loss of vision in an otherwise healthy eye is by far the most important long-term result of untreated childhood squint.

Investigation of squint

The best clinical test for eliciting the presence of true squint is the cover test. The child's attention is drawn to an interesting visual target, such as a toy or torchlight or both, and first one and then the other eye is covered either by the examiner's or mother's hand or by some form of opaque occluder, a watch being kept meanwhile on the position of the uncovered eye. If this has previously been squinting it will now move to take up fixation of the target when the other eye is covered. When children are too young or otherwise unco-operative, a simpler objective test is to view the position of the reflection of a fixation light on the cornea of each eye. When the eye is fixing the reflection is central; if the eye is not fixing the reflection is eccentric and each 1 mm deviation from the centre of the pupil indicates an angle of squint of approximately 7°. The most common error in diagnosis is to mistake epicanthic folds for manifest convergent squint. Apparent squint becomes less obvious as the child grows. However, true squints do not normally cure themselves.

It is never too early to refer a child with obvious or possible squint for full ophthalmological examination, particularly in view of the fact that the squint may in some cases be symptomatic of serious disorder. Simple clinical tests are then supplemented by other subjective tests if the child is sufficiently developed to co-operate with these. In this context the ophthalmic surgeon has the expert assistance of the orthoptic department. Orthoptists have great expertise in working with children, particularly in carrying out illiterate tests of visual acuity and tests of binocular function. Refraction under cycloplegia is carried out in the ophthalmic department. Up to the age of 3 years atropine 1 per cent is usually used either as eye drops or ointment instilled at home two or three times per day for 3 days prior to the examination. After 3 years a weaker solution such as cyclopentolate (Mydrilate®) 1 per cent instilled 30 minutes prior to the examination is usually sufficient to produce adequate relaxation of the ciliary muscles of accommodation and dilatation of the pupils. Retinoscopy will then reveal the refractive state without the risk of the child falsifying the findings by accommodating on to the examining light. An ophthalmoscopic examination of the ocular media and fundi is also undertaken to exclude the possibility of disease.

Treatment

If a significant refractive error (usually hypermetropia) is found, appropriate spectacles should be prescribed. Most children with sensible parents will co-operate with the necessary wearing of these from the age of about 18 months. If fixation of one eye is unsteady or if there is definite indication of defective vision in one eye, patching of the other eye to overcome amblyopia should be carried out under close orthoptic supervision and without delay. Up to the age of 6–8 years vision usually improves quite quickly if any significant refractive error is also corrected. Initially total occlusion of the good eye is carried out with sticky plaster patches. When a young child will not tolerate patches, instillation of atropine drops into the good eye to blur the vision is an alternative but less satisfactory method of treating amblyopia. As the amblyopia decreases varnish occlusion of a spectacle lens can be used instead of total occlusion.

If the squint is of very early onset (i.e. before the age of 1 year or so) binocular vision seldom develops whatever treatment is carried out. When the squint develops later, particularly when it is of an accommodative nature and some degree of binocular vision is already established, surgical treatment of any residual angle of squint, not controlled by spectacles alone, usually results in a complete cure of the squint. This should be undertaken without delay. Where there is no binocular vision, cosmetic squint surgery can be carried out at any convenient time but preferably at a later age when the angle of squint has stabilized.

Squint surgery involves the rearrangement of the relative actions of the ocular muscles in order to make the eyes more parallel. The common procedures are recession, a muscle weakening operation in which a rectus muscle is removed from its normal insertion and re-attached more posteriorly, and resection in which a muscle is strengthened by removing part of its length and re-attaching the cut end to the original insertion. For example, in the treatment of convergent squint a medial rectus recession is often combined with a lateral rectus resection. Absorbable sutures are used for the conjunctival incisions to save the child the discomfort of subsequent removal of stitches. In most hospitals in the UK the operation is done under inhalation anaesthesia during an admission of 48–72 hours. However, there is no compelling reason why the procedures should not be carried out on a day-case basis provided the home circumstances are satisfactory. As the results of these re-adjustments are not always entirely predictable, the parents should always be told that more than one operation may be required to produce an optimal result. Additional forms of treatment which have occasional uses are prisms in spectacles to produce a neutralization of the deviation thus compensating for a small angle of squint, and the use of strong myotic eye drops to facilitate accommodation and thus decrease the tendency to over-convergence upon near objects. Orthoptic exercises can also be used by older children to strengthen binocular fusion and the appreciation of stereopsis.

Prevalence of Visual Handicap and Frequency of Associated Disorders

In March 1975 there were 2072 children below the age of 16 years registered as blind and 2645 registered as partially sighted in England and Wales, not all of them educable. It is probable that many ineducable children who have serious visual handicaps are never registered as blind, because completion of the registration form has always been considered as related to educational requirements. The true incidence of visual handicap in that group is undoubtedly greater than it appears.

In 1968, Fine published the results of a survey of 817 children in schools for the blind and 1374 children receiving partially sighted education in England and Wales. She reported that approximately 50 per cent of the blind children studied had additional handicaps. This proportion was not significantly altered if children affected by retrolental fibroplasia were excluded from the total figures. These might be expected to show a higher frequency of other handicaps associated with premature delivery. There was an average of 1.6 additional handicaps affecting each child in the blind group. Physical disability accounted for 21 per cent of the additional handicaps, low intelligence (i.e. IQ reported as less than 70) for 20 per cent, hearing loss and/or language difficulties 9 per cent, maladjustment 9 per cent and epilepsy 8 per cent. Additional handicaps were especially common in cases of optic atrophy (40 per cent) and low in children blind as a result of ocular tumours (6 per cent) as would be expected. Forty per cent of the partially sighted children had additional handicaps (1.5 additional handicaps per child) and once again they were particularly common in cases of optic atrophy and rare in children with isolated ocular disorders such as degenerative myopia.

Children of good intelligence and with no additional handicaps are much better able to cope with partial sight in a normal school (especially one with small classes and good teachers) than are less gifted and additionally handicapped children, so that the children who attend classes or schools for the partially sighted tend to be a selected group with a lower than average intelligence.

Aetiology and Clinical Presentation

In Third World countries today (as in all countries in the past) many children are affected by uncontrolled infections, often associated with malnutrition, and severe visual handicaps are distressingly common. The great majority are due to corneal scarring from such causes as ophthalmia neonatorum, measles keratopathy and keratomalacia, often associated with destruction of the internal ocular structures and shrinkage of the eyes from previous intraocular infection or corneal perforation. Usually children so affected have no additional handicap.

With the introduction of antibiotic therapy and with improved social conditions and nutrition the incidence of blindness due to this type of disease process has decreased dramatically, as has the absolute number of blind children in populations. Consequently, the proportion of blind children who suffer from some genetically determined disorder has markedly increased. Most important among these genetic problems are Leber's amaurosis (retinal aplasia) inherited as an autosomal recessive trait, and retinoblastoma and congenital cataracts which commonly follow an autosomal dominant pattern of inheritance. At the same time recent advances in neonatal surgical and medical techniques and a higher standard of neonatal nursing care have led to the survival beyond infancy of increasing numbers of children who would previously have died; a number of these have severe visual defects which are quite commonly associated with other major handicaps. Improved neonatal care has also led to the appearance of previously unreported disorders, the most important of which is retrolental fibroplasia.

This new pattern of visual handicaps in children is well illustrated in the survey by Fraser and Friedmann (1967) of 776 children attending schools for the blind and partially sighted in England and Wales. They reported that in approximately 50 per cent of the children studied there was evidence that the cause of the visual defect was genetically determined. They also noted that perinatal difficulties had been recorded in 33 per cent of the children in their series. An association with low birth-weight was particularly common, not only in cases of retrolental fibroplasia but also in cases of congenital cataract and optic atrophy, although no differentiation was made between light for date infants and those prematurely delivered. Over two-thirds of visually handicapped children in this series suffered from one of four conditions, viz. chorio-retinal degeneration (123 cases, 16 per cent), cataracts (127 cases, 16 per cent), optic atrophy (111 cases, 14 per cent) and retrolental fibroplasia (117 cases, 23 per cent).

Since the two surveys mentioned above there have been no comparable studies. However, examination of limited school populations demonstrates a continued decrease (but not a complete disappearance) of new cases of retrolental fibroplasia and a decrease in the incidence of severely defective vision due to maternal rubella. It also seems that with the advent of a more selective policy towards early radical surgery in cases of spina bifida (p. 375), the incidence of blindness associated with paraplegia is decreasing. In other respects there has been little change in the situation.

The four commonest causes of severe visual handicap justify description in more detail.

Chorio-retinal degenerations
This is a miscellaneous group consisting almost entirely of various forms of hereditary retinal pigmentary degeneration. The most common form is Leber's amaurosis which produces congenital blindness as the result of a marked abnormality in the function of all the elements in the outer layers of the retina from the time of birth. It is inherited as an autosomal recessive defect. The

condition represents a precocious form of pigmentary retinal dystrophy closely related to retinitis pigmentosa. In later childhood a pigmentary disturbance of the retina with attenuation of retinal arteries develops. In early infancy, however, although vision is already grossly defective, the eyes may appear entirely healthy on clinical examination and the diagnosis may be confused with that of optic atrophy or cortical blindness. The technique of electroretinography enables a more exact objective assessment to be made even at a very early age. The electro-retinogram (ERG) represents the mass electrical response of the outer layers of the retina (following stimulation with a bright flash of light) which is detected, amplified and recorded by the use of a contact lens applied to the cornea. In Leber's amaurosis this response is extinguished at an early stage of the condition due to the widespread defect in function of the outer retinal layers; thus this investigation allows an exact diagnosis to be made even when the fundus of the eye appears entirely healthy on ophthalmoscopic examination.

At present no treatment is available for this condition. However, accurate genetic counselling has important preventive applications. Useful advice relies on early and exact diagnosis at the time when parents of an affected child may still wish to have further children.

In other forms of early pigmentary retinal degeneration visual symptoms usually do not appear until after the age of 5 years. In some cases, such as the lipo-fuscinoses (Spielmeyer-Vogt disease), visual symptoms may herald the onset of a combined retinal and neurological degeneration with an eventually fatal outcome.

Congenital and infantile cataract
Although cataracts occur at or shortly after birth from many causes, dominant hereditary forms are the most common. They are also a complication of some inborn errors of metabolism (recessively inherited) particularly galactosaemia. In addition cataract is the major ocular manifestation of the rubella syndrome.

Recent advances in techniques of cataract surgery in childhood, particularly the method of aspirating soft lens matter from the cataract under the high magnification of a binocular operating microscope, have led to some ameliora-tion in the visual defects which lens opacities produce. Nevertheless, the surgical treatment of congenital cataract is less successful in terms of recovery of vision than is cataract surgery in later adult life. Much more work is required to find the ideal approach to this problem, not only in terms of adequate early surgery before the onset of nystagmus (and possibly of stimulus deprivation amblyopia) limits the functional results, but also in providing a well-tolerated subsequent optical correction for the aphakic state. Constant-wear thin soft contact lenses are often prescribed, although there are enthusiastic advocates of intra-ocular lenses for young children as well as for old people.

The results of rubella cataract surgery are generally poor. Instrumentation of the lens with spillage of lens material into the eye may be followed by a chronic virus endophthalmitis, unless extremely careful and complete aspiration of the lens matter is achieved. Live rubella virus has been cultured from the cataractous lens into the third year of life in some cases.

Optic atrophy
Severe bilateral optic atrophy in early childhood has many causes and is found associated with a variety of other handicaps. In some cases the optic atrophy is an isolated defect, either hereditarily determined or resulting from an acquired disorder such as optic neuritis, drug toxicity or prolonged papilloedema. Following head injury or encephalomyelitis in childhood, optic atrophy may be associated with other defects and yet remain the dominant permanent handicap. More commonly, however, optic atrophy is only one aspect of a generalized disorder such as cerebral palsy, microcephaly or hydrocephalus. Optic atrophy may also be an important feature of craniostenosis, congenital syphilis and hereditary cerebellar degeneration.

Retrolental fibroplasia (retinopathy of prematurity)
Since its original description (Terry, 1942) this disorder has been clearly defined as an entity which occurs in prematurely delivered infants to whom oxygen has been administered in the neonatal period. The specific cause of the disorder was not determined until much later (Campbell, 1951) and the peak incidence of new cases in this country occurred between the years 1949 and 1953. Since that time sporadic cases have continued to occur.

The sequence of events which leads to the permanent cicatricial stage of the disorder is now well understood. The developing blood vessels in the peripheral part of the premature infant's retina are very sensitive to oxygen; exposure to high concentrations of this gas leads to occlusion and disintegration. As a result, when the infant is removed from an environment of high oxygen concentration the peripheral retina is relatively avascular and therefore hypoxic. The common response of the retina to chronic hypoxia is new vessel formation (as happens after central retinal vein occlusion) and this process ensues in retrolental fibroplasia. New thin walled capillaries with supporting fibrous tissue grow inwards from the retina to invade the vitreous body and the retrolental space. Recurrent vitreous haemorrhages may occur. In its most devastating form, shinkage of the mass of retrolental fibrovascular tissue in the later cicatricial stages leads to traction detachment of the retina and thus to total blindness. Lesser degrees of the disorder are recognized with localized retinal scarring only, but a long-term risk of retinal detachment formation remains and commonly there is an associated high degree of myopia.

To state that this disorder can be prevented easily by avoiding exposure to high environmental concentrations of oxygen in the neonatal period is to oversimplify the problem, for there seems little doubt that the denial of such therapy to small infants with respiratory distress increases perinatal mortality. A major advance in recent years has been the development of techniques for monitoring intra-arterial oxygen in infants rather than environmental partial pressures of oxygen in incubators. In the presence of inadequate pulmonary exchange, the arterial oxygen concentration may be abnormally low even in the presence of a very high environmental concentration. It is the former factor only which influences the development of the retinal vasculature. In the sporadic cases of retrolental fibroplasia which continue to be reported it seems likely that, with an opening of the pulmonary vascular bed and a relief of respiratory distress, there may be a sudden and possibly unrecognized increase in arterial oxygen tension. At present this can be monitored in many neonatal units by intermittent arterial pO_2 estimations, but if these are carried out at invervals of greater than 6 hours during the critical period in a child's progress, irreversible retinal vascular occlusion may result. It is to be hoped, therefore, that techniques for continuous, rather than intermittent, monitoring of intra-arterial pO_2 will become more widely available. Only then is it likely that new cases of retrolental fibrosplasia, an iatrogenic disorder which at one time became the commonest cause of infantile blindness in the Western world, will finally cease to be reported.

Diagnosis and Management

The aetiology of visual handicap in preschool children has been discussed in some detail in order to clarify the main elements of the problems of early management. The first essential is early recognition of the visual defect and prompt referral for expert examination and investigation.

The initial suspicion that a young child has a severe visual defect usually comes from the parents and particularly significant may be a history that visual responses are deteriorating after a normal early development. Comparison with peers and with siblings at a similar age is helpful in the history, as is a noted difference between poor responsiveness to visual stimuli and positive responses to sounds and touch. A thorough enquiry about the pregnancy, birth and peri-natal history as well as subsequent events is essential, as is a full family history, in view of the common hereditary tendencies already described.

Examination and further investigation
In seeking evidence of bilateral visual defects from external inspection, the presence of pendular nystagmus or of roving purposeless eye movements is particularly important. A severe defect affecting the vision of both eyes dating from birth or the early years of life usually gives rise to these involuntary move-ments, which represent a derangement of the ocular fixation reflexes. By the age of 6 weeks from birth at term, normal children have ceased to exhibit random unco-ordinated eye movements and their persistence after that age is a certain indication of poor vision.

Photophobia is also a prominent symptom in a number of serious ocular disorders in early childhood. Congenital glaucoma causes photophobia on account of corneal oedema and irritability, while for unknown reasons similar sensitivity is exhibited by many babies with Leber's amaurosis. Many blind babies rub their eyes fiercely in a characteristic fashion, probably producing pleasurable unformed visual hallucinations of retinal origin by so doing. This sign is also common in children affected by Leber's amaurosis.

An estimate of the size of the eyes on closer inspection is important. Small eyes (microphthalmos) are seen when there has been some derangement in the early stages of ocular development, such as coloboma, and when there has been intrauterine infection of the eyes as in the rubella syndrome and congenital toxoplasmosis. In the latter condition cataracts and macular scarring from chorioretinitis can cause severely defective vision. Large eyes (buphthalmos) are seen in cases of severe congenital and infantile glaucoma.

A prefocused torch is most useful in the examination of the anterior segments of the eyes, the pupillary reflexes and ocular movements. The cause of a severe bilateral visual defect may be obvious from the presence of severe corneal scarring or of dense white cataracts. Torchlight is also useful in a darkened room to assess the degree of pigmentation of the iris by transillumination. In ocular albinism cutaneous pigmentation is normal so that the diagnosis may be missed if the absence of normal iris pigmentation is overlooked.

In many cases the eyes appear normal on external examination and testing the pupillary light reflexes is helpful. As the reflex is a subcortical one, the presence of normal pupillary constriction when a bright light is shone at the eyes is not necessarily an indication of sight, for a child with complete absence of the occipital visual cortex due to porencephaly may be completely blind and yet have normal pupillary reflexes. On the other hand, the absence of responses is a very useful objective indication of a severe bilateral ocular or optic nerve disorder in a young child. The torchlight will also allow examination of the fixation of each eye, the range of ocular movements and an assessment of the presence of any squint. The latter is particularly common where the vision of one or both eyes is defective (p. 421).

It is important to assess the extent of fields of vision as well as the acuity of vision and this can be done most simply by introducing visually stimulating targets into the periphery of the visual fields from various directions, noting the refixation of the eyes upon the target when the young patient first sees it and is attracted by it. In this test it is important to use a silent target and not something like a rattle, for even a totally blind child may move the eyes towards an interesting noise using a subcortical visuostatic reflex and this can be wrongly interpreted as evidence of sight. This and other tests are described in more detail in Chapter 8.

In order to examine the internal ocular structures in any detail it is necessary to dilate the pupils. The most useful agent is a short-acting parasympatholytic drug such as cyclopentolate 0.5 per cent eye drops. Lens opacities not visible on external inspection may be revealed, as well as details of the fundus of the eye. It is impossible to describe here all the abnormalities which may be seen on ophthalmoscopy, but it is worth noting that the optic disc pallor of optic atrophy can be very difficult to distinguish from the normal range of appearances in young children. Another difficulty is that the fundi in cases of Leber's amaurosis may look entirely normal in the young child even at a stage when vision is very seriously defective.

In cases of doubt a more detailed assessment of these appearances by an experienced ophthalmologist with a special interest in paediatric ocular disorders is essential without delay. Examination may then be facilitated by a short general anaesthetic, combined with electroretinography seeking for further objective evidence of retinal dysfunction. Thorough ophthalmic examination of infants in this way requires much time and patience.

Unless there are incontrovertible signs of severe ocular disorder, the experienced clinician always hesitates to give too gloomy a visual prognosis immediately after initial examination in the neonatal period, because there are some infants who appear visually unresponsive when examined in the first weeks and months of life, who on re-examination at a later age demonstrate evidence of normal vision. This is due to lack of interest in the visual targets presented rather than to organic damage to the visual system.

Management
The aims of a meticulous examination and investigation at such an early age are to obtain an exact diagnosis and an assessment of the level of residual visual function. Unfortunately apart from cataracts and glaucoma there are few visually handicapping processes in early childhood which are at present amenable to specific treatment, but diagnosis often allows an accurate view of hereditary pattern and prognosis to be taken, so that genetic counselling can be given without delay and plans for future management and education can be made with some certainty. Even when an immediate exact diagnosis and assessment is impossible, the early detection and recognition of the handicap by professional personnel is itself a considerable step forwards, for it allows appropriate skilled help to be given to the child and to the family during the critical early stages of development.

At present the greatest problems stem from the multiplicity and the scattered and uneven distribution and quality of the agencies designed to give appropriate help in the preschool period. There is a strong argument for national rather than local solutions to these problems, especially as the number of young children affected is so small and unevenly distributed. More health visitors, social workers and infant teachers with special skills in advising the families of young blind children need to be trained and appointed to Regional or Area posts where they can act in a 'peripatetic' role, visiting and giving guidance in the homes of the families concerned. These field workers need to be in communication with the community paediatric and ophthalmic agencies. The key figures here are likely to be the paediatrician who runs the local Assessment Centre and his ophthalmic consultant colleague with a special interest in paediatric problems. They act in liaison with the Area Community Physician (Child Health), the local education authority, the headteachers of the regional schools for the blind and the partially sighted and with national agencies such as the Royal National Institute for the Blind. The RNIB already has a number of regional advisers who give an excellent peripatetic service.

Guidance to parents is initially of a very simple nature; mothers need to keep 'in touch' with their blind infants by handling and by speech and other familiar sounds. The home surroundings need to be arranged so that the child can safely explore his environment in an intimate atmosphere. It is important that nursery training for blind children should be available from an early age, so that they can be helped with learning the basic skills of walking, speech and other forms of communication. The mother should accompany the child, certainly until the age of 3 years. To allow this, social help should include facilities for siblings to be looked after during these sessions. Some additional home help may also need to be provided by the local social work department as caring for a blind child at home is exhausting and time consuming for the mother and a strain on the other members of the family. Domiciliary care is not only more successful than residential care in allowing maximum potential normal development and integration of the blind child within the family and the community, but is also cheaper even when a full range of social services is provided. Unless the home circumstances are very adverse young blind children should not be taken into residential care as they can quickly become institutionalized however dedicated and compassionate their professional protectors may be.

In planning for the child's future a team approach is essential and this has been sadly lacking in the past. This fact is highlighted in the Report of the Vernon Committee on the Education of the Visually Handicapped (Department of Education and Science, 1972). The Committee advocated that local assessment panels should be set up to discuss the future of every visually handicapped child. Each panel would comprise a developmental paediatrician, an ophthalmologist, a teacher of the visually handicapped, an educational psychologist and a representative of the social work department, all working in liaison with the child's parents and general practitioner and studying reports of the child's development and progress.

The team approach is particularly important when there are additional handicaps which render decisions about future school placement even more difficult. In general it is fairly easy to determine the group of children whose vision is so poor that they will require special whole-time education by nonsighted methods from the age of 5 years. It is difficult to predict at an early age those children who may just be unable to cope with education in a normal class on account of moderate visual defects, particularly when increasing demands are made upon visual acuity as children progress in school. In such cases it is usually best for the child to start off in the normal infants' school, the staff having been alerted to the visual problems. Reassessment of progress should be made at invervals. The child may require later transfer to a special class for partially sighted children, or remedial teaching within the present school, perhaps by peripatetic teachers of the visually handicapped.

These concepts of early notification and continued team reassessment underlie the recent decision of the Department of Health and Social Security to abolish the blind and partially sighted registration form (B.D.8) for children up to the age of 16 years and to substitute for it a form of notification of visual handicap in childhood. This is being designed at present and will include much more information concerning the child's handicaps and background. It will not involve the ophthalmic consultant, who completes the form, in giving advice in isolation regarding the child's education, as the form B.D.8 does.

There is no doubt that planning for and providing appropriate medical, social and educational facilities for visually handicapped children of all ages is a complex task. The rarity of the problem makes the logistics of delivery of adequate skilled care at a local level particularly difficult. At the preschool stage the main aim must be early notification, with exact diagnosis and expert advice in the home, with adequate back-up facilities. This requires a nationally planned framework of services and much better understanding of the existing services by the health care personnel already in the field.

Even if at present a certain amount of muddle still prevails, there is every evidence of enlightened progress being made and of the high sense of dedication of the workers involved. It is to be hoped that they can be properly rewarded by being granted the full range of facilities which is needed if the tragically handicapped children they help to care for are to have the best possible chance of developing into happy and useful members of society.

References

DEPARTMENT OF EDUCATION AND SCIENCE (1972) *The Education of the Visually Handicapped (Vernon Report)*. London: Her Majesty's Stationery Office.

CAMPBELL K. (1951) Intensive oxygen therapy as a possible cause of retrolental fibroplasia. *Medical Journal of Australia*, **2**, 48.

FINE S.R. (1968) *Blind and Partially-sighted Children. Education Survey 4. Department of Education and Science*. London: Her Majesty's Stationery Office.

FRASER G.R. and FRIEDMANN A.I. (1967) *The Causes of Blindness in Childhood*. Baltimore, Maryland: The Johns Hopkins Press.

GARDINER P., MAC KEITH R. and SMITH V. (1969) *Aspects of Developmental and Paediatric Ophthalmology, Clinics in Developmental Medicine*, No. *32*, p. 32, London: Heinemann.

TERRY T.L. (1942) Fibroplastic overgrowth of persistent tunica vasculosa lentis in infants born prematurely. *American Journal of Ophthalmology*, **25**, 1409.

CHAPTER 22

Hearing Loss

The importance of hearing impairment lies in its effects on the child's ability to share with his parents, siblings and others all those aspects of human experience which are mediated by spoken language. Deafness for a young child is not simply an inability to hear, but a failure to acquire verbal thought and verbal communication. It is difficult to imagine a more crippling handicap, but to begin with it is unobtrusive, so that early detection is rare and the number of children first referred under 1 year old remains a small proportion of the total number born deaf.

Types of Deafness

The primary anatomical classification of deafness into middle and inner ear summarizes a number of important features. Hearing loss arising within the middle ear is extremely common, usually not severe in degree and to a large extent susceptible to treatment. Deafness arising from cochlear disruption or damage to the neural pathways is infrequent, may be profound and is usually permanent.

THE MIDDLE EAR
Congenital abnormalities

These affect the structure of the middle ear and, more obviously, the pinna and the external auditory meatus. The condition may be unilateral or bilateral, with the pinna varying in appearance from normal to an irregular convoluted fold of skin. The external meatus may be well formed, narrowed or non-existent. Occasionally the only anomaly is an indisputable middle ear deafness with something not quite right in the appearance of the tympanic membrane and the disposition or shape of the malleus.

Management is determined by function rather than by appearance. If hearing is normal on one side the child will learn to talk and there will be no significant language delay. Where there is bilateral meatal atresia it is usually possible to demonstrate hearing responses at the 70 dB level. The decision to use a bone conduction hearing aid (unfortunately cumbersome and obtrusive) or to try air conduction aids, depends on the presence of a reasonable meatus which will accept and retain an ear mould. Opinion varies on the most appropriate time for surgical repair but it is probably best left until later childhood. Surgery must always be preceded by careful audiological testing and radiographic examination using polytomography, to determine the condition of the middle ear and ossicles and to exclude a non-functioning or deformed cochlea.

Secretory otitis media

This condition has a number of names, none of which is entirely satisfactory, indicating the uncertainty about its causation. It is extremely common and of considerable importance in the young child, but is easily overlooked.

The middle ear is at risk because the Eustachian tube is long, narrow and only potentially open. The lower end lies in the nasopharynx and children are especially prone to upper respiratory infections involving this region. Free passage of air to the middle ear space is impeded by any factor which prevents the lumen from being opened sufficiently, such as mucosal congestion of the tube or faulty action of the musculature attached to and acting on its walls. Following obstruction, absorption of air results in a fall of pressure in the middle ear, so that it becomes negative in comparison with normal atmospheric pressure. The tympanic membrane is flexible and moves inward to accommodate this reduction. Once the pressure on the inner and outer surfaces becomes unequal, the membrane cannot respond so sensitively to the rapid and very small changes of air pressure produced by the passage of sound. As the negative pressure increases, fluid appears in the middle ear space, either serous or mucoid, and further impairs the capacity of the membrane to vibrate freely. The child's hearing is impaired and he becomes unresponsive, distant or withdrawn and does not appear to take any interest in what is said to him. This is more likely to exasperate those around than give rise to the suspicion that his hearing is

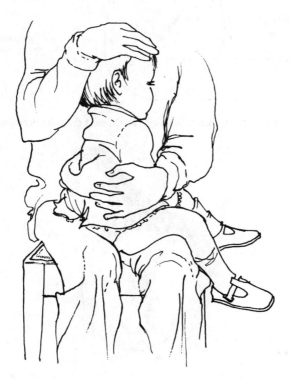

FIG. 22.1. Holding a child securely and still for examination of the ear drum.

affected. The condition may resolve spontaneously or may be prolonged and highly resistant to treatment. There is little doubt that in some infants the fluid in the middle ear cleft fails to drain and that deafness arises at birth which may persist for some time.

Of the three main ways by which the condition is detected, in the young child none of them may be at all conclusive. Thus, it is all the more important that this condition is kept in mind and any child in whom there is more than a passing middle ear hearing loss from intermittent upper respiratory infection needs detailed otological assessment.

Direct inspection of the ear drum should be a routine part of all examinations of young children and those responsible for developmental assessment need to become experienced in the use of the auriscope. It is advisable to leave this part of the examination to the end, and one must show the mother how to hold her child securely and still (Fig. 22.1). The membrane cannot be visualized in its entirety at a glance and it is necessary to scan its surface, first identifying the prominent knuckle of the lateral process of the malleus, then following

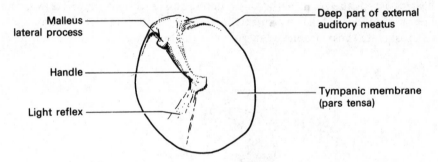

Malleus lateral process

Handle

Light reflex

Deep part of external auditory meatus

Tympanic membrane (pars tensa)

Fig. 22.2a Normal tympanic membrane, left ear, showing the more prominent landmarks.

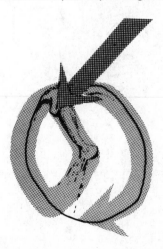

Fig. 22.2b. Examination of the tympanic membrane (for details see text).

the line of the malleus down and back, noting its inclination and colour and on past the tip of the malleus to the light reflex. Having reached the lower limit of the membrane the anterior portion of the pars tensa is studied, noting its colour and translucency, and finally the region behind the line of the malleus and light reflex (Fig. 22.2a and b). In secretory otitis media the malleus will lie more horizontally, the handle being pulled inwards and up; there may be hyperaemia over the malleus and deep meatus and the tympanic membrane loses its translucency, appearing thickened or dark. Fluid may be easy or very difficult to detect.

Hearing tests will reveal a loss, usually of the order of 35–40 dB, which may be uniform across the range or less severe in the higher frequencies. If the child has reached the age when it is possible to complete a conditioning type of test using the earphones it will be possible to determine a bone conduction threshold (Fig. 22.3). In middle ear lesions this will be normal and there will be a clear difference between the thresholds for air and bone conduction. In younger or unco-operative children this additional information will not be available and one can only note the presence and extent of hearing loss.

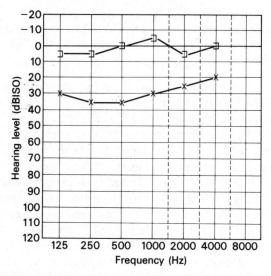

FIG. 22.3. Audiogram. Middle ear hearing loss showing air conduction (X——X) and bone conduction (]——]) thresholds for left ear.

The impedance bridge is an item of equipment which should be available in every otological and audiological clinic where the hearing of children is assessed. The principle of operation lies in measuring the amount of sound reflected back from the surface of the tympanic membrane when a low frequency tone of fixed intensity is applied (Fig. 22.4a to d). This necessitates an air tight seal of the probe in the meatal orifice and an air pump which can increase or decrease the pressure within the sealed off external auditory meatus. These pressure changes are reflected in the position of the tympanic membrane, which flexes out into

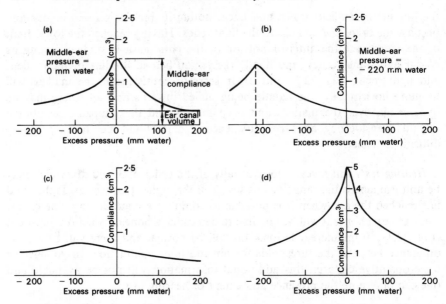

FIG. 22.4. Tympanograms. At 220 Hz: (a) normal; (b) blocked auditory tube; (c) fluid in middle ear; (d) ossicular discontinuity. Reproduced by kind permission from KNIGHT J.J. (1976). In *Acoustics and Vibration Progress*, Vol. 2, eds. Stephens R.W.B. and Leventhall. London: Chapman and Hall.

the meatus under reduced pressure, and is pushed progressively into the middle ear space when the meatal air pressure is increased. As one would expect, the most efficient position of the membrane is when the pressure in the middle and outer ears is perfectly balanced; hearing is most sensitive and the minimum amount of reflection of the probe sound occurs. As the meatal pressure is made more or less than the middle ear pressure, the stiffness of the membrane increases and a symmetrical curve can be plotted relating air pressure (changed artificially in the meatus) to the amount of sound transmitted by the membrane. By this means the middle ear pressure can be inferred, and some measure obtained of the stiffness or flexibility of the membrane and its attached ossicular chain.

There have been limitations to the use of the impedance bridge because of the laborious method of plotting the results and because the headset is woefully inappropriate for young children. Instruments designed specifically for children are now available, with a pen recorder automatically tracing the curve so that the procedure can be quickly completed. The latest instruments can also indicate the threshold of the stapedius muscle reflex, putting the loud stimulus tone (80 dB sound pressure level or more) into the ear from which the measurements are being taken. Until recently the other ear had to be used, relying on the bilateral and symmetrical reflex contraction of the stapedius muscle.

SENSORI-NEURAL DEAFNESS
Sensori-neural deafness is known also as perceptive, inner ear or nerve deafness. Surprisingly, the prevalence of this condition is unknown: the oft quoted 'one

per thousand' for severe deafness arose in the earlier years of the nineteenth century, when the pattern of disease and the standards of hygiene in the community were entirely different. In addition to those children with severe or profound loss, there are many more with lesser degrees of deafness sufficiently serious to affect their acquisition of language and educational performance.

'Congenital' deafness by custom includes children who become deaf during the perinatal period, but as in many the lesion is in fact 'acquired', it is best to consider causation on a more strictly chronological basis.

Genetic factors. There are many syndromes in which deafness is an important feature. These include abnormalities of the skin and its pigmentation and the various structures derived from it, of the skeletal tissues and of the cardio-vascular, renal and endocrine systems. None of these conditions is encountered frequently, even in specialized paedo-audiology clinics, and the diagnosis of genetically determined deafness shows unfortunate limitations.

Well-recognized syndromes, such as the Waardenberg or 'white forelock' syndrome, may be readily apparent or one or more features may be absent, including deafness. In other instances deafness may occur in the presence of atypical features which make it extremely difficult to identify the syndrome with any confidence. More frequently the difficulty lies with a severely deaf child in whom there is a complete absence of any clinically identifiable features. Not only are there no features suggestive of a syndrome, but it is not possible to identify any other cause for the deafness, that is until a second severely deaf child is born into the family. If it is not possible to identify the cause of deafness despite careful searching, it is necessary to consider the possibility of genetically determined deafness.

Intrauterine causes. Maternal infections, and in particular rubella, continue to be important in the aetiology of deafness. The features of rubella embryopathy are well known and described in detail elsewhere (Chapter 23). Confusion arises in reaching the diagnosis because of the difficulty of identifying certain types of rash. Rashes and fevers in the first 16 weeks of pregnancy are always suspect; and in a number of mothers rubella is shown to be the cause of their child's deafness in the absence of any such history, or even of contact with an infected person. It is unfortunate that the immune status of every mother is not known before conception occurs and appropriate steps taken to prevent the effects of this severely handicapping infection.

The hearing loss may vary from moderate to profound (60 dB to 90+ dB) and is usually uniform across the speech range of frequencies, or rather worse in the mid-range centred on 1000 Hz (Fig. 22.5). The majority of children are born with the damage already present in the organ of Corti; in a few the hearing loss develops subsequent to birth, reportedly as late as 4 years. With childhood deafness so inaccurately diagnosed, instances of apparent progressive hearing loss need to be greeted with some scepticism but they undoubtedly occur. Apart from the handicaps commonly associated with intrauterine rubella infection and which comprise an appalling group of learning disabilities, the hearing loss

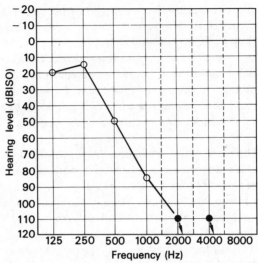

Fig. 22.5. Audiogram. Severe high frequency sensori-neural loss showing air conduction threshold for right ear.

itself may be difficult to overcome by amplification and considerable skill in hearing aid selection and fitting is required.

Perinatal causes. Chief among the causes affecting hearing function at the time of birth are anoxia and jaundice. Typically there is near normal hearing in the low frequencies and a sharp drop at 500–1000 Hz so that there may be an 80 dB loss or greater in the frequencies above (and sometimes including) 1000 Hz. Losses even of this severity may be unrecognized until well on into primary school life despite their severe effects on language learning. Speech and virtually all other sounds to which the child is normally exposed have a considerable amount of energy in the low frequency end of the range of hearing, and it is essential to distinguish between hearing components of speech and understanding spoken language. Less severe degrees of high frequency deafness (from whatever cause) may not be detected until the child of 9 years or even 11 years is failing to keep up with his peers in educational attainments.

Postnatal causes. These merge imperceptibly into all the causes of deafness known in the adult, excluding only the 'senile' deafness of presbyacusis. Meningitis is an important cause of severe deafness occurring early in life, sometimes before, sometimes after normal spoken language has begun to appear. Hearing should be assessed following recovery so that deafness may be recognized at the earliest possible moment. A number of drugs given to young children are ototoxic. Mostly they are administered under suitably controlled conditions with the additional safeguard of blood level estimation. Nevertheless, the effects of deafness on the quality of the child's whole emotional and intellectual development are so serious that the aim should be to replace every known ototoxic agent as soon as therapeutically effective alternatives become available.

Detection and Assessment of Hearing Loss

Parents' history

Parents may suspect deafness very early on the basis of a clear cut and startling failure to respond to a loud sound. Usually the presentation is less dramatic. As it is the absence of response which has to be noted, rather than an observable inappropriate reaction, it may be some time before such a negative feature is identified by parents. It is easy enough to discount failure to turn to a call, or to some loud sound, by saying that the child is engrossed in what he is doing. The failure has to be repeated many times before it is noticed to be typical of his behaviour and worth discussing with the health visitor or the doctor.

The child may be oblivious to all, or a great deal, of the sounds constantly occurring around him; mother talking, busy about her household tasks or using noisy household equipment, children playing, dogs barking, door and telephone bells ringing, all these provide countless occasions for parents to observe their child's reaction to sound. It may be possible for them to trample up and down stairs and even in and out of the room in which he is going to sleep (opening cupboards and drawers) without arousing any reaction, unless he gains information visually or by transmitted vibration about the activity going on around him. Parents may remark upon his surprise and even fear when he suddenly sees one of them standing by his cot or pram, because he has not heard the advance warnings of approach.

In the more severe forms of hearing loss the child is unable to detect any element of speech. His own vocalization will be abnormal and there will be no appearance of tuneful, inflected babble with its constant repetition of consonant and vowel, or of mimicking the essential elements of stress, rhythm, intonation and syllabic structure which in varying proportions characterizes all human speech. As the hearing loss remains undetected, so its effects on language development become more profound. The first words are delayed in their appearance perhaps for several years, or there may only be a very restricted vocabulary with no attempt at word joining.

Deafness as language disorder. The significance of deafness can only be appreciated in its entirety when it is recognized as a form of language disorder. The developmental norms of children's spoken language need to be at the fingertips of all who are responsible for their care. The child with no spoken words at 2 is in urgent need of investigation. If this failure to talk is associated with inability to make any sense of what is being said to him then deafness is the only possible diagnosis to make until detailed audiological assessment has ruled this out.

The majority of parents of hearing impaired children are aware that verbal comprehension is poor and that understanding is only achieved by pointing, or by giving the child some tangible clue of what is required of him, e.g. by handing him a cup, a duster, or his coat. The details of the child's speech and overall behaviour, elicited by careful questioning of his parents, are an essential part of the assessment, and provide an important check on the results of hearing tests. Discrepancies between the two cannot be ignored.

The use and abuse of screening tests
In the effort to obtain early diagnosis, screening tests of hearing are usually carried out at 8–10 months. The details are described elsewhere (p. 163). The concept of screening is an important one but there are many practical difficulties. The requirements are a quiet, non-reverberant room; an alert yet relaxed child; a trained tester and assistant; precisely defined acoustical stimuli, particularly with respect to loudness and to a lesser extent the frequency characteristics; the eliciting of a clearly defined response, i.e. localization of the sound source, and strict adherence to procedural details for definition of failure and of the course of action consequent upon failure. Mistakes arise under each of these headings, with serious consequences when a child with a severe hearing loss is said to be normal. Errors arise because the child can see the tester or detect her presence through shadows, reflections, touch or the glance given her by her assistant. Inadequate responsiveness is often explained away by saying that the child was too tired, too young, or not interested. The child may be incorrectly passed because the sound stimuli were too loud or because the response accepted as an indicator of hearing was not one of localization. There may be undue delay in referral through repeating the tests at monthly or 3-monthly intervals and all these problems may recur if the child health doctor, to whom the screening failures are then referred, has not been trained in these demanding and at times difficult techniques.

Assessment of degree of hearing loss
There is a wide range of audiological techniques used to assess the degree of hearing loss.

Localization techniques. Sound stimuli of increasing loudness are used in free field until a localizing response is obtained. The stimuli used include, amongst others, bells, squeaker toys, rustled paper, cup and spoon, rattles, xylophone, drum and the human voice making high and low pitched sounds. All these sounds must be constantly monitored against a sound level meter and in this way a remarkably accurate hearing threshold may be determined long before formal pure tone audiometry becomes possible. Pure tones and narrow band noise are not always as effective as the more familiar sound-producing sources in provoking a response. The former are more accurately specified stimuli but the free field audiometer's output is frequently inadequate, if limited to 80 dB SPL (Sound Pressure Level).

Conditioning techniques. The child is first encouraged to respond to a sound, the loudness of which is well above his threshold. The stimulus may be a drum beat or chime bar with the added advantage of the visual component (which is removed by subsequently working out of the child's field of vision), the voice or the free field pure tone audiometer. Some 2-year-old children are able to grasp the requirements of this technique, though such a response is not common under the age of 3 years. It should be performed in free field without earphones and with a very simple test response, not requiring absorbing manipulation by the child. As the child becomes older earphones can be tried and the bone conduction transducer used. Children who cannot or will not co-operate should have their hearing assessed by localization techniques. A preliminary assessment by this latter method will often prevent errors arising in children who are over anxious to co-operate in conditioning audiometry, producing spuriously good hearing thresholds.

Verbal recognition and speech tests. It is essential to determine the child's hearing for speech and the vocabulary used should bear some relationship to the child's age and experience. A picture card test in a 5-year-old may produce results which mislead one into thinking the child's hearing for speech is normal, because the task is too easy linguistically. For the young child household objects and toys are useful; later, picture cards representing single syllable words are used in groups of 12 to 16. A preliminary vocabulary check is essential, each object or picture being presented to the child one at a time so that he can name it or his mother can state whether or not he knows the name. The advantage of using objects and pictures is that the child is not forced into talking and is more likely to point than to repeat the word. A trial run is advisable with the tester sitting in front of the child and using an adequately loud voice. Next, lip reading is eliminated by going round beside or behind the child, with the speaking voice maintained well above threshold until confidence is gained. The loudness of the voice is then dropped until errors and hesitancies appear. After noting a failure it is important, particularly in the insecure or poorly co-operative child, to reinforce his response by making the voice sufficiently loud again for him to hear and succeed. A sound level meter placed beside the child but visible to the speaker is essential. With practice the voice can be controlled to produce 5 dB changes of loudness for the vowel sounds. Word lists using single syllable words, spondees and sentences are used with co-operative children who are prepared to repeat out loud what they have just heard.

The stapedial reflex threshold. Reflex contraction of the stapedius muscle occurs when the subject is exposed to sounds of about 80 dB SPL or more. The muscle is attached to the neck of the stapes and its contraction restricts movement of the ossicle. This increase of stiffness is transmitted to the ossicular chain and the tympanic membrane and can be detected by using the impedance bridge. The membrane is first balanced at its most flexible point by equalizing the pressure of air on either side and the tone then switched on. Normal hearing can be determined for the usual range of frequencies in children in whom it would otherwise be very difficult. Any abnormality of the reflex response necessitates detailed audiological and otological examination.

Electrophysiological tests of hearing. However experienced the clinician testing a child's hearing, there will always be occasions when it is impossible to gain an adequate estimate of the auditory threshold. There are many features of a child's behaviour and organic disability which contribute to this. It is unforgivable for bias and misconception to replace precise and rigorous measurement.

If a child's hearing cannot be assessed, this is not an admission of incompetence but is a factual observation of the difficulty encountered. Nevertheless, it remains essential to obtain an accurate indication of the threshold and without further delay.

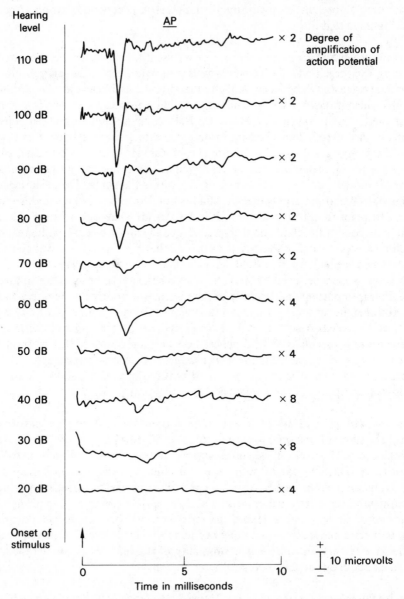

FIG. 22.6. Compound action potentials recorded by transtympanic electrocochleography. The traces show the threshold, estimated at 25 dB, for wide band clicks delivered by a loud-speaker at a distance of 0.5 m, the child being under light general anaesthesia. The subject was a very disturbed, mentally retarded, 4-year-old boy with gross limitation of language development.

Out of a range of procedures the most satisfactory at the present time is the transtympanic electrocochleogram. The technique provides a measure of the compound action potential in the auditory nerve, this neural activity being induced synchronously in as many nerve fibres as possible by the use of clicks. The changes of electrical current are in microvolts and are picked up by a needle electrode inserted through the tympanic membrane. A series of rapidly repeated clicks is used and the minute electrical responses processed by a small averaging computer. When activity is present a wave form of the type shown in Fig. 22.6 appears. The intensity of the clicks is reduced after each positive response until normal threshold is reached or no visible response is obtained. The electrical activity originates from that part of the cochlea nearest to the tip of the electrode and represents mostly high frequency response. It is not possible to obtain a conventional threshold audiogram and, though accurate for higher frequencies, no direct information on the low frequency end of the hearing range can be gained. Another drawback is the necessity for light general anaesthesia, but this is less of a disadvantage than might appear at first sight, since the children in whom it is used are often hyperactive and unable to concentrate or listen. The procedure is time-consuming and costly in terms of personnel and apparatus. It should never be used routinely but reserved for the difficult child and disputable diagnosis, when it becomes indispensable.

A number of other techniques have been and are in use, including evoked response audiometry (involving the monitoring of electroencephalographic activity) and certain tests dependent upon reflex auditory pathways. Each has its place in detailed description of the auditory threshold, or as a screening procedure but none is yet in a suitable state of development for more widespread paedo-audiological use.

Once the hearing loss has been established, its pattern and degree, and the probable cause, it is necessary for the child to have his overall developmental status assessed and the visual acuity measured, if these have not already been carried out.

The child with other handicaps
Each of the causes of middle ear and sensori-neural deafness considered earlier puts the child at risk of a hearing loss which will affect the normal development of spoken language. Many of the conditions associated with other forms of handicap involve the possibility of deafness. It is too often assumed that the child with cerebral palsy or mental handicap is not able to talk because of his predominant handicap and no effort made to assess hearing, which can in any case prove to be an extremely difficult undertaking. The general use of the impedance bridge to measure the stapedial reflex threshold would provide an essential screening tool and overcome much of the preliminary difficulty in determining whether a particular handicapped child hears normally or not. Every child who is under consideration for any form of special education should have a competent otoscopic examination and hearing assessment.

Principles of Management

It is important to reach a decision about the child's hearing without delay. Either the child's hearing is within normal limits or it is not and the sooner the question is resolved one way or the other, the better for the child, his parents and those responsible for his care. In the presence of language delay there is no way forward until the hearing status of the child has been unequivocally determined and the overall pattern of attainments and disabilities explained in non-speculative terms. The danger lies in putting a child whose language development is already impaired, if not severely retarded, into a diagnostic limbo where hearing loss, auditory imperception, autism, receptive aphasia, emotional disturbance and mental retardation all compete for the label depending on the particular bias of the person completing the assessment. The possibility of diagnostic error must always be borne in mind and this puts considerable demands on the clinician primarily responsible for planning the child's management.

Parents' questions

With the diagnosis of hearing loss established the parents will want a number of questions answered. This is natural; it is they who will carry the burden of care of their child and they need to be given all the information that will enable and encourage them to be colleagues able to carry out the task competently. The invariable questions are: what sort of hearing loss, what degree of loss, when will it get better, can it be cured, what caused it and will my child be able to talk? All those involved with the child's care must be prepared to spend time discussing these and many other questions as they arise. The doctor has an important role, but the greater amount of explanation and guidance will come from the health visitor and especially the peripatetic teacher of the deaf.

Surgical intervention

If there is any otological abnormality it is necessary to seek surgical advice so that the middle ear can be restored to maximum efficiency. If all the hearing loss can be attributed to the middle ear it will be sufficient in most instances to review the child's progress in acquiring language. If middle ear loss of 30 dB or more persists despite therapy, it will be necessary to consider a hearing aid. Hearing loss in children with good low frequency hearing but a loss in the higher frequencies (and the rare children in whom this pattern is reversed) present considerable problems which can only be solved on an individual basis. The main consideration is the child's ability to recognize spoken words and understand the meaning of what is said to him.

Hearing aids

As soon as it has been decided that a child will benefit from amplification, arrangements should be put in hand for hearing aids to be supplied and fitted without delay. Impressions are taken for earmoulds which will adapt the receiver heads of the aids to the child's ears. These need to be comfortable, carefully made and well fitting so that advantage can be taken of the acoustical power in the hearing aid. The factor which all too frequently limits the total output of the aid, and the gain to the child, is not the aid itself but poorly fitting earmoulds; the gain control cannot be turned up sufficiently before acoustic feedback from the ear to the microphone of the aid produces the characteristic howl.

There are three main types of hearing aid; the body worn, the ear level or post-aural, and the radio-microphone aids. Within each category there is a bewildering variety of possibilities of combinations of response characteristics. The main factors to be considered in selecting an aid are:

the acoustic gain, i.e. the output of the aid to the ear compared to the input of a tone of say 1000 Hz at 60 dB;

the maximum amplification;

the overall range of frequencies covered and the gain for each frequency band;

the inclusion or not of circuitry for damping down or curtailing sudden loud noises, of particular importance when recruitment is suspected with intra-cochlear lesions and,

electronic arrangements designed to maintain a reasonably constant volume of the spoken voice despite variation of the distance of the child from the speaker.

Apart from these technical factors there are other important considerations:

the design of the controls and ease of operation;

the cost of the aid and the cost of running the aid in terms of battery consumption;

its robustness and ability to stand up to undue wear and tear;

the ease of servicing and promptness of return by the repairing agency.

The pure tone audiogram, or any other threshold measure of hearing, is at best an imperfect guide to hearing aid selection and gives little information on how the child can use his residual hearing between threshold and the level at which loudness discomfort creates tolerance problems. Nor is there any indication of how sharply defined or blurred and indistinct are sounds, or the competing effect of two or more sounds occurring simultaneously. It cannot be assumed that any particular child can automatically hear properly with a hearing aid. Children with similar pure tone losses may have very different patterns of cochlear and neural damage and very different abilities to discriminate and perceive complex sounds at the appropriate rate.

Some indication of the suitability of a particular aid will be given by measuring the child's threshold in free field, under standard conditions, using pure tones or narrow band noise and measuring it again with the hearing aids *in situ*. When the child has sufficient vocabulary to participate, speech tests carried out in free field, and monitored by a sound level meter if non-recorded material is being used, are a useful indication. There is a wide deviation in the accuracy of speech discrimination scores, and differences of less than 10 per cent between two scores cannot be considered significant in choosing between two aids. It is not in the child's interest to keep changing the aids in the hope that one or other model may be a little better.

It is customary to provide body-worn aids for younger children since they are less vulnerable to damage than ear-level aids, which can easily become dislodged in play. The cost factor, which cannot be avoided, combined with the prior availability and long standing use of body-worn aids has determined the main criterion of selection. For the less severely deaf, the National Health Service OL56 and 57 body-worn aids, and the ear level BE11 and 12 models are invaluable. An important feature is the acoustic gain, which may be insufficient even in the most expensive ear-level aids. Ear-level aids have the advantage of being in the correct position to receive sound so that head movement comes naturally into play; they cannot be covered up with several layers of clothing, so reducing gain and increasing adventitious noise; and the child does not hear his own voice at unduly high levels of amplification, which may in some instances exert an inhibiting effect on speech.

Hearing aid selection is a series of compromises between these competing factors, combined with the increasing demands of parents for children to have ear-level aids fitted. As the child himself gets older the emotional resistance to body-worn aids increases and from the age of 9–10 years onward it is this rather than any other factor which may determine the necessity to fit ear-level aids. However, if comparison with the body-worn aids in use shows the latter to be indubitably better, the child will usually accept the result.

It is necessary for the parents and teachers to check the child's use of his aids routinely, to make sure that they are in good repair, the batteries are not run down and earmoulds fit well. It is essential to ensure that the child is using his hearing; simply applying a hearing aid is no guarantee that he will learn to listen and to perceive speech, even when useful gain can be demonstrated on pure tone testing. It is salutary to remember, however, that some children are given aids with which it is not possible to demonstrate any useful gain.

The peripatetic teacher of the deaf
Every child who has a hearing aid should be supervised regularly at home and, if appropriate, at school by a trained teacher of the deaf. This function usually falls to the peripatetic teacher who has the dual role of supervising the auditory training of the child and his development of vocalization and language, and of counselling the parents in all aspects of management of their child. This includes training them to become adept at stimulating their child's understanding of the world around him and his ability to communicate within the family. It will be found that long, continued, patient explanation of the nature of the handicap is necessary, and of its effect on development of the child's language, personality and behaviour. The deaf child has significant effects on other members of the family, with the attendant difficulties of parental acceptance of the handicap, intolerance of his stranger behaviour and resentment at the time devoted specially to him. It needs skilful handling to overcome such problems and the majority of parents need detailed advice and support.

The hearing impaired child needs to mix with normally hearing children and playschools, day nurseries and nursery schools have an important part to play in encouraging normal social behaviour, self-confidence and communication skills. The community paediatrician, the peripatetic teacher of the deaf or the family doctor need to discuss the problems of the child with the person in charge of the nursery and encourage individual adult members of staff to participate in helping the child learn to talk.

Assessment of progress
The child's progress must be watched carefully and he should be reassessed at regular 3–4 monthly intervals. The points to remember are the condition of the child's ears, the hearing threshold, the fit of the earmoulds, the functioning of the hearing aids, their suitability for his type and level of hearing loss and his language development.

A speech therapist trained and experienced in assessing childhood language has a vital contribution to make at these review clinic visits. Assessment of linguistic progress includes vocabulary size, the way in which words are joined together to form sentences, the intelligibility of his speech and attendant factors such as control of volume and pitch, patterns of intonation and the range and type of consonants present. Even more important is the child's understanding of what is said to him. What does he hear, how much better (if at all) can he manage with his aids on, what can he understand and by what means? Can he carry out tasks when he cannot see the speaker's face and hands, does he need the additional clues provided by lip-reading (or does he rely on this) or will he only respond to gestures such as pointing by hand or a glance of the eye?

School placement
As school age approaches at 5 years, a decision has to be reached on the most appropriate form of placement. This decision does not depend only upon the audiometric loss, but also upon the child's understanding and use of language. If verbal comprehension and expression are less than a year behind his age level, it is difficult to see why he should not be placed in the ordinary school, whatever his hearing loss. Children with severe losses may do surprisingly well so long as they have understanding and sympathetic teachers and the full support of their families.

The possibility that children with severe difficulties in acquiring language may have other learning difficulties should always be borne in mind and psychological assessment using non-verbal scales and sub-sections of standard instruments will be required.

If the hearing loss is severe or profound and if language development is so seriously retarded in the 5-year-old that it is appropriate to a child of less than 2 years, he is clearly experiencing great difficulty and it will be necessary to consider the advisability of placement in a school for the deaf. There is opportunity in some schools of exposure to methods of language training which include certain forms of manual communication, such as the traditional sign system with finger spelling, or more recent developments such as the Paget Gorman Sign System or Cued Speech. Advantage should always be taken of the residual hearing as auditory clues, however minimal, are essential to the child's appreciation of speech patterns and to his developing control of voice quality and intonation contours. Group training aids will help this process.

The majority of children will fall between these two extremes. They will have a partial hearing loss which is fairly or well compensated by hearing aids. These children are best helped by being placed in special units in ordinary schools. The so-called Partially Hearing Units provide the opportunity of integration with ordinary children for certain periods during the day, combined with the more intensive and personal care of a teacher of the deaf who has a small number of children to look after (usually with additional help) and a classroom which is suitably treated to reduce ambient noise and reverberation, with the provision of further amplification devices such as the loop and the group aid.

The parents' desire not to have their child away from home at boarding school, or subjected to long journeys to a special school or unit, introduces constraints which cannot be ignored and which may suggest the desirability of a trial period within a particular mode of education which is not the first choice of their advisers. The child's placement should not be looked upon as static and immutable. His progress should be under regular review and watched carefully. This is more important because for many children placement is a compromise between what is most appropriate and what is available.

Further Reading

BALLANTYNE J. and GROVES J. (1971) *The Ear. Scott-Brown's Diseases of the Ear, Nose and Throat, Volume 2*, 3rd Ed. London: Butterworth.

DALE D.M.C. (1967) *Deaf Children at Home and at School*. London: University of London Press.

EWING A. and EWING E.C. (1971) *Hearing Impaired Children under Five. A guide for parents and teachers*. Manchester: Manchester University Press.

GERBER S.E. (1974) *Introductory Hearing Science*. London: W.B. Saunders.

HINCHCLIFFE R. and HARRISON D. (1976) *Scientific Foundations of Otolaryngology*. London: Heinemann.

TOWER D.B. (1975) *Human Communication and its Disorders, Volume 3 The Nervous System*, ed. Eagles E.L. New York: Raven.

WATSON T.J. (1967) *The Education of Hearing-Impaired Children*. London: University of London Press.

WHETNALL E. and FRY D.B. (1964) *The Deaf Child*. London: Heinemann.

CHAPTER 23

The Deaf-blind Child

The deaf-blind child was defined by Davis (1961) as one 'whose combination of auditory and visual handicap is such that he cannot be educated adequately in a normal program for deaf or blind children'.

The rarity of this condition is illustrated by the fact that in the series of 11 865 children aged 10–12 years reported by Rutter, Graham and Yule (1970) there were no deaf-blind children although the incidence of blindness and deafness was 1.3 and 1.2 per 1000 respectively.

Several authors have considered populations of visually handicapped or hearing handicapped children and have reported the incidence of the other sensory handicap in these groups. Fraser and Friedmann (1967) found that 47 out of 776 (6.06 per cent) of visually handicapped children in educational establishments had an additional defect of hearing; Fine (1968) found that this occurred in 133 (6.07 per cent) of 817 blind and 1374 partially sighted children. If these figures are applied to the incidence of blindness found in the Isle of Wight, this would give an incidence of approximately 7.8 deaf-blind children per 100 000. Jensema and Mullins (1974) reporting from the USA found that 7 per cent of a very large population of deaf children had a visual problem and if this proportion is the same in Britain, this would give an incidence of approximately 8.4 deaf-blind children per 100 000.

Aetiology

As with other handicaps in childhood, the deaf-blind syndrome may be genetic in origin or may be acquired as the result of pre-, peri-, or postnatal hazards.

The comparative rarity of the combined handicap means that there is considerable difference in aetiology in many of the reported series; a few families with a genetic disorder or a local outbreak of rubella will significantly alter the ratio of genetic to acquired causes. Similarly, the presentation of the visual and auditory handicaps may be exceedingly variable in different series. Moreover, the two conditions may not be manifest at the outset. For instance in the rubella syndrome, it is usual for the auditory handicap to be detected much later than the other disabilities (Borton and Stark, 1970; Forrest and Menser, 1970), whereas in Usher's syndrome the auditory handicap is detected early whilst vision may remain apparently normal until teenage (McLeod et al., 1971).

GENETIC CONDITIONS

Rare genetic disorders are responsible for approximately one-third of cases (27 per cent, Fraser and Friedmann, 1967; 42 per cent, Bergstrom, 1973). Bergstrom (1973) listed 27 possible conditions in which deaf children might have a visual disorder and Kaplan in the same publication cited 14 conditions in which deafness was frequently associated with eye defects and 25 in which it occasionally occurred. Most of the syndromes described are eponymous, so far the enzyme defect having been determined in very few of the presumed metabolic disorders.

A comprehensive account of neuroretinal disorders is given by Vinken and Bruyn (1972) and cases involving hearing defect are included. Pigmentary retinopathy is associated with deafness in Usher's and Hallgren's syndromes and also in Refsum's syndrome (with ataxia and polyneuritis) and the Laurence–Moon–Biedl syndrome (with obesity, hypogonadism and mental retardation). Neuroretinal degeneration occurs in the Alstrom and Cockayne syndromes. In all these cases the deafness is sensori-neural.

Optic atrophy may occur as a primary condition but is more often secondary to lesions of the skull, as in Apert's syndrome (acrocephalosyndactyly), Crouzon's disease (craniofacial dysostosis) and Albers-Schönberg disease (osteopetrosis). Often in these cases the deafness is also secondary and conductive in nature.

Other conditions not affecting the nervous system directly may affect the structure of the eye and the auditory conductive pathways. The visual defect may be due to lesions of the cornea (as in the mucopolysaccharidoses), the lens (as in Alport's syndrome and the ectodermal dysplasias), or associated with retinal detachment (Roaf's syndrome) or colobomata (Goldenhar's and Treacher Collins syndromes). The associated deafness may be conductive or sensori-neural and other structural abnormalities may be associated with the primary defect.

Other handicaps should always be sought in children who present with visual or auditory disabilities which are genetic in origin.

ACQUIRED CONDITIONS

Prenatal rubella
In all published series prenatal rubella infection is the commonest single cause of the deaf-blind syndrome. Fraser and Friedmann (1967) report 34 per cent, Budden *et al.*, (1974) 46 per cent, Bergstrom (1973) and Jensema and Mullins (1974) 58 per cent. Prospective studies have shown variation in the type of lesions which occur and in the severity of handicap.

All workers are agreed that the most severe manifestations of prenatal rubella infection follow when maternal infection occurs during the first trimester (Dudgeon, 1967, 1969; Borton and Stark 1970; Peckham, 1972). The incidence and combination of effects shows a range from fetal loss through abortion or stillbirth to a number of single or multiple handicaps in survivors.

From Australia, Forrest and Menser (1970) found that 7/41 affected children

(17 per cent) had a single handicap only and 27/41 (66 per cent) had a combined audiovisual handicap, with or without other disabilities: from Britain, Gumpel (1972) reported a single handicap in 14/83 (17 per cent) and 47/83 (57 per cent) deaf-blind with or without other disabilities.

The commonest ocular lesions are cataract and pigmentary retinopathy. These may occur together or as single defects in one or both eyes. The presence of a cataract may make it difficult to observe the retinopathy, the appearance of which is diagnostic of rubella, although the condition itself is frequently symptomless. Other lesions which occur on their own or in association with the above, are glaucoma, microphthalmia or anophthalmia.

Hearing loss may be peripheral (due to cochlear destruction and less commonly to middle ear abnormalities) or central. Central auditory imperception is defined as inability to respond appropriately to sound on a cortical level. In a series of 112 rubella syndrome children with significant speech delay (Ames *et al.*, 1970) the primary cause of failure to develop speech was peripheral hearing loss in 35 per cent, central auditory imperception in 27 per cent, these conditions combined in 12 per cent and mental retardation or cerebral palsy in 9 per cent. The remaining 17 per cent were typical deaf-blind children with peripheral loss in two-thirds and CAI in one-third. Most investigators find the auditory lesion to be progressive and in any suspected case serial auditory testing is essential (Borton and Stark, 1970; Forrest and Menser, 1970; Gumpel *et al.*, 1971; Peckham, 1972).

The audiovisual handicaps described are the result of direct attack of the virus on the eye and the brain and in some children this may cause additional disorders, such as cerebral palsy and/or mental retardation (De Long, 1971). Cardiac lesions are also common.

The diagnosis of rubella embryopathy rests upon clinical confirmation of rubella in the mother at the appropriate stage of pregnancy, presence of one or more of the classical signs in the child and positive serological status of the child and mother. In this respect it is useful to remember that the incidence of rubella infection in preschool children is low, less than 7 per cent up to the age of 4 years (Gumpel *et al.*, 1971), and therefore a significant rubella titre up to that age indicates the probability of previous intrauterine infection. Changes in antibody levels in fetus, infant, child and mother are reported in detail by Dudgeon, Marshall and Soothill (1969).

Prevention of rubella by vaccination of susceptible females of appropriate age is now possible (Peebles, 1971). If a pregnant woman, who is in contact with rubella during her pregnancy and is thought to be susceptible, wishes the pregnancy to continue to term, Peckham (1972) has shown that administration of pooled gamma globulin is effective in preventing the most serious effects of intrauterine rubella infection.

Perinatal
The main perinatal factors which lead to a combined audiovisual handicap are prematurity, anoxia or both. Retrolental fibroplasia occurs only in small premature infants and is associated with inadequately controlled administration

of oxygen (p. 426). Fraser and Friedmann found that 8/177 (4 per cent) of children with retrolental fibroplasia had a hearing loss and Fine found 28 out of 317 (9 per cent). Other visual defects associated with prematurity are cataracts or severe errors of refraction. Anoxia may cause cataracts, optic atrophy or cerebral blindness.

Auditory handicaps may arise from the effects of prematurity, anoxia or kernicterus damaging the cochlear nucleus (Hall, 1964).

Both prematurity and anoxia may be associated with cerebral palsy or mental handicap, so that in some children the sensory handicaps are a component of a more global disorder.

Postnatal

Later acquired causes of audiovisual handicap are less common but may arise from road traffic and other accidents and non-accidental injury; from infections such as meningitis, encephalitis or autoimmune disorders, or from cardiac arrest.

Assessment

The purpose of comprehensive assessment is 'to discover the medical, social and educational needs of handicapped children and to bring such appropriate facilities that exist to their aid' (Moore, 1973). For most children the assessment services provided in the paediatric department of the district general hospital are adequate to fulfil this. However, the deaf-blind child poses a problem of such rarity and complexity that local facilities may not always suffice to unravel the closely woven strands of multiple handicap. Davis (1961) describes the dilemma of the deaf-blind child as follows: 'When both sensory defects are present in an individual, although many of the characteristics of the deaf child and of the blind child may be present, the end result is not a simple combination of characteristics; it is a personality structure that is unique and exceedingly complex and the range of variation within the group is greater than the addition of the ranges of variation for the two separate groups.'

It is clearly essential to make skilled and accurate assessments of the degree and type of visual and auditory handicap and to effect correction of either or both as far as this can be achieved. In addition, attention must be given to any associated disabilities whether these are motor, perceptual, emotional, behavioural or intellectual. This will entail prolonged observation and evaluation by an experienced multidisciplinary team and will probably need to be undertaken in a residential setting.

Ophthalmic assessment

The tests to be used are no different from those described in Chapters 8 and 21 but additional skills are necessary to elicit the child's participation. Much will depend on his ability to communicate. Play activities which involve procedures such as attachment of scalp electrodes should be initiated whenever possible in order to facilitate the fixing of leads for later testing of cortical evoked responses. For other procedures (e.g. electroretinography, electro-oculography, funduscopy, retinoscopy and refraction) general anaesthesia may be required, preferably undertaking all necessary investigations at one session.

Auditory assessment

Audiometricians and audiologists are accustomed to evaluating the hearing of difficult children, whether shy, timid, obstreperous or handicapped in other ways, but the blind child presents the greatest challenge. Hearing tests must be carried out on a conscious child, so that it is not possible to have recourse to anaesthesia. Problems arise first in the audiometric screening tests carried out by health visitors as infants with visual handicap may not locate sounds. It is important that those who fail the test should be referred immediately to an expert hearing centre. The conditioning techniques used for mentally handicapped children may be adapted for deaf-blind children. Play techniques need to be used prior to evoked response audiometry as for visual evoked responses. Positive auditory evoked responses do not necessarily mean that the child hears normally, but may help to differentiate between sensori-neural deafness and central auditory imperception thus affording guidance in management (Ames *et al.*, 1970). Even when there is a positive response in early testing it is essential that this should be repeated at regular invervals in view of the progression of auditory handicap in many children with the rubella syndrome.

Evaluation of the child's global ability

Even if it has been possible to make some assessment of the child's visual and auditory competence, there still remains the problem of the child's overall mental ability. The extreme sensory deprivation suffered by a child with a combined visual and auditory handicap is bound to cause delay in the acquisition of many skills and may at times lead to symptoms of withdrawal with features of autism. Milburn (1967) discusses in detail the utilization of other sensory modalities in blind persons and affords an insight into some of the difficulties likely to face children who are also deprived of auditory information. Gross motor development may be affected by lack of sensory stimulation or by the delay in maturation described by De Long (1971) and in some children there may be specific defects in motor pathways causing cerebral palsy. Over-protection by parents and family is commonplace and the child's lack of experience may affect both his mobility and his social competence. As there are no formal test procedures available, the child's response to skilled training affords the best means of evaluating future potential and of deciding appropriate educational methods. Usually it will be necessary to place the child in an optimal environmental programme, which may be residential, so that he is helped and encouraged by staff who are experienced in dealing with all disabilities.

Management

Principles for management of a particular handicap are governed by the general and specific needs of the child and the response that these demand from the parents and the professionals who are helping them.

The deaf-blind baby starts with a double disadvantage. He may be in intensive care by reason of prematurity, rubella infection or the effects of a difficult delivery and therefore, it is not possible to establish from the outset the close physical contact between mother and baby, desirable for all nursing couples, but particularly essential for the deaf-blind. In addition, the mother expects positive information, particularly with regard to diagnosis, prognosis and management, and in the case of many, if not most, deaf-blind babies this cannot be offered immediately.

In view of these difficulties, emotional and psychological support should be started in the maternity unit and carried on in the community from the most suitable source, whether health visitor, family doctor, community child health doctor or the paediatric hospital service. Freeman (1975) describes most vividly the difficulties for a mother handling a deaf-blind child during the early months of life and later. She describes the early techniques which she used to help and train her own child. Bumbalo and Seidel (1975) report how these techniques can be fostered and encouraged by community nurses visiting the homes regularly and initiating the techniques for encouragement of communication, mobility and social skills described below. Although the training and provision of specialist community nurses/health visitors, as recommended by Fox (1974), is not universal in Britain, some area health authorities have already created such posts. At this stage care and support of this kind does not require accurate diagnosis or comprehensive assessment of future needs.

Early management has two main objectives, establishment of communication and attainment of social independence. Handling the baby is all-important for the inception of these. Normal babies who receive visual and auditory clues from their surroundings soon begin to anticipate being picked up from cot or pram for feeding or changing. Such clues cannot be given to the deaf-blind child who must make use of olfactory and tactile senses. Therefore the mother and other attendants should use consistent cues, olfactory (perfume and soap) and tactile (touch on the hand, forehead or elsewhere) prior to picking up the baby and should always do so gently and slowly.

Freeman (1975) gives detailed guidance on the attainment of mobility, social independence and communication.

Mobility

Children with useful residual vision and normal motor ability may not need additional skilled help to attain mobility; visual goals provide adequate motivation and the child is able to move his body in response. Those children with a severe visual handicap, or whose motor control is poor or abnormal, benefit from the help of a physiotherapist trained in developmental methods. Children who are pleasurably accustomed to movement and handling will respond more rapidly to mobility training and to learning social skills.

Social skills

The young child needs to be positively involved as soon as possible and a sign system built up to be used consistently with all routines. Freeman (1975) suggests that in most situations in the early years one should consider what information a seeing-hearing child would derive from familiar routines and then set about ways of giving the deaf-blind child the same information in a different form.

Bathing and washing should mean splashing in warm water, prior to the use of soap. Babies should always be cued before being lifted out and like normal children who enjoy their bath their protests should thereafter be ignored. Feeding should mean favourite food in the fingers which hopefully will go to the mouth and drinking should mean hands round cup or bottle. Undressing should begin by guiding hands to hat and shoes with the adult always at the back of the child so that the guided movements are in the correct direction; dressing should begin by tapping the limb to be offered for garments to be put on.

Communication
To begin with communication will be largely idiosyncratic as mother and baby begin to make contact, but this should be gradually extended to a wider circle, father, siblings, grandparents and supporting professionals. The family sign language should then be gradually carried over to one of the established forms such as Paget Gorman*, or the manual alphabet for the child with little or no vision but adequate mental function and motor control.

Concurrently with the general home management of the child which is helping him to discover himself as a personality, specialist skills and experience should be given to the correction, where possible, of the sensory disabilities and to the training of the child in the use of residual and alternative sensory input. Therefore ophthalmological treatment (Chapter 21) and audiological treatment (Chapter 22) should be pursued with vigour, as for children with a single handicap. Educational advisers for blind children and peripatetic teachers of the deaf will need to be members of the team helping the mother and working with other on-the-spot professionals.

When the time comes for formal education the child will almost certainly need to attend a special unit for the deaf-blind in which the teaching staff, whenever possible, are doubly qualified for children with auditory and visual handicaps. In some children the overall handicap will be so severe that they cannot respond to such special education and they may be placed in a unit for mentally handicapped children. In this situation the staff of the unit will need help from appropriate specialist teachers. Aspects of educational assessment and instruction were covered by a number of contributors at the Fourth International Conference on Deaf-Blind Children to which the reader is referred (De Long and Peebles, 1971).

* Particulars of the Paget Gorman sign system, produced by the Association for Experiment in Deaf Education, London, can be obtained from A.E.D.E. Publications Committee, c/o 13 Ashbury Drive, Tilehurst, Reading, Berkshire.

References

AMES M.D., PLOTKIN S.A., WINCHESTER R.A. and ATKINS T.E. (1970) Central auditory imperception. *Journal of the American Medical Association*, **213**, 419

BERGSTROM LaV. (1973) The ear specialist's role in management of the deaf blind child. In *Diagnosis and Evaluation of Deaf Blind Children*, eds. Moriarty D.F., Smith W.J. and Horsley J.L. Denver, Colorado: Colorado Department of Education.

BORTON T.E. and STARK E.W. (1970) Audiological findings in hearing loss secondary to maternal rubella. *Pediatrics*, **45**, 225

BUDDEN S.S., ROBINSON G.C., MACLEAN C.D., CAMBON K.G. (1974) Deafness in infants and preschool children. *American Annals of the Deaf*, **119**, 387.

BUMBALO J.A. and SEIDEL M.A. (1975) Identifying and serving a multiple handicapped population. *Nursing Clinics of North America*, **10**, 341.

DAVIS C.J. (1961) The deaf-blind child: diagnosis and evaluation. *Proceedings of the Convention of American Instructors of the Deaf*, **40**, 69.

DE LONG G.R. (1971) Possible contributions from paediatric neurology and neuropathology to the understanding and management of congenital rubella children. In *4th International Conference on Deaf Blind Children*. Watertown, Mass.: International Council of Educators of Blind Youth.

DUDGEON J.A. (1967) Maternal rubella and its effect on the foetus. *Archives of Disease in Childhood*, **42**, 110.

DUDGEON J.A. (1969) Congenital rubella. Pathogenesis and immunology. *American Journal of Diseases of Children*, **118**, 35.

DUDGEON J.A., MARSHALL W.C. and SOOTHILL J.F. (1969) Immunological responses to early and late intrauterine virus infections. *Journal of Pediatrics*, **75**, 1149.

FINE S.R. (1968) *Blind and Partially Sighted Children. Education Survey 4.* London: Her Majesty's Stationery Office.

FORREST J.M. and MENSER M.A. (1970) Congenital rubella in school children and adolescents. *Archives of Disease in Childhood*, **45**, 63.

FOX A.M. (1974) *They Get this Training but they Don't Really Know how You Feel.* London: National Fund for Research into Crippling Diseases.

FRASER G.R. and FRIEDMANN A.I. (1967) *The Causes of Blindness in Childhood.* Baltimore: Johns Hopkins Press.

FREEMAN P. (1975) *Understanding the Deaf–Blind Child.* London: Heinemann.

GUMPEL S.M. (1972) Clinical and social status of patients with congenital rubella. *Archives of Disease in Childhood*, **47**, 330.

GUMPEL S.M., HAYES K. and DUDGEON J.A. (1971) Congenital perceptive deafness: role of intrauterine rubella. *British Medical Journal*, **2**, 300.

HALL J.G. (1964) The cochlea and the cohlear nuclei in neonatal asphyxia. *Acta Oto-laryngologica*, Suppl. **194**, 1.

JENSEMA C. and MULLINS J. (1974) Onset, cause and additional handicaps in hearing impaired children. *American Annals of the Deaf*, **119**, 701.

KAPLAN M. (1973) The role of the ophthalmologist in the diagnosis and evaluation of deaf-blind children. In *Diagnosis and Evaluation of Deaf-blind Children* eds. Moriarty D.F., Smith W.J. and Horsley J.L. Denver, Colorado: Colorado Department of Education.

McLEOD A.C., McCONNELL F.E., SNEENEY A., COOPER M.C. and NANCE W.E. (1971) Clinical variation in Usher's syndrome. *Archives of Otolaryngology*, **94**, 321.

MILBURN W.O. (1967) Utilization of sensory information with special reference to blindness. In *Visual and Auditory Defects Accompanying Mental Retardation*, eds. Cawley J.F. and Matkin N.D. Connecticut: University of Connecticut.

MOORE J.R. (1973) Comprehensive Assessment. In *The Young Retarded Child*, ed. Griffiths M.I. Edinburgh: Churchill Livingstone.

PECKHAM C.S. (1972) Clinical and laboratory study of children exposed in utero to maternal rubella. *Archives of Disease in Childhood*, **47**, 571.

PEEBLES T.C. (1971) Prevention and treatment of the rubella syndrome. In *4th International Conference on Deaf-Blind Children*. Watertown Mass.: International Council of Educators of Blind Youth.

RUTTER M., GRAHAM P. and YULE W. (1970) *A Neuropsychiatric Study in Childhood. Clinics in Developmental Medicine. Nos. 35/36*. London: Heinemann.

VINKEN, P.J. and BRUYN G.W. (1972) Neuroretinal degenerations. In *Handbook of Clinical Neurology*. Amsterdam: North Holland Publishing Company.

CHAPTER 24

Speech Disorders

The development of a child's language and speech provides an absorbing and rewarding study. Psychologists, phoneticians, linguists and psycholinguists have all made major contributions to our understanding of normal and abnormal development patterns. Perhaps the major clinical advance in recent years has been the growing understanding by the clinical specialists (audiologists, speech therapists and paediatricians) of their respective roles in the assessment and management of children with language disorders. This has led to an increasing trend towards combined clinics, which can only be of benefit to the children, their families and to the professionals themselves.

There is little that gives greater pleasure to parents than hearing their child's first words. Conversely great disappointment is caused by the child who does not talk, or talk 'properly'. When a child is slow to walk this is more easily dismissed as due to laziness, obesity or being 'just like his father', but when a child is slow to talk, most people think this means low intelligence. Parental anxiety is often suffered in silence until brought out into the open by a comment from relative or friend. Unfortunately simplistic explanations and 'cures' are usually suggested such as tonsillectomy, division of a tongue tie or a visit to the doctor to see if he is 'all right'. If a visit to the family doctor does take place (often after some delay to see whether 'he will start talking by himself') the parents may be told that the child will grow out of it or they are regaled with anecdotal recollections about other late talkers. If the child is referred further this is as likely to be to an ENT clinic as to a speech clinic. The number of children who have had their tonsils and adenoids removed before referral to speech clinics is still inordinately high.

Thus when a child first presents at a speech clinic it is not unusual to find that there has been a long time lag since the parents first became concerned at the child's slow or disordered speech development. Too often the delay itself has heightened the anxieties and disappointment at the child's performance, especially if hopes of an instant cure have been unwisely encouraged. By this time the child himself is frequently on the defensive or has reacted with a frank behaviour problem.

In areas where development screening of total infant and young child populations is in operation, speech delays and disorders are likely to be identified earlier and more often referred directly to speech clinics. However, if the more usual course of events is not borne in mind when evaluating the parents' account of the child's problem or when assessing the child himself, then the attempt to reach a diagnosis may be seriously impeded from the outset.

Examination and Investigation

Children who present with speech and language problems form a motley group. Among those who present as late or poor talkers I find many with associated developmental disorders as well as psychiatric and social pathology. Perhaps it is because speech problems are regarded as 'respectable' that many parents first appear with their children complaining of poor speech rather than other difficulties. Hence the necessity for a complete and wide-ranging assessment of the child's development as well as a detailed investigation of his speech and language. The paediatrician is in the best position to complete the former and the speech therapist the latter.

The examination and assessment takes time and the white-tiled clinical atmosphere of many out-patient departments is not ideal. Many teams find that it is best for the speech therapist to see the child and his parents first in a relaxed atmosphere, where she can play informally with him. Put at ease in a play situation the child is more likely to participate verbally than if confronted immediately with a formal test situation (p. 172). After this the paediatrician can join in the play session or the child, parents and therapist can move into the paediatrician's office, where again a variety of toys provides opportunity for spontaneous play.

History. The paediatrician begins by taking a detailed history. When talking about the family history, social background and the sequence of the child's language development the parents' other concerns are likely to emerge. During this time the doctor also has an excellent opportunity to assess the normality or otherwise of the child–parent relationship, the degree of concern (and the direction of that concern) and to observe the child's behaviour.

Particular emphasis should be placed on a history of speech disorders in the immediate family and in second degree relatives. The history of pregnancy, labour and delivery can often throw light on the origin of the child's basic disorder. Mother's health during the puerperal period may give an indication of the initial bonding process. The early feeding pattern and responses of the child are usually remembered well, particularly if there were difficulties. Most parents do not understand the significance of these for the child's later speech production, just as they do not recognize that a 'good baby' who gives no trouble might in fact be showing an abnormality of development.

It may be better to obtain the detailed history of motor, adaptive and social development before going on to take a detailed history of the child's language development, as the former is less prone to interpretative influences. The child's past health history, particularly of convulsions and recurrent upper respiratory tract infections, is most important. The latter may well have been complicated by otitis media with intermittent episodes of deafness or the more chronic condition of secretory otitis media or 'glue ear' (p. 433).

Physical examination. The physical examination should include a complete neurological examination. This may show previously unsuspected abnormality of the cranial nerves, mild forms of neurological syndromes such as ataxia or asymmetry, signs of delayed maturation as detected by the Oseretsky test of motor maturation (Oseretsky, 1931; Doll, 1976) or associated movements as described by Fog and Fog (1963).

Examination of the lips, gums, teeth, tongue, palate, nose and ears is essential to detect any structural abnormality or functional difficulty.

Developmental assessment. The third aspect of the paediatrician's investigation is a general developmental assessment (Chapter 4). This must include screening tests for visual acuity and visual fields as well as tests of hearing (Chapter 8). Short attention span and hyperactivity will also be noted.

By this time a reasonably accurate picture will have been built up of the child's ability to communicate and understand and of his willingness to make contact with strangers, all of which may be very important in determining whether further investigations and referral are required. The initial team of speech therapist and paediatrician may then ask for the help of an audiologist, otolaryngologist or other professionals, such as an educational psychologist or psychiatrist, to enlarge the picture further.

Classification and Presentation of Speech and Language Disorders

It is important to have a classification of children's speech and language disorders not just to satisfy the doctor's diagnostic instincts but to give a guide to necessary investigations, treatment and likely prognosis. The clinical classification described by Ingram (1959) has been shown to be very useful and has stood the test of time (Table 24.1).

Dysphonia

The only common impairment of voicing in young children is hoarseness. It is often difficult to know exactly why this occurs but it is probably on the basis of a chronic laryngitis. Dysphonia is known to be associated with large families and to be commoner in poor homes. In these groups a child is liable to have more respiratory tract infections and may require to shout against the babble of voices, which in turn are in competition with the radio and television. A clinical point often made by parents is that voice quality varies a good deal from day to day and from situation to situation.

As inflammatory changes (including nodules) are often present on the vocal cords, referral to an otolaryngologist is usually necessary. Asking a young child to rest his voice is unreasonable but the parents can be asked to reduce noise level in the home and speak quietly themselves. If the child attends a play group this may need to be discontinued for a period because of the high noise level pertaining in these groups.

Dysrhythmia

This heading covers the whole range of 'non-fluencies' and refers to blocking of speech as much as stammering. Children are commonly referred with this sort of problem at the play group stage (i.e. 3 years or older), at which age excitement

TABLE 24.1. Clinical classification of speech disorders.

Disorders of voicing (dysphonia)

Disorders of respiratory co-ordination (dysrhythmia)

Disorders of speech sound production with demonstrable dysfunction or structural abnormalities of tongue, lips, teeth or palate (dysarthria)

Due to local abnormalities of:

jaws and teeth

tongue

lips

palate

pharynx

mixed

Due to neurological abnormalities:

upper motor neurone lesions

nuclear agenesis

lower motor neurone lesions

abnormal movement patterns

Disorders of speech sound production not attributable to dysfunction or structural abnormality but associated with other disease or adverse environmental factors (secondary speech disorders)

Associated with:

mental defect

hearing defect

true dysphasia

psychiatric disorders

adverse environmental factors

combinations of the above

The developmental speech disorder syndrome

(specific developmental speech disorders)

Mixed speech disorders comprising two or more of the above categories

---

tends to exaggerate a physiological dysrhythmia. The term 'clutter', in common use amongst paediatricians and speech therapists, helps to differentiate these milder dysrhythmias from the prognostically more significant stammer or stutter. Cluttering may be accentuated by the habit parents (and often grandparents) have of asking the child to stop what he is saying, repeat and start again speaking slowly. This inevitably results in frustration in the child.

Temporary non-fluencies are quite common in older children but only 1 per cent of children have a persistent speech dysrhythmia (Andrews and Harris, 1964). These authors noted a strong family predisposition and suggested that 'stuttering may be transmitted as a single dominant gene, the penetrance being modified by other genetic and environmental factors'. The psychological stress that so frequently accompanies stutter is more likely to be a result rather than the cause.

Early management should be indirect and should concentrate on working with the parents, teachers and others involved with the child, encouraging them to detract rather than attract attention to his difficulties. Later treatment involves a marked investment of the child's time, energy and application to ensure success and is usually reserved until the early teens. The most commonly used technique is that of syllable timed speech.

Dysarthria

Many parents attribute their child's speech difficulty to structural abnormality and hope for a quick success following surgical treatment. While paying attention to the various structures and functions of the speech apparatus, it ill behoves the doctor to build up hopes which cannot be fulfilled in practice. For example, tongue tie is very common but it is extremely rare for a child's speech defect to be caused by this. The speech therapist will be able to detect any lack of mobility of the tongue, particularly in the formation of tongue tip sounds.

Apart from the hypernasality produced by major forms of cleft palate, nasal escape can also be caused by sub-mucous cleft. This is usually associated with a bifid uvula and is felt (by a carefully inserted finger) as a V formation of the posterior hard palate, instead of the normal midline single knob at the junction of the hard and soft palate.

Palatal disproportion is another cause of nasal escape. Here the palate moves normally but the naso-pharyngeal aperture is abnormally large and closure is not achieved. These children have a rather typical appearance in profile with a long protruding maxilla. Nasal escape is detected by holding a finger under the child's nose while he says 'ee'. Unilateral or bilateral nasal escape is detected by hot air blowing on the examining finger. Function of the palate can be further demonstrated by a palatogram, in which the soft tissues of the pharynx are visualized on x-ray at rest, while the child is saying 'ee' (for palatal closure) and 'nn' (for palatal opening).

There is controversy about thumb-sucking and consequent protrusion of the upper incisors as a cause of dysarthria particularly lisp. In this author's experience this is rarely the only cause of lisp, which is more likely to be caused by persistence of the infantile form of tongue thrust. Little can be done to prevent early thumb-sucking but orthodontic treatment may be indicated later. This also has a pleasing cosmetic result.

Secondary speech disorders

Mental defect. When slow speech development is associated with commensurate slow development in all other fields mental retardation is the most likely diagnosis (p. 80). It should be remembered that such children are at risk of other problems related to the cause of their mental retardation, e.g. high tone deafness in children with congenital rubella.

Hearing defect. Normal hearing is of critical importance for the acquisition of language. Unlike the older child, the very young child cannot indicate that he is not hearing properly as he is unaware, in terms of experience, that his auditory environment should be otherwise. Hearing loss is extremely common in childhood (p. 4). Mild to moderate degrees of hearing loss are very difficult to identify and diagnose in the early years.

Dysphasia. It is probable that true (acquired) dysphasia is not so uncommon in early childhood as is usually thought. It may not be recognized because the complete picture of aphasia is not produced in a child who is still in the process of developing language. Acquired dysphasia may follow some febrile convulsions and the para-infectious encephalopathies.

Psychiatric disorders. The serious (and rare) condition of infantile autism (p. 487) presents as severe language retardation in association with severe behavioural and emotional problems. A significant feature is the child's inconsistent response from infancy to sounds of any kind.

Children subjected to psychosocial deprivation tend to have poor speech and show poor use of language and reading skills as they grow older. However, psychosocial deprivation is an uncommon cause of a marked delay in speech development (Rutter and Mittler, 1972). When it does occur comprehension of language is not retarded to the same extent as spoken language and production of word sounds. Another feature is that gesture is used little by these children.

Speech disorders in children with cerebral palsy

When large numbers of children with cerebral palsy are studied, at least one-half are found to have significant speech defects (Ingram, 1964). These arise from a complex variety of causes which are often compounded in an individual child. Even children whose control of the bulbar musculature is not affected may suffer from dysphasia, defective hearing and attention or from global retardation. In addition there are the deprivations of sensori-motor and language stimulation so common in cerebral palsy (p. 322) and the difficulties arising from inadequate, inappropriate or multiple changes in the child's speech therapy and early education programmes.

Bilateral hemiplegia and dyskinetic cerebral palsy. In some children there is actual paresis and in others inco-ordination of the bulbar musculature (i.e. the muscles which control movements of the lips, jaws, tongue, palate and vocal cords). Typically bulbar paresis is seen in children with bilateral hemiplegia and inco-ordination and involuntary movements in those with dyskinesia. Often there is a history of severe feeding difficulty in infancy, with persistence of bite reflex or tongue thrust and continuous drooling of saliva. While children with bilateral hemiplegia are frequently mentally retarded (and thus non-speaking), those with dyskinesia are more likely to be of normal intelligence but may be further handicapped by hearing defect. The dyskinetic's speech has a marked fluctuation in tone and rhythm, largely due to involuntary movements which disrupt the utterances and even the individual words. There tends to be marked heightening of anxiety and increase in spasmodic movements as the child attempts to get over each individual difficulty. Consequently, relieving tension, minimizing the gross movements and increasing the efficiency of rhythm of breathing and voicing are obvious objectives for therapy.

Hemiplegia. Children with congenital hemiplegia often have a normal pattern of speech development. If they do show a disorder then a simple retardation is the most common. If the hemiplegia is acquired then, as would be expected, children with right-sided hemiplegia will have more difficulty with speech than those with left hemiplegia (p. 289). As complete dominance of one cerebral hemisphere is not usually achieved till the age of 8 years or over, the timing of the acquired insult will largely determine the severity of the defect and the prognosis for further acquisition of speech and language.

Diplegia. The likelihood of diplegic children having speech defects largely depends on the extent of the cerebral palsy and whether or not there is associated mental retardation. Those with minimal upper limb involvement are unlikely to have much difficulty with articulation, whereas those with more marked involvement of the upper limbs may have bulbar paresis and are also more likely to be mentally retarded. Nevertheless, in groups of diplegic patients the commonest pattern is again simple retardation of speech development.

Ataxic cerebral palsies. In ataxic cerebral palsies the scanning speech of adult cerebellar disease is occasionally heard. However, simple retardation is a much more frequent pattern. Although these children may show little actual paresis, they frequently exhibit marked inco-ordination of the movements of lips, tongue and palate. The delay in speech development is often quite marked in the first few years of life, but when speech does appear it may develop rapidly and eventual prognosis be good. However, speech therapy is often required for articulation defects in the early school years.

Basics of management. The implications for management are obvious. As children with cerebral palsy have a high incidence of speech defects, these can be anticipated and early advice on management given to the parents when they are attending for physiotherapy for the more obvious early motor defect. If the child has a marked bite reflex, desensitization techniques are required. If the child has a marked tongue thrust, or gaping mouth with drooling, the early feeding techniques of the Bobath method should be applied. As with any child, contact with normal children and normal verbal contact with adults should be encouraged and indeed exaggerated. In this way the secondary adverse environmental effects can be minimized and appropriate speech therapy techniques be initiated at the right time, thus avoiding the too common delays in seeking and obtaining skilled help.

The developmental speech disorder syndrome

Children of normal intelligence, who have no anatomical or physiological difficulty associated with speech production nor any of the secondary problems mentioned previously, but who show a pattern of slow speech development, are considered to suffer from the developmental speech disorder syndrome. This is an umbrella term which covers a range of disorders from relatively mild delays of speech development to severe language and speech retardation. In its milder degrees it represents the commonest cause of referral to speech clinics. It is found more commonly in boys and there is often a strong family history of similar slow speech development and also of left handedness, ambidexterity and reading and writing difficulties.

In *mild* cases there is no retardation of language development but articulation is unclear due to omissions and substitutions of consonants. This is particularly noticeable with the later acquired consonants and in consonant clusters. Typically, the child speaks with the clarity to be expected 12–18 months earlier. The mother often volunteers that she was the first to understand what the child said, followed by his father and, only after some time, close friends and relatives. Perhaps because of the attention drawn to his difficulty, the child is often inhibited in using speech to strangers.

If parents are made aware of the excellent prognosis in children who have this pattern of speech development, this in itself has a therapeutic effect. Thereafter they must be encouraged to engage in play activities with the child in which he gets the maximum reward for using speech. These include stories and games in which the child takes part as well as using books and picture cards. Often the most striking improvement takes place when the child joins a play group or nursery class with children of his own age.

In *moderate* degrees, the child has retardation in the development of language as well as in the development of articulation (Ingram, 1969). He is slow in reaching the early speech milestones and subsequent lack of clarity is more severe than in the milder form described above.

As speech development in these children progresses at a much slower rate than normal, speech therapy is frequently required in the first few years at school. Much patience from family members and speech therapist as well as from teacher and classmates is needed in handling such children. Progress may seem to take place in fits and starts and it is not infrequent for the child to get 'fed-up' with speech therapy at some stage. In this event it is often wise to discontinue formal therapy for a period of several months and start again when the child is more co-operative. At school the child may be slow to start to read and write and this can add further stress to management.

When the problem is *severe*, children not only have expressive difficulties, but also difficulties in comprehension. Parents are often puzzled by the child's apparent ability to hear sounds other than speech perfectly well but not to understand or respond to name or simple requests. Typically these children gesture and point a great deal and often show marked attention to the movement of a speaker's face and lips. The various terms used to describe the severe form are: developmental receptive dysphasia, word deafness, auditory imperception and central deafness. The exact diagnosis of this rare condition may take some time to establish and must necessarily involve the audiologist and teacher for the deaf as well as the speech therapist and paediatrician.

In such children special techniques used for management of the young deaf child must be employed. In each case an individual plan of regular assessment must be evolved to review the effect of any form of therapy and rate of progress. The latter will give the best indication of prognosis but it must be remembered that a large proportion of severely affected children will not catch up even in the later school years, nor as adults develop ready verbal fluency or manage more than the elementary levels of reading and spelling. At present, only a small number of boarding schools exist for the education of such children.

Lastly it must be remembered that educational intelligence tests in common use discriminate unfairly against children with moderate or severe degrees of the developmental speech disorder syndrome. Even tests which contain only performance items usually require an intact comprehension of language. Hence these children are often regarded as having low intellectual potential. Their actual potential can be gauged only after repeated assessment by a skilled psychologist.

R.J. PURVIS

The Role of the Speech Therapist in Management

The child who is under 3 years of age is not given exercises. The overall aim is to help the child to develop skills which will increase his ability to cope with the difficult stages in normal language development. Even with the older child attempts are made to keep treatment informal and enjoyable.

Developmental language problems
The child with an apparently mild language problem, who does not improve with general advice to mother and admission to play group, will require an individualized programme to stimulate co-ordination, auditory perception and imitation of speech sounds, the whole worked into games.

The child needs to focus his attention on what he hears and to learn to listen if he is to articulate new sounds, correct substitutions and become aware of syntactic rules. Initially, with the young child, concentration can be encouraged by using sound-making toys such as rattles, whistles and drums. These are placed on a table in front of him and he identifies the different sounds with his eyes closed. Even young children can learn to cover their own eyes in this play situation. The next step is to introduce objects beginning with the same sound, e.g. bell, bus, baby, bed, bird and bottle. The child must be prevented from lip reading in this game which is intended to make him use his auditory perception. When the child has learnt to cope with objects, pictures can be introduced. For example, the child of 3 years enjoys playing with sets of pictures of graded phonic difficulty. He is asked to identify pictures with sounds which commonly cause confusion in speech handicapped children. These games can be played at home with parents and siblings.

When the child has reached school age, phonetic symbols can be introduced to reinforce auditory perception work and articulatory exercises. It may be helpful to begin treatment by using a sound already used correctly, so providing the child with success. A scrap book can be kept and the child can be encouraged to find pictures illustrating a particular sound. The relationship between the parent and the child must be a happy one if it is to withstand the effort of learning new and difficult speech sounds over a number of years and therefore success should be fostered. Various aids may be used to make treatment interesting, such as a sound activated mechanism (SAM), a mirror, tape recorder and a language master. Work will inevitably become more formal as the child grows older.

Similarly parents are encouraged to play games to develop conceptual skills. Picture matching helps the young child to cope with symbols and picture lotto can be enjoyed by all the family.

If the child continues to make mistakes after a programme of auditory perception exercises, another cause may be receptive dysphasia. A child with this disorder usually has the ability to communicate with gestures and responds to the spoken word like a partially hearing child by trying to lip read.

Generalized developmental delay

The Dorchester Assessment Unit activity group provides for such children aged 12 months to 3 years approximately. The group is run by an occupational therapist, a physiotherapist and a speech therapist working as a team with the help of an aide. The role of the occupational therapist is to stimulate an awareness of the child's individuality and to develop his relationships with others, the physiotherapist encourages his normal physical development and mobility, while the speech therapist stimulates pre-linguistic and linguistic skills.

The mothers bring the children once a week and although they leave the group for part of the session, they return to join in various activities and watch the therapists working with the children.

Some children bombarded with speech which is beyond their comprehension stop responding. For the mother of such a child it is important for the therapist to encourage her to use language specifically suited to the needs of her child. After listening to exaggerated intonation patterns used on simple phrases by the therapist, the young child may introduce similar cadences in his jargon. Increasing the child's awareness of speech sounds can be achieved by imitating sounds in games with his mother and these may appear later superimposed on the cadences.

The child who is concentrating on acquiring the skills of standing and walking has difficulty in developing another complicated motor skill. He seems unable to progress significantly in expressive speech until he has learned to walk successfully. It is nevertheless important that the child with a developmental speech disorder should be stimulated and the input of language encouraged. There is a risk that a mother may stop talking to a child from whom there is no feedback. The group situation helps to counteract this.

The relaxed setting in the activity group gives rise to the spontaneous exchange of ideas between the therapists and the mothers. It is often found that the supportive role of the group is the most important aspect of treatment especially when this is prolonged.

The children usually progress to a preschool play group. It is therefore important that the therapists liaise with the play group leaders. The purpose of attendance at a nursery school or play group is to allow the child to develop in a normal environment where attention to the handicap is minimal.

Moderate or severe retardation

Very young children suffering from, e.g. Down's syndrome, benefit from the form of group treatment described above where the emphasis is on encouraging the normal stages of development. Retarded children have difficulty in mastering the deeper structure of language as they grow older. The aim is to stimulate them in their early years when their ability to acquire new speech and language patterns is at its optimum.

The early diagnosis of the child with moderate or severe mental retardation is very important especially if he seems unable to benefit from a preschool play group. The mildly retarded child may be able to develop speech and integrate socially but the more severely retarded child may begin to show antisocial behaviour unless he receives specialized help.

One general characteristic of the severely subnormal child is his almost complete dependence on adults to initiate new learning (Department of Education and Science, 1975). Because of this reliance on adult help, speech therapy needs to be carefully programmed beginning with simple exercises to encourage comprehension, imitation and cognitive skills.

Language stimulation can be started with games to achieve communication. Sometimes this involves teaching a child meaningful gestures, such as shaking hands for 'hello' and waving for 'bye-bye'. The severely subnormal child may be unable to communicate in even the most simple way with those around him. Such a child can be shown later how to follow simple commands and recognize and manipulate miniature toys, thus developing his understanding. It is often difficult for parents to appreciate that the child's comprehension must be developed before his expressive ability can improve. However, once a simple action is explained and followed through with some success, structured programmes for language stimulation can be attempted.

A series of programme sheets to help parents continue therapy at home has been introduced in the Dorchester Assessment Unit (Appendix 24.1). There are 12 programme sheets which can be individually tailored for each child. The early exercises range from games to encourage communication (e.g. peep-bo), to exercises to strengthen the articulatory mechanism (e.g. blowing and licking).

The severely subnormal child may not be able to progress through all the programme sheets and it may be helpful to introduce a structured mime system (if ability to gesture is adequate) of the type described by Levitt (1970). This is adapted from the Paget–Gorman system (p. 455) and can work well if used in a simple form. It is readily understood by most people as many of the gestures are self-explanatory. A more complicated system is being developed but this may mean that the child has a code which is restricted to communication with those who have learnt the gestures. The more severely mentally handicapped child may have to use eye pointing to help make his needs known. However, this has limited use and the child should always be encouraged to develop as much speech as is possible. Communication problems of retarded children are discussed further elsewhere (p. 253).

The autistic child has some of the characteristics of the child with receptive dysphasia but does not use gesture and does not show the same desire to communicate. Since autistic children are thought to lack inner language and seem to have a global language deficit the therapist may help these children to symbolize.

Cerebral palsy

In the child with cerebral palsy (as in the severely mentally handicapped child) the basic skills of drinking and eating efficiently may not have been acquired. He may not have progressed from primitive suckling to sucking or learned normal chewing. Since the same muscles are used for speaking as for eating, the child will be unable to produce intelligible speech sounds later if these immature patterns persist. Excessive drooling is common. This is due to difficulty in controlled swallowing and lip closure and to insensitivity of the circumoral area to saliva.

The transition from feeding therapy to speech therapy is gradual. The young spastic child is unable to inhibit primitive reflexes and this results in his speech remaining integrated with movements of the rest of his body. The whole body reacts when he attempts to speak, often causing exaggerated movements. In contrast the floppy child has diminished tone, often leaving him unable to make the first movements necessary for speech. A speech and language programme should begin as soon as possible to prevent delay in the onset of vocalization and to prevent grotesque movements becoming integrated with speaking.

Speech impairment in the cerebral palsied child is due to several factors. His facial and oral musculature may be affected and his breathing and phonation may be dominated by the over or under functioning of the respiratory muscles. The child should be treated therefore in positions which particularly suit his needs and where his muscle tone is as near normal as possible. The reflex inhibiting postures (RIP) used by the physiotherapist can be adapted for speech therapy. The first pre-linguistic skill to be encouraged will be babbling, using sounds the child is already making. Careful observation of the child's breathing is necessary to see if it is too shallow or irregular, as this will affect his ability to vocalize. Rhythmic massage of the rib cage, passively regulating the child's breathing within the RIP, will often produce good vocalization. The therapist may then superimpose passive movements on the lips, producing a [p] sound and then progress through other sounds, so giving the child a tactile as well as an auditory impression.

The cerebral palsied child in a reflex inhibiting posture can more easily listen to and watch an adult talking to him, whereas if he is left to move freely he may be unable to maintain eye-contact or hold his head still to listen to speech. It is important therefore, that the child should spend as much time as possible in controlled positions and his parents should be shown how to stimulate him in these positions.

As the child progresses it is hoped that the facilitated babbling will come under his control and the first meaningful speech will appear. Once the child has mastered speech in controlled positions, he may be able to maintain fluency in the freedom of a chair and a therapy programme can follow more orthodox lines.

If the cerebral palsied child reaches school age and a severe speech disability

* *Bliss System. Information Officers*, Miss J. Hammond and Mrs. T. Bailey, Heathfield School, Fareham, Hampshire.
Publications Officer, Miss A. Paterson, Scottish Council for the Care of Spastics, 5 Rillbank Terrace, Edinburgh.

persists, other means of communication may be needed to supplement speech. The Bliss symbolic language system* (Hammond & Bailey, 1976) is one method by which children with understanding but virtually no speech can learn to communicate. A simpler picture board may be used successfully by non-speaking mentally handicapped children. A child with reasonable hand control may be able to operate an electric typewriter, possibly with an extended keyboard and a child with any voluntary function of mouth (suck and blow), head or limbs can be trained to use a typewriter with a Possum (patient operated selector mechanism) control. Great satisfaction is found in expressing views on paper which cannot be said fluently in conversation.

S. GOODWIN

Appendix 24.1

Speech and Language Programme Achievement Cards

I.   (1) Sucking: with help/against gravity
      (2) Lip exercises (blowing): feather through straw, whistle or mouth organ, match or candle, bubbles
      (3) Tongue exercises: licking food off spoon, corners of mouth, upper and lower lips, roof of mouth, upper teeth; chewing toffee/gum all around the mouth

II.   (1) Pre-trial eye contact: on adult, on object
      (2) Attention: pointing to object, with/without help
      (3) Response to instructions: 'don't touch', 'listen', 'give me the —— please'
      (4) Gestures: goodbye, hello, very good, good boy/girl, please, thank you

III.   (1) Listening and recognizing: bell, drum, rattle
      (2) Discriminating between pairs
      (3) Listening to words and recognizing (by responding to 'show me'/'give me'): ball, baby, car, boat, bus, comb, shoe, hat, box, table, chair, floor

IV.   (1) Animal sound imitation: cat, dog, duck, cow
      (2) Imitation of motor behaviour: e.g. shut your eyes, touch your nose, stand up, clap, etc.
      (3) Auditory perception: pick out object/picture from similar sounding ones in sets of 2, 4, 6

V.   (1) Selecting correct object from 2 (e.g. ball/*baby*) or 3 (e.g. baby/*boat*/bus)
      (2) Recognizing 'listen', looking at adult and responding to spatial instructions: e.g. put the ball *in* the box, put the box *on* the floor
      (3) Recognizing key words: own name, No, come here, don't touch, hot, sit down, potty
      (4) Saying words with meaning: e.g. bye-bye, hello
      (5) Saying 4 'listening' words (III, 3)
      (6) Naming an object from a choice of 4

VI.   (1) Placing missing objects: 2–5
      (2) Naming missing objects: 1–5
      (3) Finding objects on the table: 1–10
      (4) Finding hidden object: 1–5
      (5) Finding pairs of objects: 1–5 pairs
      (6) Picture matching: point to 6/12 pictures
      (7) Picture lotto: 6/12 pictures

VII.   (1) Using 'listening' words: saying word from object
      (2) Saying word from picture

VIII.   (1) Phrases (using objects as above), point and say: e.g. baby's nose, table and chair
      (2) Common phrases: stand up, sit down, oh dear!
      (3) Rhymes: copying actions/words

IX.   (1) Colours (red, yellow, blue, green, black, white): recognizing from choice of 2/3/6
      (2) Pairing colour with object: e.g. red bus, green ball

X.   (1) Recognizing difference between 'describing' words: big/little, fast/slow, fat/thin, hot/cold, round/square, hard/soft
      (2) Saying describing words
      (3) Pairing adjective and object: e.g. big book, round ball

XI.   Using a bag or box: place 1–5 objects in bag: ask: where is it? what is it? whose is it? To assist learning adult points to object and names, points to object and asks question

XII.   (1) Describing action pictures with full sentence: e.g. the girl is washing her hands. To teach simple sentence formation ask what is the girl *doing*? what is the girl doing? *who* is washing her hands and repeat full sentence
      (2) Show 2 pictures: pick out the one described

The cards are suitable for home programmes of speech and language stimulation for mildly and more severely retarded preschool children. They are listed roughly in ascending order of difficulty. The therapist selects the card most appropriate to the child and if necessary alters it to suit special needs. Space is provided to date first attempt and achievement, and for parents to write comments. Older children and those of normal mental ability are treated in ways suggested by Fraser and Blockley (1973).

The idea of achievement cards came from Mrs. M. Rees, L.C.S.T., Adviser for the Mentally Handicapped, Exeter, to whom I am indebted for much assistance and encouragement.

References

ANDREW G. and HARRIS M. (1964) The phenomenon of stammering. In *The Child who does not Talk*, eds. Renfrew C. and Murphy K. *Clinics in Developmental Medicine. No. 13.* London: Heinemann.

DEPARTMENT OF EDUCATION AND SCIENCE (1975) *Educating Mentally Handicapped Children.* London: Her Majesty's Stationery Office.

DOLL E.A. (1976) Oseretsky Motor Proficiency Tests. Editor and sponsor. In *Catalogue of Psychological Tests and Clinical Procedures.* London: National Foundation for Educational Research.

FOG E. and FOG M. (1963) Cerebral inhibition examined by associated movements. In *Minimal Cerebral Dysfunction*, eds. Bax M. and Mac Keith R. *Clinics in Developmental Medicine No. 10.* London: Heinemann.

FRASER G.M. and BLOCKLEY J. (1973) *The Language Disordered Child.* London: National Foundation for Educational Research.

HAMMOND J. and BAILEY P. (1976) An experiment in Blissymbolics. *Special Education*, **3**, 21.

INGRAM T.T.S. (1959) A description of classification of common disorders of speech in childhood. *Archives of Disease in Childhood*, **34**, 444.

INGRAM T.T.S. (1964) The complex speech disorders of cerebral palsied children. In *The Child who does not Talk*, eds. Renfrew C. and Murphy K. *Clinics in Developmental Medicine No. 13.* London: Heinemann.

INGRAM T.T.S. (1969) Language development in children. In *Manual of Child Psychology*, ed. Carmichael L, 2nd Ed. London: Chapman Hall.

LEVITT L.M. (1970) *A Method of Communication for Non-speaking Severely Retarded Children.* Cambridge: Heffer.

OSERETSKY N. (1931) Psychomotorik methoden zur untersuchung der motorik. *Zeitschrift fur Angewandte Psychologie (Leipzig)*, **17**, 1.

RUTTER M. and MITTLER P. (1972) Environmental influences on language development. In *The Child with Delayed Speech*, eds. Rutter M. and Martin J.A.M. *Clinics in Developmental Medicine No. 43.* London: Heinemann.

Further Reading

BLOCKLEY J. and MILLER G. (1971) Feeding techniques with cerebral palsied children. *Physiotherapy*, **57**, 300.

BRAY J. (1976) Cutting the wires: remote control links for Possum equipment. *Action, National Fund for Research into Crippling Diseases.* July 10.

CRICKMAY M. (1972) *Speech Therapy and the Bobath Approach to Cerebral Palsy.* Springfield, Illinois: C. Thomas.

GWYNNE-EVANS E. (1951) The organisation of the oro-facial muscles in relation to breathing and feeding. *British Dental Journal*, **91**, 135.

INGRAM T.T.S. (1969) Developmental disorders of speech. In *Handbook of Clinical Neurology*, eds. Vinken P.J. and Bruyn G.W. Vol. 4. Amsterdam: North-Holland Publishing Company.

JEFFREE D. and McCONKEY R. (1976) *Let Me Speak.* London: Souvenir Press.

MARLAND P. (1953) Speech therapy for cerebral palsy based on reflex inhibition. *Journal of the College of Speech Therapists*, **17**, 65.

MOLLOY J. (1969) *Teaching the Retarded Child to Talk*. London: Unibooks, University of London Press.

RYAN M. (1976) *Feeding can be Fun*. London: Spastics Society.

CHAPTER 25

Behaviour Disorders

Problems Reaching the Family Doctor and Paediatrician

The majority of behaviour problems in the preschool period are exaggerations or inappropriate prolongations of normal behaviour patterns, relatively uncomplicated and likely to resolve with the passage of time with or without some alterations in management. When the child's behaviour is bizarre (i.e. would be considered abnormal at any age even in a modified form), is causing family disruption (even if the behaviour in itself seems insufficient to account for parental reaction) or is developmentally or socially incapacitating (i.e. is interfering with opportunities for learning and social interaction), psychiatric referral is indicated. In this section common behaviour problems are considered which can usually be managed adequately by family doctor or paediatrician.

From the parents' point of view a behaviour problems is any behaviour which they feel to be abnormal or which causes them anxiety or embarrassment. If the mother is sufficiently concerned to seek advice the problem merits attention, explanation and counselling, even if the doctor considers the behaviour normal and characteristic for age. In other situations, particularly when the child is subject to regular developmental checks (as in a screening programme) the medical adviser sees a problem where the mother does not. Whether or not a behavioural aberration is seen as a problem by parents and if it is, their reaction to it and consequent handling of the child, depends on their personalities, upbringing, life experiences and expectations and on the social, economic, domestic and emotional circumstances pertaining in the home.

A medical adviser who sets out to counsel parents about upbringing and behaviour must take account of the complex factors that determine interactions between parents and children and provide the rationale for different patterns of parental management. Too often explanations and recommendations, understandable to and applicable by middle class parents in comfortable circumstances are presented to those from a totally different social and cultural setting where 'ideal' solutions may be completely unrealistic because of adverse circumstances that cannot be removed and only with difficulty modified. In addition, too often there is unwarranted interference with child rearing practices which, though not typical of middle class mores, have not been shown to have any harmful effect on the child. The wide gap between theory, advice and actual practice is vividly illustrated in the Newsons' Nottingham study (Newson and Newson 1963, 1968). Attitudes and criticisms that lower the mother's self-confidence and self-esteem will not be helpful in the common situation of some disturbance in the mother–child relationship initiating or perpetuating irritating forms of behaviour.

There is no ideal method of child rearing which will avoid the common behaviour problems of early childhood. Temperamental differences in children are apparent from birth. Within one family one baby may be easy to handle, content and responsive and another, equally wanted, be cranky, over-reacting and unrewarding. When a mother and child seem to be interacting poorly, one should consider whether maternal mishandling is responsible for troublesome behaviour or results from it or, as most often is the case, the one is reinforcing the other and vice versa. Certainly some children are constitutionally more endearing than others, whilst some mothers are temperamentally calm and loving and others are 'worriers' by nature.

BODY MANIPULATIONS AND OTHER HABITS

Sucking thumbs and other objects
Sucking thumbs, fingers, dummies and 'suck rags' is a universal form of infant behaviour. Thumb sucking persists into the second and third years, when many who seldom suck by day continue to do so when going off to sleep. At the same time the child may rub his cheek with a woolly toy or piece of cloth, pull at an ear lobe or lock of hair or indulge in some other individual repetitive activity. Some children suck when tired, bored or unsure of themselves. Some revert to thumb sucking after the birth of a sibling or other unsettling change in routine and stop again when the period of uncertainty is past. The habit is prolonged if the child is nagged, reprimanded or ridiculed. If ignored (and there are no continuing tensions in the home or undue pressures being put on the child) most thumb-suckers have largely stopped sucking by day by 3–4 years and at night by 5–6 years.

Malocclusion of the permanent dentition has been reported in a few of those children who continue to thumb-suck after the age of 6–7 years.

Dummies. There is no evidence to support the widespread condemnation of this type of comforter which is used by two-thirds of all children under 2 years of age (Spence *et al.*, 1954; Newson and Newson, 1963). The dinkie feeder or Dormel (a small plastic bottle containing some sweetened liquid) given to the young child to suck on is harmful because constant sucking of sweetened substances leads to early caries of incisor teeth. The same danger applies when the dummy is dipped in sugar or syrup.

Handling the genitals
The baby boy discovers and grabs hold of his penis rather earlier than he grabs his toes; both actions have similar significance. Erection of the penis is common in young infants especially when passing urine. Neither of these behaviours has erotic significance. Masturbation, which is a rhythmic stimulation of the genital area with preoccupation, excitement and satisfaction, is seen from about 6 months. The baby rubs his thighs together in a variety of rocking movements,

the toddler may rub the genital area against some part of the furniture and the older child (usually 2–3 years or more) may use his hands. The habit may start with some local irritation, the baby rubbing himself to relieve itching. Masturbation is seen more often at bedtime, when it appears to be a manoeuvre to induce relaxation and sleep and when the child is bored and has nothing else to do, e.g. when the toddler, who is not tired, is put in his cot for an afternoon nap.

Apart from simple distraction the habit should be ignored. After the age of 3–4 years the child can appreciate that this activity is not socially acceptable in public places.

In a few cases the rhythmic activities, flushed or pale face, fixed stare and lack of response may suggest an epileptic manifestation and EEG investigation be needed to exclude that diagnosis.

The habit does no harm to the child apart from the effects of parental reaction. When parents feel excessive anxiety or shame and find it difficult to talk about their earlier experiences from which these feelings stem, psychiatric advice may be indicated.

Head banging, head rolling and rocking

These annoying but harmless habits are usually seen first in the second 6 months of life. The 9-month baby may roll his head from side-to-side when lying supine, to the extent that he wears his hair away leaving a bald patch. He may bang his head on the mattress or cot sides when put down to sleep and may rock himself and the cot with such energy that he succeeds in moving it across the room. The 1 to 2-year-old may bang his head on the floor or against the wall. This may be a manifestation of temper or attention seeking but often there is no obvious cause.

Parents are concerned because they associate such habits with retardation, fear damage to the head with banging and because of disturbance to family and neighbours caused by cot rocking.

Head banging does not seem to harm the child in any way and has usually disappeared by 2 years unless the habit is perpetuated as an attention-seeking device. Padding cot sides may help mother if not the child. Rocking causes less noise if castors are removed and the cot stood on a soft rug. As soon as he is old enough the child should be transferred to a low bed, though the habit may well have been discontinued by then.

PROBLEMS OF MANAGEMENT

Feeding, toiletting and sleeping battles are common in the second and third years of life when the child is going through the negative stage. The first two are preventable being largely due to mishandling. Sleeping problems afflict some parents whose management cannot be faulted.

Feeding problems

Early feeding battles and food refusal result from parental anxiety about food intake and from food forcing.

The complaints are various: the baby of 9–15 months wants to feed himself; he is not allowed to do so because of the mess and refuses to eat altogether. This child has what mother considers to be a very small appetite, that one is excessively faddy. Mother has fixed ideas about the amount the child should eat and what foods are good for him. The dawdler of 18 months to 2 years insists on feeding himself but instead of getting on with the job turns his food over and over with his spoon, gets his hands into the mess and smears it over his face. When food forcing is employed the child refuses to chew, spits the food out, stores it up in his mouth to be disposed of later, chokes and vomits. The child is coaxed, bribed, distracted, threatened, punished, rewarded, all to no avail. Every meal time becomes a confrontation.

Feeding problems quickly resolve when food in small amounts and attractively prepared (with due attention to reasonable likes and dislikes) is put down in front of the child; utensils and remainders being removed without comment after a suitable interval. In practice it is often very difficult to persuade mothers to adopt such a regime. The mother may regard food offered to the child as an expression of her love and rejection of food as a rejection of herself. The stratagem of removing the child for a period to a neutral atmosphere may be unhelpful as it may reinforce the mother's feeling of rejection if it is demonstrated that the child will eat for someone else but not for her.

Feeding battles like other problems of management and behaviour are much increased in the offspring of over-anxious and over-protective mothers, in those who are too strict and rigid, and those whose handling is inconsistent, sometimes indulgent and sometimes punitive (Drillien, 1964).

Pica or persistent dirt eating is uncommon. It is most often seen in deprived or retarded children and is one cause of lead and other poisoning.

Toilet training problems

Toiletting problems reported by mothers are as diverse as are training practices. They range from those of the mother who has confused early conditioning with voluntary control to those of the professional wife who believes that toilet training before 2 or 3 years is positively harmful and then discovers that her child, still in nappies, is not acceptable in play group.

Many young babies empty bowel and bladder immediately after feeding, and potting for a few minutes at these times can save much laundering. There is no evidence that early potting is associated with later toiletting battles or other behaviour problems, when the increased proportion of over-anxious and rigid mothers engaging in rigorous toilet training is taken into account. Maternal attitudes, not the training procedures, are linked with problem behaviours.

Toilet problems are unlikely to arise or be perpetuated if the child is potted regularly, for short periods, starting some time after he is able to sit securely on his pot and if the pot is discarded without fuss during temporary periods of resistance. Mothers need to understand the urgency of the early period of voluntary control; that learning to hold on and then being unable to let go (the child performing as soon as he is lifted from the pot) is a normal stage in developing control and that there are constitutional maturational differences in the ages of acquiring sphincter control that have nothing to do with moral worth of the child or competence of the mother.

Stool smearing is not uncommon in normal children between 12 and 18 months. With tact and distraction it may be avoidable, but may continue as an attention-seeking device if seen to cause adult anxiety or disgust.

Faeces retention is a more serious problem. Frequently this begins with pain on defaecation due to an anal fissure. Prompt treatment with local anaesthetic ointment and a stool softener may effect a rapid cure. More rarely, deliberate withholding appears to be a reaction to maternal anxieties and pressures on the child to produce daily an adequate stool in the appropriate receptacle, or an extreme form of negative behaviour, or an irrational fear of the action and its product. Marked tension and disruption can ensue with the whole household revolving around the state of the child's bowels.

With prolonged retention the rectum becomes filled with hard faecal masses which cannot be passed, while faecal soiling with liquid matter from higher up the bowel occurs continuously. In severe cases hospital admission may be necessary for rectal washout and re-education of the bowel with laxatives and also to remove the child from emotional tensions and to allow the mother time to express her feelings and problems, possibly in a psychotherapeutic interview.

It should not be forgotten that although Hirschsprung's disease most often presents in the first week of life, some cases present with increasing constipation at later ages. A full rectum makes that diagnosis unlikely.

Nocturnal enuresis. Some children become dry at night before the age of 2 years, most achieve this between 2 and 4 years and about 1 in 10 (in UK samples) is still wet more often than not at 5 years. Constitutional differences in maturation of the necessary mechanisms appear to exist. Boys tend to be later to acquire sphincter control than girls. A history of bedwetting in parents and siblings of enuretics is common. Bakwin (1971) reported that concordance for enuresis (defined as bed-wetting after 4 years) was twice as high in monozygotic as in dizygotic twins. External influences also affect the age of achieving night-time continence, particularly stress and anxiety in the third and fourth years of life (Douglas, 1973). Mac Keith (1973) considers that nocturnal bladder control emerges spontaneously, without being learned, when maturation occurs, that this has occurred in nearly all children by 5 years but in a minority emergence of consequent dryness is inhibited by anxiety and defeatism. He concludes that with a low anxiety system of toilet training, enuresis can be prevented in 98.5 per cent of children.

Sleeping problems

Sleeping problems are common in the first 3 years of life. They are demoralizing and exhausting for parents and difficult to treat. Although sleeping problems are increased in the offspring of over-anxious and rigid mothers, in many instances it is difficult to pinpoint any adverse factors in maternal attitudes or handling.

There is a wide variation in the sleep requirements of young children and some problems arise because parents have rigid ideas about how much sleep is necessary for good health. If the child is reluctant to lie down but is content to talk to himself, sing or play with toys no problem should exist. Early morning waking does not usually persist after 3 years; if it does the child can usually appreciate that he should not disturb his parents. Before that age mother's schedule may need to be adjusted to fit in with early rising.

Problems arise when the child not only is unready for sleep (even by the time his parents wish to retire) but screams persistently when left in his cot, becomes hysterical or makes himself sick. Other children settle happily to sleep but wake a few hours later fully refreshed and start screaming to be lifted. Frequently the problems are exacerbated by circumstances that cannot be altered such as inadequate housing, complaints from neighbours and sleep requirements of siblings.

Since children who cry at night are usually immediately restored to good humour when lifted, one presumes that some part of the problem is separation anxiety or attention seeking. Thus a first line in management would be to try to ensure that during the day the child is receiving attention and affection. Regular and pleasant routines, at a bed-time dictated by the child's sleep requirement rather than parental convenience, are helpful, though prolongation of putting to bed rituals should be avoided.

In some instances lifting the child, bringing him downstairs and thereafter totally ignoring him (mother busying herself with a household chore) proves effective after a few nights' trial.

Leaving the child to cry, albeit with his door ajar and mother looking in from time to time, works with some but is often impracticable for the domestic reasons mentioned above. Recourse to drugs may be unavoidable; these should be given before the child starts to cry and in adequate dosage. Chloral is the drug of choice, e.g. increasing dosage up to a maximum of 15 ml (1500 mg) triclofos elixir at 1 to 2 years. Promethazine hydrochloride (Phenergan elixir up to 10–15 ml, 10–15 mg) is another useful drug though generally if one hypnotic is ineffective others will be equally so. Drug therapy should be tried for 3–4 weeks and then gradually withdrawn in the hope that an acceptable sleeping pattern will have become established. Many parents finally resort to taking the child into their own bed. If this proves effective (and usually it does) the doctor's disapproval should be restrained if he has been unable to produce an alternative solution.

Fear of the dark and night terrors. Fear of the dark, like other fears, is most common after 2 years. The child's fears are very real to him and as far as is possible the frightening situation should be removed and only gradually reintroduced, as the child can tolerate this.

Night terrors are commoner after 3 years. They occur during arousal from slow wave sleep. The child wakens terrified and screaming, efforts to rouse him may fail and next morning he cannot recollect the incident. The episodes may mimic nocturnal psychomotor seizures and EEG may be required to eliminate this possibility. The child with night terrors seldom shows other behaviour problems of any degree and parental mishandling is not obvious. With frequent night terrors a mild sedative may be indicated.

DISTURBANCES OF SOCIAL BEHAVIOUR

Negative behaviour and attention seeking

Negative behaviour is a normal stage in growing up and away from total dependence on the mother. It is apparent from 1–3 years and at its height between 18 and 30 months. Manifestations vary with individual temperament of the child and maternal management. Many of the battles that ensue during this period could be avoided with tact and reasonable latitude on the part of care-takers, and recognition of the inadvisability of having a fight over inessentials with a child of this age, if for no other reason than that the child is likely to win.

Attention-seeking devices are manifold over the same age range; many have been mentioned. Temper tantrums are a normal reaction to the many frustrations of this age, when ambition outstrips capabilities or conflicts with adult sanctions. Tantrums and negative behaviour are increased when the child (or his mother) is tired, hungry or unwell. Temper should only be considered a problem when tantrums occur daily and on minor provocation. Excessive negativism, marked attention seeking and frequent tantrums may result from the child's experience that only when he is 'naughty' does he receive attention. The technique of behaviour modification, in which desirable behaviours are noted with apprecia-tion and approval and undesirable behaviours are ignored, is most helpful during this stage of normal development.

Breath-holding. Attacks may start in the second 6 months of life but are most common between 1 and 3 years. The child starts to cry, then holds his breath before expiration. He goes red in the face, followed by a bluish tinge around the lips sometimes with pallor. After a few seconds he lets his breath out with a sigh and is fully recovered. Occasionally breath-holding is prolonged, cyanosis is marked and the child loses consciousness, when immediately he starts to breathe again. Very rarely a short clonic convulsion occurs. With severe breath-holding attacks the question of seizures may arise and EEG be indicated. However, usually the history clearly indicates provoking factors of temper, minor injury or fear.

Aggression and jealousy

Some degree of aggressive behaviour, hitting, kicking and biting playmates and siblings, is to be expected in 2–4-year-olds. Rivalry for possession of a toy or for parental attention leads to sudden eruptions of aggressive temper. Sheridan (1975) described the egocentric philosophy of the 2-year-old in a co-operative play situation as 'I come, I see, I grab and what I have I hold'. By 3 years the desire for approval is beginning to outweigh the need for instant gratification, though quarrels are still frequent, particularly with siblings.

Jealousy, particularly manifest with the birth of a sib, is most common between 18 months and 3–3½ years. At younger ages the child is unlikely to pay more than passing attention to the intruder though he may be distressed at separation from mother (especially if this has been prolonged on account of obstetric complications) and be excessively clinging on her return. At older ages the child can be included in caretaking responsibilities.

Jealousy is greatly aggravated and prolonged by favouritism.

Shyness
Most children pass through a shy stage between 9 and 18 months. Other children are more persistently shy, sometimes only with strange adults but often with other children as well. This is likely to be an inborn trait of temperament which the child, and also his parents, have to learn to live with.

Some of the behaviour problems, briefly described above, are likely to be manifest to some degree in all normal children and to be at their height in the second and third years of life. Often all that is needed is an opportunity for the mother to discuss the problems with an informed and understanding listener. With multiple problems and obvious mishandling expert psychiatric advice may be needed, particularly to help the mother (or both parents) understand and acknowledge the basis of their feelings about the child and his behaviour.

C.M. DRILLIEN

A Child Psychiatric Approach

The doctor approaching the assessment and treatment of a serious behaviour problem in a preschool child will inevitably and appropriately begin his appraisal with a set of different assumptions and expectations from those adopted in a child with an undoubted physical problem such as epilepsy or cerebral palsy. Emotional and behaviour problems in the young child occur as a result of an interaction between the temperament of the child and the environment, particularly the family environment, whereas with disorders of physical causation, psychosocial disability is seen as mainly secondary to the existence of the child's handicap. A neurodevelopmental approach which puts primary emphasis on what is wrong 'within the child' will therefore be less helpful as far as psychiatric disorders are concerned, for here the presenting symptom in the child is likely to be at least as much a reflection of family tension as of a biological defect. The previous section contains a discussion of mainly reactive behaviour disorders and management problems occurring in relatively normal family situations. Behaviour problems in retarded children are considered elsewhere (p. 251). In the present section a brief account will be given of the prevalence of emotional and behaviour disorders and their associated factors in the general child population and this will be followed by a discussion of the management of more severe disorders occurring within children and parents.

FREQUENCY OF DISORDERS IN THE PRESCHOOL PERIOD

The great majority of emotional and behaviour problems in this age group need to be considered as extreme versions of the sorts of ordinary difficulties which most children have, rather than as disease entities in their own right. In determining the prevalence of such problems, it is therefore necessary to establish arbitrary criteria which take into account the amount of suffering shown by the child and the family, together with the severity and persistence of the difficulty.

Using such an approach with a standardized behaviour screening questionnaire, Richman *et al.* (1975) found the rate of moderate and severe disorders in a total population of 3-year-old children living in a North London borough to be 7 per cent. Mild disorders accounted for a further 15 per cent so that about one in five children in this population must be regarded as having shown some significant and persistent problem over the year in question. Girls were affected to the same degree as boys and there was no clear tendency for more disorders to occur in lower socio-economic groups. By comparing the children identified as disturbed with a control group matched for sex and social class, it was possible to examine the importance of a number of associated factors. These could be divided into three main groups. Family relationship factors were prominent. Thus, depression in mothers and parental marital discord were present to a significantly greater degree in the disturbed group. Social and environmental factors were also found in the children with difficulties. They were more likely to be living in high rise flats and there were more of other types of social stresses, such as financial hardship. Finally, factors within the child were also associated with behaviour disorders. Disturbed children were much more likely to show a significant delay in language development and, incidentally, children with serious language delay were also found to have a very high rate of behaviour problems. Although temperamental factors were not examined in this study, other studies (e.g. Thomas *et al.*, 1968) have demonstrated that adverse temperamental characteristics are probably of considerable importance in determining which children show difficulties. There appear to be some children who, from an early age, perhaps the first few months of life, cry more easily and more intensely, are irregular and inconsistent in their sleeping and feeding patterns and are more generally unadaptable, and these tend to show more behaviour problems later on (p. 340).

Finally in this brief account of the occurrence of psychological disorders in the preschool group, it should be emphasized that these are neither trivial nor transient disorders. In the Richman study, approximately two-thirds of disturbed children were still showing significant difficulties a year later and it is more than possible that some of these disorders persist in different forms into school and later adult life.

ASSESSMENT AND MANAGEMENT OF DISORDERS IN PARENTS AND CHILDREN

In assessing a child with an overtly psychiatric disorder or a physical symptom for which no organic cause has been found, the paediatrician or other doctor providing health care will need to have the skills to elicit both individual psychopathology in the parents and disturbances in family relationships, at least to a degree which will enable him or her to understand how best to help the child. This is not a straightforward matter. The child has been presented as showing the problem, not the parents or the family. The doctor will not, at least in the initial stages, be aware of the extent to which the family have already considered the possibility that stress or psychological factors are important in the development of the child's problem. He will therefore need to be cautious, for if he is insensitive to the fears the parents may have that their own behaviour has produced distress and suffering in their child, he will merely increase their defensiveness and prolong the period during which it is impossible to look at the family's wider functioning in relation to the child's symptoms.

A cautious approach will require time, as well as skill and patience, and this is not an easy matter within a busy out-patient department. Some paediatricians, clinic and family doctors do, however, manage to organize their work so as to provide time when this situation arises, and Goodall (1976) has described how one general paediatrician has managed to achieve this very effectively. She has arranged to put aside a full afternoon twice monthly for further assessment of such problems, with not more than four children booked for each session. If such planned appointments are possible, it is also likely to be more feasible for fathers to be present. In the UK, the attendance of fathers will not often occur unless it is specifically suggested that this would be helpful.

A discussion of family functioning, when it is the child who has presented with a problem, is most easily initiated by taking some aspect of the child's functioning and asking how this has affected the family. For example, when asking about early feeding, it is natural to enquire how the mother herself was feeling at the time, for it is well known and acceptable that many women are emotionally labile during the puerperium. If the mother admits to having felt low, she can then be asked whether she got over this, or whether it is still a problem. She can also be asked if she was under any pressure at that time (e.g. cramped housing or seeing little of her husband) and if so, it is easy to ask whether such pressures are still operating and whether other difficulties in the family have arisen since. Other leads into the way the family works include asking what impact the child's problem has on the family. Sometimes, when children show these difficulties, it leads to arguments between parents over what to do. Has that happened in this family? The taking of a family history, for example of a child showing clumsiness, may also be used as a means of obtaining information about relationships. The parents may be asked if either of them had any problems in doing up buttons or learning to read as children, and whether they did or not, they may still be asked who they think the child takes after in other ways, such as his personality. Finally, the parents may be asked directly if they have had any physical or nervous trouble in their lives.

The information so obtained may, of course, reveal an immense variety of situations and the paediatrician will need to consider carefully how he can use this information as helpfully as possible. In this he has a duty to the whole family as well as to the child. Indeed, if he sees his duty as entirely resting with the child's interests, he will often fail to obtain relevant information. When a mother perceives her child's behaviour as highly persecutory to her, she is unlikely to confide easily in a paediatrician or other doctor who seems to be allying himself with her tormentor.

By the end of his diagnostic appraisal (and this may take more than one session) the doctor should have some idea of the answers to the following questions:

Is there a significant handicapping behavioural or emotional problem in the child?

Is there a significant psychiatric disorder in one or both parents?

If there is no problem with the child but there does exist a problem within the parents, the great majority of paediatricians and child health doctors would feel that their responsibility ended with communicating this fact to the family doctor or referral agency (who is quite likely to be aware of the fact anyway).

A 4-year-old boy was referred to a paediatrician by his family doctor because of food refusal. He was brought by his father who explained that the boy was now eating well. However, he had been through a period of quite serious anorexia for a week about a month previously, at the time when he had been referred. This had occurred when his mother had temporarily left the home following her fourth overdose, a fact the referring doctor had not mentioned in his letter. The child was now eating well, and after a period of withdrawal was beginning to want to play again with his friends in the neighbourhood. His mother, who was staying with her own mother, was on the point of return. She had always refused psychiatric treatment. The child showed in his drawings that he regarded it as possible that he was responsible for his mother leaving home, but at his age this must be regarded as a normal fantasy. Otherwise the child had no problems. The most appropriate course here, following discussion with the child, was felt to be communication with the family doctor and the social service department, but it was not felt appropriate to continue with child-centred treatment and no further appointments were made.

If, however, there is a problem both within the child and within one or both parents, a further question needs to be asked:

Can the disorder within either parent or child be regarded as almost certainly primary, the other disorder being secondary and still reactive?

If the parental disorder (most commonly depression or personality disorder) can be seen as clearly primary then, assuming the parents are insightful and prepared to accept that judgment, referral to an appropriate adult agency, (the family doctor or adult psychiatrist) will be indicated. On the other hand, if the parents are defensive about this possibility, then the child health doctor or paediatrician may need to provide ongoing care to help them gradually to accept this possibility, at which point appropriate referral can be made.

In some cases, however, the child's disorder may be seen as clearly primary, and this is most likely to be the case where the child is showing a clear-cut hyperkinetic syndrome or autism.

A 3-year-old boy presented with severe overactivity, frequent outbursts of screaming and tantrums. He was destructive and unable to concentrate on anything. The health visitor confirmed that he had been an extremely difficult child from the early weeks. His mother was at her wits end with him and found herself frequently crying and wishing she were dead. She was spending sleepless nights tossing and turning, wondering how she was going to continue to cope with him. She had no previous history of psychiatric illness and the marital relationship was good though it had recently become strained. The child was referred to, and treated by, a child psychiatrist and the parents received support and advice from both the psychiatrist and psychiatric social worker.

However, if as is very commonly the case, neither the disorder in the child nor that in the parents can be regarded as clearly primary but there is a complex interaction between the two, then it is usually more appropriate for a child-centred agency to remain involved. Adult facilities are rarely as well geared to the needs of children and their families as child-centred facilities are suited to the needs of parents and families. The paediatrician with his medical social worker should be capable of helping families to improve their ability to talk about their difficulties, and this in itself is often a vital step in improvement in family functioning generally. Nevertheless, some such problems prove intractable to simple advice and guidance and do need referral or specialized psychiatric help.

A 3-year-old girl with a serious sleep problem, who had been waking her parents several times a night for several months, had failed to respond to chloral and Phenergan® or to advice from doctors and paediatricians that she 'must never be left at night' or that she 'should be left to cry it out'. Her mother was depressed secondarily, but it was also felt that she had a rather rejecting attitude towards the child. The child was referred to a psychiatric facility and the situation improved when the parents were able to talk to a social worker (in front of the child) about their own marital difficulties, which had started when the mother had become pregnant with the child whose problem was now so prominent. Presumably the child had been waking and was unable to return to sleep because of feelings of insecurity in relation to her parents.

PSYCHIATRIC DISORDERS ARISING MAINLY FROM 'WITHIN THE CHILD'

The hyperkinetic syndrome
Overactivity in children arises for a variety of reasons, all of which need to be considered as possible aetiological factors when children present with this problem.

Level of activity is partly determined as a *temperamental characteristic*. Some children are inherently more active than others and these differences are likely to show themselves most obviously in the second and third years of life when children become more mobile.

Some children become more active when they are *anxious*. Whereas in a new situation most young children withdraw and become relatively immobile, some become much more active and tear about until they are used to the place. This can give a misleading impression to a doctor who may assume that the overactivity of a youngster in his consulting room is characteristic of his general behaviour rather than specific to a new situation.

Finally, severe overactivity may occur as part of a rather poorly differentiated cluster of symptoms, the *hyperkinetic syndrome*, in which, in the absence of severe social stress (and in addition to overactivity), there may be impersistence, lack of concentration, short attention span, distractibility, impulsiveness, and lack of social inhibition. These problems are generalized and not situation specific although they will be less marked in some situations than others, e.g.

when a child is enjoying a one-to-one relationship in a quiet consulting room compared to when the child is in a crowded, noisy classroom. These defects may be accompanied by language delay and there may be secondary behaviour and learning problems.

Although this syndrome is commonly thought of as a manifestation of minimal brain damage or dysfunction, there are a number of disadvantages in accepting this assumption. Often there is no good evidence of brain damage, and even if there is a history of birth trauma or an excess of slow wave activity in the electroencephalogram, it is impossible to link these events or findings with even a low level of certainty to the behavioural syndrome in an individual child. The diagnosis of the hyperkinetic syndrome is therefore a clinical one, made on the basis of the child's behaviour rather than on the history or the results of special investigations.

Treatment is symptomatic. The parents should be given a careful explanation which puts emphasis on the fact that their child's troubles are mainly physiologically determined. If the term 'brain damage' or 'brain dysfunction' are used, then it will be important to monitor what meaning these terms have for the parents. Although these children do have a physiologically determined problem, they are nevertheless very responsive to environmental changes and parents should be encouraged to note for themselves situations in which the child behaves best. Most hyperactive children are able to be more relaxed in a relatively unstimulating environment without too many toys or distracting material around. In an educational setting they cope best when not expected to sustain attention for too long and are provided with different tasks at regular intervals. Behaviour modification techniques, in the form of operant conditioning with positive reinforcement (reward) for gradually achieving longer periods of concentration and task orientation, may achieve some success and should be undertaken if a psychologist with interests and skills in this area is available.

Finally, stimulant drugs sometimes have a paradoxical calming effect on such children and, if the child is severely affected, are well worth a trial. From the age of 4 years upwards, dexamphetamine sulphate in an initial dose of 2.5 mgs *mane* can be given and the dose gradually built up over a week to about 5 mg morning and lunchtime (higher doses can be used in older children). A related drug, methylphenidate (Ritalin®), can be given starting with 5 mg morning and noon and increasing every 3 days until benefit is evident or side-effects appear, up to a maximum of 20 mg twice daily at 4–6 years. Habituation may occur and the drugs are often most effective when a child is given a break at weekends and during the school holidays. Side-effects are not uncommon. The child may become even more overactive or depressed and apathetic, in which case the drug should be stopped. Long-term administration also produces some stunting of growth, perhaps related to appetite suppression, so that continuous medication needs to be carefully monitored. However, catch-up growth occurs when the drugs are stopped. If the stimulant drugs are ineffective, but the problem remains severe, it is also worth while trying the effect of haloperidol (0.05 mg/kg body weight/day, in two divided doses) combined with an anti-Parkinsonian agents such as benzhexol. Finally it should be mentioned that the symptoms these children present do pose considerable burdens on the parents who need to have a supportive relationship with an informed professional: family doctor, paediatrician, psychiatric social worker, psychologist or child psychiatrist.

The prognosis of the severe form of the hyperkinetic syndrome is not good. Although the overactivity usually diminishes, such children often present with quite severe problems of behaviour and learning difficulties later in their school careers.

Childhood autism

Apart from the rare organically determined dementias, this is virtually the only type of psychosis occurring in the first 5 years of life. An excellent account of the condition is provided by Wing (1976), and the following description is necessarily brief and incomplete.

The child may be abnormal from birth or may have a period of normal development up to 2 or 2½ years. Often the first manifestation is a lack of social responsiveness, the child being slow to smile, very slow to recognize his mother as different from other people, and averse to physical contact and cuddling. He may avoid eye-to-eye contact. Characteristically this occurs in the context of normal motor development. As the child grows older he may go through a much delayed period of separation anxiety (at about 4–5 years) but his social relationships are likely to be permanently uneasy and strained. Language development is always delayed and about half the children currently diagnosed as autistic are not speaking at all by the age of 5 years. Characteristically when they do talk these children echo speech in a mechanical fashion over a prolonged period of months or even several years and they have particular difficulty in the use of pronouns. Associated problems include the presence of mannerisms, resistance to change and attachment to unusual objects.

The relationship of the condition to mental retardation has been a matter of controversy, but is now clearer. It seems that most autistic chidren do have a degree of mental retardation even in their non-verbal abilities, and about half of them are in the severely subnormal range. Where autism is associated with this serious degree of mental retardation, the main handicap lies in the subnormality of intelligence.

The aetiology of autism is almost always undetermined. However, there are various pointers to suggest that the condition is primarily physiologically rather than psychologically determined, though it is possible that in some extremely vulnerable children psychological stress does play an important part. As the children get older they seem to share more and more in common with developmentally aphasic youngsters. Further, the incidence of epilepsy is high, approximately one-fifth of autistic children having at least one epileptic fit. Finally, exhaustive investigation of parental personality and attitudes have failed to demonstrate any unusual degree of psychopathology.

The prognosis of the condition is poor with only a small minority of children being able eventually to lead independent lives, and these are the most intelligent and least affected by the manifestations of autism. No medical treatment is available, but the children can certainly be helped by special education and sometimes also by psychological techniques aimed at improving language development or breaking down maladaptive behaviour patterns. Again parents of such children need support and guidance from someone experienced in the management of this condition and this help will usually be most appropriately provided by a child psychiatrist.

THE CHILD PSYCHIATRIST AND CHILDREN WITH NEURODEVELOP-MENTAL PROBLEMS

The role of the child psychiatrist in the assessment and management of young children with developmental problems cannot be clearly specified because it depends so much on the professional interests and attitudes of the paediatrician and child psychiatrist and their capacity to work together. Certainly, when child psychiatric teams are available, one would think they should have a part to play in those situations described above, i.e. the child with a severe management problem whose difficulty does not resolve with simple measures, and children with the hyperkinetic syndrome and autism, but the role of the child psychiatrist and his or her team need not end there. Child psychiatrists are in some places involved in postnatal counselling to groups of mothers with handicapped children, in helping to detect children at risk of battering in special care units and in guiding and counselling nursing and medical staff of wards to which young children are admitted. They may also work with paediatricians and others in assessment centres to which children with developmental retardation are referred, so that the family crises which referrals to such centres sometimes precipate can be dealt with as helpfully as possible.

P.J. GRAHAM

References

BAKWIN H. (1971) Enuresis in twins. *American Journal of Diseases of Children*, **121**, 222.

DOUGLAS J.W.B. (1973) Early disturbing events and later enuresis. In *Bladder Control and Enuresis*. ed. Kolvin I., Mac Keith R.C. and Meadow S.R. *Clinics in Developmental Medicine Nos. 48/49*. London: Heinemann.

DRILLIEN C.M. (1964) Behaviour in the pre-school and early school age periods. In *The Growth and Development of the Prematurely Born Infant*. Edinburgh: Churchill Livingstone.

GOODALL J. (1976) Opening windows into a child's mind. *Developmental Medicine and Child Neurology*, **18**, 173.

MAC KEITH R.C. (1973) The causes of nocturnal enuresis. In *Bladder Control and Enuresis*. eds. Kolvin I., Mac Keith R.C. and Meadow S.R. *Clinics in Developmental Medicine Nos. 48/49*. London: Heinemann.

NEWSON J. and NEWSON E. (1963) *Infant Care in an Urban Community*. London: Allen and Unwin.

NEWSON J. and NEWSON E. (1968) *Four Years Old in an Urban Community*. London: Allen and Unwin.

RICHMAN N., STEVENSON J.E. and GRAHAM P. (1975) Prevalence of behaviour problems in 3 year old children: an epidemiological study in a London borough. *Journal of Child Psychology and Psychiatry*, **16**, 277.

SHERIDAN M.D. (1975) The importance of spontaneous play in the fundamental learning of handicapped children. *Child: care, health and development*, **1**, 3.

SPENCE J., WALTON W.S., MILLER F.J.W. and COURT S.D.M. (1954) *A Thousand Families in Newcastle-upon-Tyne*. London: Oxford University Press.

THOMAS A., CHESS S. and BIRCH H.G. (1968) *Temperament and Behaviour Disorders in Children*. London: University of London Press.

WING L. (1976) *Early Childhood Autism*, 2nd Ed. Oxford: Pergamon Press.

Further Reading

RUTTER M. (1975) *Helping Troubled Children*. Harmondsworth, Middlesex: Penguin Education.

STONE F.H. (1976) *Psychiatry and the Paediatrician*. London: Butterworth.

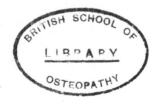

INDEX